THIS IS YOUR **PASSBOOK**® FOR ...

COMMISSION ON GRADUATES OF FOREIGN NURSING SCHOOLS QUALIFYING EXAM (CFGNS)

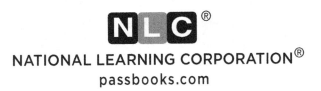

NATIONAL LEARNING CORPORATION®
passbooks.com

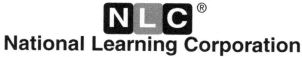

PASSBOOK® SERIES

THE *PASSBOOK® SERIES* has been created to prepare applicants and candidates for the ultimate academic battlefield – the examination room.

At some time in our lives, each and every one of us may be required to take an examination – for validation, matriculation, admission, qualification, registration, certification, or licensure.

Based on the assumption that every applicant or candidate has met the basic formal educational standards, has taken the required number of courses, and read the necessary texts, the *PASSBOOK® SERIES* furnishes the one special preparation which may assure passing with confidence, instead of failing with insecurity. Examination questions – together with answers – are furnished as the basic vehicle for study so that the mysteries of the examination and its compounding difficulties may be eliminated or diminished by a sure method.

This book is meant to help you pass your examination provided that you qualify and are serious in your objective.

The entire field is reviewed through the huge store of content information which is succinctly presented through a provocative and challenging approach – the question-and-answer method.

A climate of success is established by furnishing the correct answers at the end of each test.

You soon learn to recognize types of questions, forms of questions, and patterns of questioning. You may even begin to anticipate expected outcomes.

You perceive that many questions are repeated or adapted so that you can gain acute insights, which may enable you to score many sure points.

You learn how to confront new questions, or types of questions, and to attack them confidently and work out the correct answers.

You note objectives and emphases, and recognize pitfalls and dangers, so that you may make positive educational adjustments.

Moreover, you are kept fully informed in relation to new concepts, methods, practices, and directions in the field.

You discover that you arre actually taking the examination all the time: you are preparing for the examination by "taking" an examination, not by reading extraneous and/or supererogatory textbooks.

In short, this PASSBOOK®, used directedly, should be an important factor in helping you to pass your test.

COMMISSION OF GRADUATES OF FOREIGN NURSING SCHOOL QUALIFYING EXAMINATION

Preparing for the exam

The best way to prepare for the CGFNS Qualifying Exam® is to review what you learned in your basic nursing education program. Study these areas: adult (medical and surgical) nursing, maternal/infant nursing, nursing care of children and psychiatric/mental health nursing. You also can benefit from reviewing the nursing process and patient needs as they are taught in the United States.

The NLC CGFNS Passbook®

NLC has developed this passbook® to help you identify your strengths and weaknesses in nursing knowledge by providing hundreds and hundreds of sample questions in the subjects tested on the exam.

Examination Modules

Safe, Effective Care Environment test

The questions on the Safe, Effective Care Environment test center on two main areas: management of care and safety and infection control. The nurse must be able to manage the care of patients in a cost-effective manner and does so by coordinating, supervising and/or collaborating with members of the multidisciplinary health care team. This test will focus on such concepts as advocacy, advance directives, case management, client rights, confidentiality, and continuity of care, delegation, and information technology, legal/ethical aspects of care, quality improvement and setting priorities.

The second aspect of providing a safe, effective care environment is protecting clients and health care personnel from environmental hazards. The nurse must provide care that prevents accidents and injuries, promotes institutional and home safety for the client, and addresses emergency response planning. Content in this section will focus on such concepts as disaster planning, error prevention, handling of hazardous/infectious materials, medical and surgical asepsis, reporting of adverse incidents, safe use of equipment, standard precautions and use of restraints and other security devices.

Health Promotion and Maintenance test

The nurse assists clients and their families through the normal and expected stages of growth and development from conception through advanced old age and provides care that promotes the client's ability to achieve optimum health. The questions on the Health Promotion and Maintenance emphasize promoting health, preventing illness and detecting health problems early in the process.

Content will focus on such concepts as aging, ante/intra/postpartum and newborn care, developmental stages and transitions, body image changes, family planning, family systems, and human sexuality. Test questions also will address disease prevention, health and wellness, health promotion programs, health screening, high-risk behaviors, immunizations, lifestyle choices, self-care and techniques of physical assessment.

Psychosocial Integrity test

The questions on the Psychosocial Integrity test center on two major areas: providing nursing care that promotes the client's ability to cope, adapt and/or problem solve situations related to illnesses or stressful events and managing and providing care for clients with acute or chronic mental illnesses. The nurse creates a therapeutic environment that supports the client's health and wellbeing.

Content in this test will focus on such concepts as abuse and neglect, behavioral interventions, chemical and other dependencies, coping, crisis intervention, cultural diversity, family dynamics, grief and loss, religious and spiritual influences on health, sensory and perceptual alterations, stress management, support systems and therapeutic communication.

Physiological Integrity test

The Physiological Integrity test comprises four sections: basic care and comfort, pharmacological and parenteral therapies, reduction of risk potential and physiologic adaptation The nurse provides comfort and assistance in the performance of activities of daily living; manages and provides care related to the administration of medications and parenteral therapies; reduces the likelihood that clients will develop complications or health problems related to existing conditions, treatments or procedures; and manages and provides care to clients with acute, chronic or life-threatening physical health conditions.

Content in this test will focus on the following areas:

Basic care and comfort: assistive devices, elimination, mobility/immobility, non-pharmacological comfort interventions, nutritional and oral hydration, personal hygiene, and rest and sleep.

Pharmacological and parenteral therapies: Adverse effects/ contraindications/interactions, blood and blood products, central venous access devices, chemotherapy, dosage calculation, expected actions and outcomes, intravenous therapy, medication administration, parenteral and intravenous therapies, pharmacological pain management and total parenteral nutrition.

Reduction of risk potential: Changes and abnormalities in vital signs, diagnostic tests, laboratory values, potential alteration in body systems, potential for complications of diagnostic tests, treatments and procedures, potential for complications from surgical procedures and health alterations, system-specific alterations and therapeutic procedures.

Physiologic adaptation: Alterations in body systems, fluid and electrolyte imbalances, hemodynamics, illness management, medical emergencies, pathophysiology and unexpected response to therapies.

Question format
Multiple-choice questions

The CGFNS Exam is primarily of the multiple-choice type. This means choosing a correct answer from several choices. The multiple-choice questions generally describe a patient, the symptoms, the treatments or the nursing care the patient will receive contains all the information you need to choose the correct answer. The Exam takes approximately three hours to complete.

———

HOW TO TAKE A TEST

You have studied long, hard and conscientiously.

With your official admission card in hand, and your heart pounding, you have been admitted to the examination room.

You note that there are several hundred other applicants in the examination room waiting to take the same test.

They all appear to be equally well prepared.

You know that nothing but your best effort will suffice. The "moment of truth" is at hand: you now have to demonstrate objectively, in writing, your knowledge of content and your understanding of subject matter.

You are fighting the most important battle of your life—to pass and/or score high on an examination which will determine your career and provide the economic basis for your livelihood.

What extra, special things should you know and should you do in taking the examination?

I. YOU MUST PASS AN EXAMINATION

A. WHAT EVERY CANDIDATE SHOULD KNOW
Examination applicants often ask us for help in preparing for the written test. What can I study in advance? What kinds of questions will be asked? How will the test be given? How will the papers be graded?

B. HOW ARE EXAMS DEVELOPED?
Examinations are carefully written by trained technicians who are specialists in the field known as "psychological measurement," in consultation with recognized authorities in the field of work that the test will cover. These experts recommend the subject matter areas or skills to be tested; only those knowledges or skills important to your success on the job are included. The most reliable books and source materials available are used as references. Together, the experts and technicians judge the difficulty level of the questions.

Test technicians know how to phrase questions so that the problem is clearly stated. Their ethics do not permit "trick" or "catch" questions. Questions may have been tried out on sample groups, or subjected to statistical analysis, to determine their usefulness.

Written tests are often used in combination with performance tests, ratings of training and experience, and oral interviews. All of these measures combine to form the best-known means of finding the right person for the right job.

II. HOW TO PASS THE WRITTEN TEST

A. BASIC STEPS

1) Study the announcement

How, then, can you know what subjects to study? Our best answer is: "Learn as much as possible about the class of positions for which you've applied." The exam will test the knowledge, skills and abilities needed to do the work.

Your most valuable source of information about the position you want is the official exam announcement. This announcement lists the training and experience qualifications. Check these standards and apply only if you come reasonably close to meeting them. Many jurisdictions preview the written test in the exam announcement by including a section called "Knowledge and Abilities Required," "Scope of the Examination," or some similar heading. Here you will find out specifically what fields will be tested.

2) Choose appropriate study materials

If the position for which you are applying is technical or advanced, you will read more advanced, specialized material. If you are already familiar with the basic principles of your field, elementary textbooks would waste your time. Concentrate on advanced textbooks and technical periodicals. Think through the concepts and review difficult problems in your field.

These are all general sources. You can get more ideas on your own initiative, following these leads. For example, training manuals and publications of the government agency which employs workers in your field can be useful, particularly for technical and professional positions. A letter or visit to the government department involved may result in more specific study suggestions, and certainly will provide you with a more definite idea of the exact nature of the position you are seeking.

3) Study this book!

III. KINDS OF TESTS

Tests are used for purposes other than measuring knowledge and ability to perform specified duties. For some positions, it is equally important to test ability to make adjustments to new situations or to profit from training. In others, basic mental abilities not dependent on information are essential. Questions which test these things may not appear as pertinent to the duties of the position as those which test for knowledge and information. Yet they are often highly important parts of a fair examination. For very general questions, it is almost impossible to help you direct your study efforts. What we can do is to point out some of the more common of these general abilities needed in public service positions and describe some typical questions.

1) General information

Broad, general information has been found useful for predicting job success in some kinds of work. This is tested in a variety of ways, from vocabulary lists to questions about current events. Basic background in some field of work, such as sociology or economics, may be sampled in a group of questions. Often these are principles which have become familiar to most persons through exposure rather than through formal training. It is difficult to advise you how to study for these questions; being alert to the world around you is our best suggestion.

2) Verbal ability

An example of an ability needed in many positions is verbal or language ability. Verbal ability is, in brief, the ability to use and understand words. Vocabulary and grammar tests are typical measures of this ability. Reading comprehension or paragraph interpretation questions are common in many kinds of civil service tests. You are given a paragraph of written material and asked to find its central meaning.

IV. KINDS OF QUESTIONS

1. Multiple-choice Questions

Most popular of the short-answer questions is the "multiple choice" or "best answer" question. It can be used, for example, to test for factual knowledge, ability to solve problems or judgment in meeting situations found at work.

A multiple-choice question is normally one of three types:

- It can begin with an incomplete statement followed by several possible endings. You are to find the one ending which *best* completes the statement, although some of the others may not be entirely wrong.
- It can also be a complete statement in the form of a question which is answered by choosing one of the statements listed.
- It can be in the form of a problem – again you select the best answer.

Here is an example of a multiple-choice question with a discussion which should give you some clues as to the method for choosing the right answer:

When an employee has a complaint about his assignment, the action which will *best* help him overcome his difficulty is to
A. discuss his difficulty with his coworkers
B. take the problem to the head of the organization
C. take the problem to the person who gave him the assignment
D. say nothing to anyone about his complaint

In answering this question, you should study each of the choices to find which is best. Consider choice "A" – Certainly an employee may discuss his complaint with fellow employees, but no change or improvement can result, and the complaint remains unresolved. Choice "B" is a poor choice since the head of the organization probably does not know what assignment you have been given, and taking your problem to him is known as "going over the head" of the supervisor. The supervisor, or person who made the assignment, is the person who can clarify it or correct any injustice. Choice "C" is, therefore, correct. To say nothing, as in choice "D," is unwise. Supervisors have and interest in knowing the problems employees are facing, and the employee is seeking a solution to his problem.

2. True/False

3. Matching Questions
Matching an answer from a column of choices within another column.

V. RECORDING YOUR ANSWERS

Computer terminals are used more and more today for many different kinds of exams.

For an examination with very few applicants, you may be told to record your answers in the test booklet itself. Separate answer sheets are much more common. If this separate answer sheet is to be scored by machine – and this is often the case – it is highly important that you mark your answers correctly in order to get credit.

VI. BEFORE THE TEST

YOUR PHYSICAL CONDITION IS IMPORTANT
If you are not well, you can't do your best work on tests. If you are half asleep, you can't do your best either. Here are some tips:

1) Get about the same amount of sleep you usually get. Don't stay up all night before the test, either partying or worrying—DON'T DO IT!
2) If you wear glasses, be sure to wear them when you go to take the test. This goes for hearing aids, too.
3) If you have any physical problems that may keep you from doing your best, be sure to tell the person giving the test. If you are sick or in poor health, you relay cannot do your best on any test. You can always come back and take the test some other time.

Common sense will help you find procedures to follow to get ready for an examination. Too many of us, however, overlook these sensible measures. Indeed, nervousness and fatigue have been found to be the most serious reasons why applicants fail to do their best on civil service tests. Here is a list of reminders:

- Begin your preparation early – Don't wait until the last minute to go scurrying around for books and materials or to find out what the position is all about.
- Prepare continuously – An hour a night for a week is better than an all-night cram session. This has been definitely established. What is more, a night a week for a month will return better dividends than crowding your study into a shorter period of time.
- Locate the place of the exam – You have been sent a notice telling you when and where to report for the examination. If the location is in a different town or otherwise unfamiliar to you, it would be well to inquire the best route and learn something about the building.
- Relax the night before the test – Allow your mind to rest. Do not study at all that night. Plan some mild recreation or diversion; then go to bed early and get a good night's sleep.
- Get up early enough to make a leisurely trip to the place for the test – This way unforeseen events, traffic snarls, unfamiliar buildings, etc. will not upset you.

- Dress comfortably – A written test is not a fashion show. You will be known by number and not by name, so wear something comfortable.
- Leave excess paraphernalia at home – Shopping bags and odd bundles will get in your way. You need bring only the items mentioned in the official notice you received; usually everything you need is provided. Do not bring reference books to the exam. They will only confuse those last minutes and be taken away from you when in the test room.
- Arrive somewhat ahead of time – If because of transportation schedules you must get there very early, bring a newspaper or magazine to take your mind off yourself while waiting.
- Locate the examination room – When you have found the proper room, you will be directed to the seat or part of the room where you will sit. Sometimes you are given a sheet of instructions to read while you are waiting. Do not fill out any forms until you are told to do so; just read them and be prepared.
- Relax and prepare to listen to the instructions
- If you have any physical problem that may keep you from doing your best, be sure to tell the test administrator. If you are sick or in poor health, you really cannot do your best on the exam. You can come back and take the test some other time.

VII. AT THE TEST

The day of the test is here and you have the test booklet in your hand. The temptation to get going is very strong. Caution! There is more to success than knowing the right answers. You must know how to identify your papers and understand variations in the type of short-answer question used in this particular examination. Follow these suggestions for maximum results from your efforts:

1) Cooperate with the monitor
The test administrator has a duty to create a situation in which you can be as much at ease as possible. He will give instructions, tell you when to begin, check to see that you are marking your answer sheet correctly, and so on. He is not there to guard you, although he will see that your competitors do not take unfair advantage. He wants to help you do your best.

2) Listen to all instructions
Don't jump the gun! Wait until you understand all directions. In most civil service tests you get more time than you need to answer the questions. So don't be in a hurry. Read each word of instructions until you clearly understand the meaning. Study the examples, listen to all announcements and follow directions. Ask questions if you do not understand what to do.

3) Identify your papers
Civil service exams are usually identified by number only. You will be assigned a number; you must not put your name on your test papers. Be sure to copy your number correctly. Since more than one exam may be given, copy your exact examination title.

4) Plan your time
Unless you are told that a test is a "speed" or "rate of work" test, speed itself is usually not important. Time enough to answer all the questions will be provided, but this

does not mean that you have all day. An overall time limit has been set. Divide the total time (in minutes) by the number of questions to determine the approximate time you have for each question.

5) Do not linger over difficult questions

If you come across a difficult question, mark it with a paper clip (useful to have along) and come back to it when you have been through the booklet. One caution if you do this – be sure to skip a number on your answer sheet as well. Check often to be sure that you have not lost your place and that you are marking in the row numbered the same as the question you are answering.

6) Read the questions

Be sure you know what the question asks! Many capable people are unsuccessful because they failed to *read* the questions correctly.

7) Answer all questions

Unless you have been instructed that a penalty will be deducted for incorrect answers, it is better to guess than to omit a question.

8) Speed tests

It is often better NOT to guess on speed tests. It has been found that on timed tests people are tempted to spend the last few seconds before time is called in marking answers at random – without even reading them – in the hope of picking up a few extra points. To discourage this practice, the instructions may warn you that your score will be "corrected" for guessing. That is, a penalty will be applied. The incorrect answers will be deducted from the correct ones, or some other penalty formula will be used.

9) Review your answers

If you finish before time is called, go back to the questions you guessed or omitted to give them further thought. Review other answers if you have time.

10) Return your test materials

If you are ready to leave before others have finished or time is called, take ALL your materials to the monitor and leave quietly. Never take any test material with you. The monitor can discover whose papers are not complete, and taking a test booklet may be grounds for disqualification.

VIII. EXAMINATION TECHNIQUES

1) Read the general instructions carefully. These are usually printed on the first page of the exam booklet. As a rule, these instructions refer to the timing of the examination; the fact that you should not start work until the signal and must stop work at a signal, etc. If there are any *special* instructions, such as a choice of questions to be answered, make sure that you note this instruction carefully.

2) When you are ready to start work on the examination, that is as soon as the signal has been given, read the instructions to each question booklet, underline any key words or phrases, such as *least, best, outline, describe*

and the like. In this way you will tend to answer as requested rather than discover on reviewing your paper that you *listed without describing*, that you selected the *worst* choice rather than the *best* choice, etc.

3) If the examination is of the objective or multiple-choice type – that is, each question will also give a series of possible answers: A, B, C or D, and you are called upon to select the best answer and write the letter next to that answer on your answer paper – it is advisable to start answering each question in turn. There may be anywhere from 50 to 100 such questions in the three or four hours allotted and you can see how much time would be taken if you read through all the questions before beginning to answer any. Furthermore, if you come across a question or group of questions which you know would be difficult to answer, it would undoubtedly affect your handling of all the other questions.

4) If the examination is of the essay type and contains but a few questions, it is a moot point as to whether you should read all the questions before starting to answer any one. Of course, if you are given a choice – say five out of seven and the like – then it is essential to read all the questions so you can eliminate the two that are most difficult. If, however, you are asked to answer all the questions, there may be danger in trying to answer the easiest one first because you may find that you will spend too much time on it. The best technique is to answer the first question, then proceed to the second, etc.

5) Time your answers. Before the exam begins, write down the time it started, then add the time allowed for the examination and write down the time it must be completed, then divide the time available somewhat as follows:
   • If 3-1/2 hours are allowed, that would be 210 minutes. If you have 80 objective-type questions, that would be an average of 2-1/2 minutes per question. Allow yourself no more than 2 minutes per question, or a total of 160 minutes, which will permit about 50 minutes to review.
   • If for the time allotment of 210 minutes there are 7 essay questions to answer, that would average about 30 minutes a question. Give yourself only 25 minutes per question so that you have about 35 minutes to review.

6) The most important instruction is to *read each question* and make sure you know what is wanted. The second most important instruction is to *time yourself properly* so that you answer every question. The third most important instruction is to *answer every question*. Guess if you have to but include something for each question. Remember that you will receive no credit for a blank and will probably receive some credit if you write something in answer to an essay question. If you guess a letter – say "B" for a multiple-choice question – you may have guessed right. If you leave a blank as an answer to a multiple-choice question, the examiners may respect your feelings but it will not add a point to your score. Some exams may penalize you for wrong answers, so in such cases *only*, you may not want to guess unless you have some basis for your answer.

7) Suggestions
  a. Objective-type questions
    1. Examine the question booklet for proper sequence of pages and questions
    2. Read all instructions carefully
    3. Skip any question which seems too difficult; return to it after all other questions have been answered
    4. Apportion your time properly; do not spend too much time on any single question or group of questions
    5. Note and underline key words – *all, most, fewest, least, best, worst, same, opposite,* etc.
    6. Pay particular attention to negatives
    7. Note unusual option, e.g., unduly long, short, complex, different or similar in content to the body of the question
    8. Observe the use of "hedging" words – *probably, may, most likely,* etc.
    9. Make sure that your answer is put next to the same number as the question
    10. Do not second-guess unless you have good reason to believe the second answer is definitely more correct
    11. Cross out original answer if you decide another answer is more accurate; do not erase until you are ready to hand your paper in
    12. Answer all questions; guess unless instructed otherwise
    13. Leave time for review

  b. Essay questions
    1. Read each question carefully
    2. Determine exactly what is wanted. Underline key words or phrases.
    3. Decide on outline or paragraph answer
    4. Include many different points and elements unless asked to develop any one or two points or elements
    5. Show impartiality by giving pros and cons unless directed to select one side only
    6. Make and write down any assumptions you find necessary to answer the questions
    7. Watch your English, grammar, punctuation and choice of words
    8. Time your answers; don't crowd material

8) Answering the essay question

Most essay questions can be answered by framing the specific response around several key words or ideas. Here are a few such key words or ideas:

M's: manpower, materials, methods, money, management
P's: purpose, program, policy, plan, procedure, practice, problems, pitfalls, personnel, public relations
a. Six basic steps in handling problems:
    1. Preliminary plan and background development
    2. Collect information, data and facts
    3. Analyze and interpret information, data and facts
    4. Analyze and develop solutions as well as make recommendations

5. Prepare report and sell recommendations
6. Install recommendations and follow up effectiveness

b. Pitfalls to avoid
1. *Taking things for granted* – A statement of the situation does not necessarily imply that each of the elements is necessarily true; for example, a complaint may be invalid and biased so that all that can be taken for granted is that a complaint has been registered
2. *Considering only one side of a situation* – Wherever possible, indicate several alternatives and then point out the reasons you selected the best one
3. *Failing to indicate follow up* – Whenever your answer indicates action on your part, make certain that you will take proper follow-up action to see how successful your recommendations, procedures or actions turn out to be
4. *Taking too long in answering any single question* – Remember to time your answers properly

EXAMINATION SECTION

EXAMINATION SECTION
TEST 1

DIRECTIONS: Each question or incomplete statement is followed by several suggested answers or completions. Select the one that BEST answers the question or completes the statement. *PRINT THE LETTER OF THE CORRECT ANSWER IN THE SPACE AT THE RIGHT.*

Questions 1-10.

DIRECTIONS: Questions 1 through 10 are to be answered on the basis of the following information.

Ms. Martha McCarthy, 32 years old, is brought to the emergency unit on a stretcher. Ms. McCarthy was in an automobile accident and is conscious upon admission. X-rays show that she has considerable vertebral damage at the level of T-6. The surgical unit is notified that Ms. McCarthy will be brought directly from the x-ray department.

1. Which of the facts about Ms. McCarthy, if obtained when she is admitted to the hospital, would MOST likely require early intervention?
She

    A. is a vegetarian
    B. last voided 7 hours ago
    C. smokes 2 packs of cigarettes a day
    D. is menstruating

1. _B_

2. Twelve hours after admission, Ms. McCarthy begins to develop some difficulty in breathing.
In addition to obtaining a respirator and calling the physician, the nurse would show the BEST judgment by

    A. turning Ms. McCarthy onto her abdomen to promote drainage from the mouth and throat
    B. encouraging Ms. McCarthy to exercise her upper extremities at intervals
    C. elevating the foot of Ms. McCarthy's bed
    D. bringing pharyngeal suction equipment to Ms. McCarthy's bedside

2. _D_

3. Considering the level of Ms. McCarthy's injury (T-6), it is MOST justifiable to assume that her respiratory difficulty is due to

    A. edema of the cord above the level of injury
    B. hemorrhage into the brain stem due to trauma
    C. movement of the parts of the fractured vertebrae
    D. severing of the nerves that activate the diaphragm

3. _A_

4. The nurse can prevent Ms. McCarthy's lower extremities from rotating externally by placing

    A. her feet against a footboard
    B. pillows against her calves

4. _D_

C. trochanter rolls along the inner aspects of her knees
D. sandbags against the outer aspects of her thighs

5. Ms. McCarthy is to have a laminectomy.   5. B
   The CHIEF purpose of a laminectomy for her is to

   A. realign the vertebral fragments
   B. relieve pressure on the cord
   C. repair spinal nerve damage
   D. reduce spinal fluid pressure

6. Ms. McCarthy is highly susceptible to the development of decubitus ulcers because   6. A

   A. an intact nervous system is necessary for maintenance of normal tone of blood
      vessels
   B. flexor muscles have a greater loss of tone than extensor muscles
   C. decreased permeability of the capillary walls results from central nervous system
      damage
   D. atonic muscles have an increased need for oxygen

7. Ms. McCarthy has a laminectomy and spinal fusion. The physician tells her that she will   7. A
   not be able to walk without the use of supportive devices.
   Before surgery, Ms. McCarthy should have been informed that the bone to be used as
   a graft for a spinal fusion is MOST likely to be obtained from the

   A. posterior iliac crest   B. adjacent sacral vertebrae
   C. humerus   D. sternum

8. The nursing staff notices a pronounced change in Ms. McCarthy's behavior after the phy-   8. C
   sician discusses her prognosis with her. She is now overtly rebellious, responding nega-
   tively to personnel, to treatments, and to nursing measures.
   The interpretation of her behavior is that she is

   A. unable to face the prospect of a long rehabilitative program
   B. projecting her own unhappiness onto others
   C. reacting to the change in her body image
   D. seeking punishment for feelings of guilt about her injury

9. A rehabilitative program is started for Ms. McCarthy. She is to wear leg braces.   9. B
   When applying Ms. McCarthy's leg braces, it is ESSENTIAL for the nurse to consider
   that Ms. McCarthy

   A. cannot move her lower extremities
   B. has no sensation in her lower extremities
   C. can flex her knees to a 45-degree angle
   D. cannot fully extend her hip joints

10. To achieve success in a rehabilitation program for Ms. McCarthy, the MOST important   10. B
    information about Ms. McCarthy is her

    A. knowledge of services available to her
    B. personal goals
    C. being encouraged by her family
    D. relationship with members of the health team

Questions 11-16.

DIRECTIONS: Questions 11 through 16 are to be answered on the basis of the following information.

Ms. Beth Marks, a 21-year-old college student, sustains a head injury as a result of a fall down a flight of stairs. She is brought to the emergency room with a pronounced swelling of the forehead. She is admitted to the hospital for observation.

11.   On admission, Ms. Marks' blood pressure was 110/80, her pulse rate was 88, and her respiratory rate was 20.
It would be MOST indicative of increasing intracranial pressure if her blood pressure, pulse, and respirations were, respectively,

    A.   90/54; 50; 22   B.   100/66; 120; 32
    C.   120/90; 96; 16   D.   140/70; 60; 14

11. ___D___

12.   Ms. Marks' condition worsens. She has a craniotomy, and a hematoma is removed. Her postoperative orders include elevation of the head of her bed, and mannitol.
When Ms. Marks reacts from anesthesia, she is put in a semi-reclining position to

    A.   increase thoracic expansion and facilitate oxygenation of damaged tissue
    B.   provide adequate drainage and prevent fluid accumulation in the cranial cavity
    C.   decrease cardiac workload and prevent hemorrhage at the surgical site
    D.   reduce pressure in the subarachnoid space and promote tissue granulation

12. ___B___

13.   It is CORRECT to say that in this case mannitol is expected to

    A.   decrease body fluids
    B.   elevate the filtration rate in the kidney
    C.   control filtration of nitrogenous wastes
    D.   increase the volume of urine

13. ___D___

14.   The PRIMARY purpose of administering mannitol to Ms. Marks is to

    A.   promote kidney function
    B.   prevent bladder distention
    C.   reduce cerebral pressure
    D.   diminish peripheral fluid retention

14. ___C___

15.   Eight hours after surgery, Ms. Marks' temperature rises to 104° F. (40° C.), and a hypothermia blanket is ordered for her.
Ms. Marks' temperature elevation is MOST likely due to a(n)

    A.   accumulation of respiratory secretions resulting from inadequate ventilation
    B.   alteration of metabolism resulting from pressure on the hypothalamus
    C.   increase in leukocytosis resulting from bacterial invasion
    D.   constriction of the main artery in the circle of Willis resulting from a ventricular fluid shift

15. ___B___

16.   Following a craniotomy, a patient may be given caffeine and sodium benzoate to

    A.   lessen cerebral irritation by depressing the cerebrum
    B.   improve the sense of touch by blocking spinal nerve reflexes

16. ___D___

C.   enable commands to be followed by activating the medullary cells
D.   increase mental alertness by stimulating the cerebral cortex

Questions 17-25.

DIRECTIONS: Questions 17 through 25 are to be answered on the basis of the following information.

Mr. Paul Peters, 61 years old, is admitted to the hospital. Vascular occlusion of his left leg
is suspected, and he is scheduled for an arteriogram.

17.   The nurse is to assess the circulation in Mr. Peters' lower extremities.   17.A
Which of these measures would be ESPECIALLY significant?

A.   Comparing the pulses in the lower extremities
B.   Comparing the temperatures of the lower extremities
C.   Noting the pulse in the left leg
D.   Noting the temperature of the left leg

18.   Which of these symptoms manifested in Mr. Peters' affected left extremity would indicate   18.C
that he has intermittent claudication?

A.   Extensive discoloration
B.   Dependent edema
C.   Pain associated with activity
D.   Petechiae

19.   Following Mr. Peters' admission, an IMMEDIATE goal in his care should be to   19.D

A.   improve the muscular strength of his extremities
B.   achieve maximum rehabilitation for him
C.   prevent the extension of his disease process
D.   protect his extremities from injury

20.   During the night following his admission, Mr. Peters says that he can't sleep because his   20.C
feet are cold.
The nurse should

A.   offer Mr. Peters a warm drink
B.   massage Mr. Peters' feet briskly for several minutes
C.   ask Mr. Peters if he has any socks with him
D.   place a heating pad under Mr. Peters' feet

21.   Information given to Mr. Peters about the femoral arteri-ogram should include the fact   21.A
that

A.   a local anesthetic will be given to lessen discomfort
B.   there are minimal risks associated with the procedure
C.   the radioactive dye that is injected will be removed before he returns to his unit
D.   a radiopaque substance will be injected directly into the small vessels of his feet

4

22. When Mr. Peters is brought back to his unit following the arteriogram, which of these actions would be appropriate?

    22.___C___

    A. Encourage fluid intake and have him lie prone
    B. Apply heat to the site used for introducing the intravenous catheter and passively exercise his involved extremity
    C. Limit motion of his affected extremity and check the site used for the injection of the dye
    D. Restrict his fluid intake and encourage him to ambulate

23. The results of Mr. Peters' arteriogram revealed a marked narrowing of the left femoral artery. He has a venous graft bypass performed. Following a stay in the recovery room, he is returned to his room.
The postoperative care plan for Mr. Peters should include which of these notations?

    23.___B___

    A. Keep the affected extremity elevated
    B. Check the pulse distal to the graft site
    C. Check for color changes proximal to the proximal site
    D. Check for fine movements of the toes

24. During the first postoperative day, Mr. Peters is kept on bed rest.
Which of these exercises for Mr. Peters would it be APPROPRIATE for the nurse to initiate?

    24.___D___

    A. Straight leg raising of both lower extremities
    B. Range of motion of both lower extremities
    C. Abduction of the affected extremity
    D. Dorsiflexion and extension of the foot of the affected extremity

25. When Mr. Peters returns to bed after ambulating, it would be MOST important for the nurse to check

    25.___D___

    A. his blood pressure
    B. his radial pulse
    C. the temperature of his affected extremity
    D. the pedal pulse of his affected extremity

KEY (CORRECT ANSWERS)

1.	B	11.	D
2.	D	12.	B
3.	A	13.	D
4.	D	14.	C
5.	B	15.	B
6.	A	16.	D
7.	A	17.	A
8.	C	18.	C
9.	B	19.	D
10.	B	20.	C

21.	A
22.	C
23.	B
24.	D
25.	D

TEST 2

DIRECTIONS: Each question or incomplete statement is followed by several suggested answers or completions. Select the one that BEST answers the question or completes the statement. *PRINT THE LETTER OF THE CORRECT ANSWER IN THE SPACE AT THE RIGHT.*

Questions 1-8.

DIRECTIONS: Questions 1 through 8 are to be answered on the basis of the following information.

Three days ago, Susan Cooper, 4 years old, was admitted to the hospital with a diagnosis of heart failure. She was digitalized the day of her admission and is now to receive a maintenance dose of digoxin (Lanoxin) 0.08 mg. p.o.b.i.d. Susan has been under medical supervision for cystic fibrosis and has severe pulmonary involvement.

1. The stock bottle of Lanoxin contains 0.05 mg. of the drug in 1 cc. of solution. How much solution will contain a single dose (0.08 mg.) of the drug for Susan? _____ cc.

   A. 0.06   B. 0.6   C. 1.6   D. 2.6

   1. C

2. Prior to the administration of a dose of Lanoxin to Susan, the nurse should take her _____ pulse.

   A. femoral   B. apical
   C. radial   D. both apical and radial

   2. B

3. The nurse would be CORRECT in withholding Susan's dose of Lanoxin without specific instructions from the doctor if Susan's pulse rate were below beats per minute.

   A. 100   B. 115   C. 130   D. 145

   3. A

4. Which of these measures is likely to be MOST helpful in providing for Susan's nutritional needs while she is acutely ill?

   A. Serving her food lukewarm
   B. Giving her only liquids that she can take through a straw
   C. Offering her small portions of favorite foods frequently
   D. Mixing her foods together so that they are not readily identifiable

   4. C

5. Because Susan has symptoms of acute cardiac failure, her oral feedings will DIFFER from the feedings of a normal child the same age in the

   A. size of the feedings *only*
   B. rapidity and size of the feedings
   C. frequency and rapidity of the feedings
   D. size, rapidity, and frequency of the feedings

   5. D

6. All of the following information is part of Susan's health history. Which fact relates MOST directly to a diagnosis of cystic fibrosis?

   A. Emergency surgery as a newborn for intestinal obstruction
   B. Jaundice that lasted 4 days during the newborn period

   6. A

C.   A temperature of 104° F. (40° C.) followed by a convulsion when she was 6 months old

D.   A left otitis media treated with antibiotics when she was 12 months old

7.   Susan is placed in a mist tent in order to

    A.   increase the hydration of secretions
    B.   prevent the loss of fluids through evaporation
    C.   aid in maintaining a therapeutic environmental temperature
    D.   improve the transport of oxygen and carbon dioxide

7.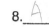

8.   Susan is receiving pancreatin replacement therapy to promote the absorption of

    A.   protein
    B.   carbohydrate
    C.   vitamin C (ascorbic acid)
    D.   sodium

8. A

Questions 9-13.

DIRECTIONS: Questions 9 through 13 are to be answered on the basis of the following information.

Ms. Leslie Browne, a 21-year-old college student, is seen by a physician because of fatigue and weight loss. Physical examination reveals slight enlargement of her cervical lymph nodes. Ms. Browne is admitted to the hospital for diagnostic studies.

9.   Ms. Browne states that she has had a low-grade fever. Which of these questions pertaining to Ms. Browne's low-grade fever should the nurse ask INITIALLY?

    A.   When did you first notice that your temperature had gone up?
    B.   Has your temperature been over 102 degrees?
    C.   Have you recently been exposed to anyone who has an infection?
    D.   Do you have a sore throat?

9. A

10.   Ms. Browne is to have a chest x-ray and is to be transported to the x-ray department by stretcher. All of the following actions may be taken by the nurse when sending Ms. Browne for the x-ray. Which action is ESSENTIAL?

    A.   Strap Ms. Browne securely to the stretcher.
    B.   Place Ms. Browne's chart under the mattress of the stretcher.
    C.   Ask Ms. Browne to remove her wristwatch.
    D.   Assign a nurse's aide to accompany Ms. Browne.

10. A

11.   The results of diagnostic tests establish that Ms. Browne has Hodgkin's disease with involvement of the cervical and mediastinal nodes. She is to have an initial course of intravenous chemotherapy with mechlorethamine (Mustar-gen) hydrochloride. The Mustargen that Ms. Browne receives is administered to her through the tubing of a rapidly flowing intravenous infusion.
The purpose of this method of administration is to

    A.   reduce the half-life of the medication
    B.   minimize the side effects of the medication

11.

C. decrease irritation of the blood vessel by the medication
D. control the rate of absorption of the medication

12. While Ms. Browne is receiving Mustargen therapy, she is MOST likely to develop   12. D

A. alopecia   B. fecal impactions
C. temporary neuropathy   D. transient nausea

13. The insertion site of Ms. Browne's intravenous infusion is edematous.   13. B
Which of these actions should the nurse take?

A. Lower the height of the infusion container
B. Discontinue the infusion
C. Flush the infusion tubing with 5 ml. of isotonic saline solution
D. Reduce the rate of infusion

Questions 14-25.

DIRECTIONS: Questions 14 through 25 are to be answered on the basis of the following information.

Mr. Robert Dine, a 66-year-old widower who has diabetes mellitus, is admitted to the
hospital in metabolic acidosis. He has gangrene of the great toe of his left foot and ulceration
of the heel.

14. Immediately after Mr. Dine's admission, the nurse places him on his side and then at fre-   14. C
quent intervals turns him from side to side.
The CHIEF purpose of these actions is to

A. reduce the possibility of pulmonary embolism
B. insure maximal circulation in the gangrenous extremity
C. promote the exchange of oxygen and carbon dioxide
D. facilitate the breakdown of lactic acid

15. Because Mr. Dine has a gangrenous toe and a heel ulcer, which of the following equip-   15. D
ment is ESSENTIAL to his care?

A. Sheepskin pad   B. Heat lamp
C. Bed board   D. Cradle

16. The physician has ordered warm saline dressings to be applied to Mr. Dine's heel ulcer   16. A
for 20 minutes twice a day. A nurse observes another staff nurse preparing a clean basin
and a washcloth to carry out the treatment. Which of these approaches by the nurse who
makes the observation would be APPROPRIATE?

A. Interrupt the nurse assembling supplies to discuss the procedure
B. Present the situation for discussion at a team conference
C. Do nothing, as the procedure is being done using correct technique
D. Do nothing, as each nurse is accountable for her or his own actions

17. Mr. Dine's lesions have not responded to conservative medical therapy. He is scheduled   17. _A_
to have a below-the-knee amputation of the affected extremity. Mr. Dine's orders include
administration of regular insulin on a sliding scale. Mr. Dine, who received isophane
(NPH) insulin prior to his admission to the hospital, has been on regular insulin since
admission. Regular insulin is to be continued for him until after his recovery from surgery.
Mr. Dine asks what the reason is for this order. Which of the following information would
give Mr. Dine the BEST explanation?

    A.   When complications are present, diabetes is more manageable with regular insu-
lin.
    B.   During the first week after a patient recovers from an episode of diabetic acidosis,
the likelihood of a recurrence is greatest.
    C.   Diminished activity intensifies the body's response to long-acting insulin.
    D.   Diabetic acidosis causes a temporary increase in the rate of food absorption.

18. Mr. Dine asks why he cannot be given insulin by mouth. He should be informed that insu-   18. _A_
lin is NOT given by mouth because it

    A.   is destroyed by digestive enzymes
    B.   is irritating to the gastrointestinal tract
    C.   is detoxified by the liver
    D.   cannot be regulated as it is absorbed

19. Mr. Dine is receiving an intravenous infusion of 5% glucose in distilled water. Regular   19. _A_
insulin is administered intravenously every two hours.
The purpose of the insulin is to

    A.   enhance carbohydrate metabolism
    B.   promote conversion of fat to glycogen
    C.   stimulate gluconeogenesis
    D.   assist in the regulation of fluid absorption

20. Regular insulin is given to Mr. Dine on a sliding scale to   20. _B_

    A.   lengthen its peak action
    B.   minimize the risk of hypoglycemia
    C.   prolong glyconeogenesis
    D.   prevent the rapid release of glucagon

21. Mr. Dine has a below-the-knee amputation. Following recovery from anesthesia, he is   21. _C_
brought back to the surgical unit. Because Mr. Dine has diabetes mellitus, he is susceptible to the development of a wound infection postoperatively.
Mr. Dine's care plan should include measures that will overcome the fact that patients
with diabetes mellitus have

    A.   ketone bodies excreted into their subcutaneous tissue
    B.   a greater insensitivity to antibiotics
    C.   decreased ability to combat pathogens
    D.   a larger number of microscopic organisms on their skin

22. To prevent the deformities to which Mr. Dine is particularly susceptible, his affected limb should be placed with the hip

    22. _D_

    A. flexed and the knee extended
    B. rotated outwardly and the knee flexed
    C. extended and the knee flexed
    D. and knee extended

23. Mr. Dine's condition improves. Physical therapy treatments are begun for him. He is to be taught crutch-walking. After returning from his first treatment, Mr. Dine begins to cry. The nurse's attempts to explore with Mr. Dine the reasons for his crying have been unsuccessful. Under these circumstances, it would be justifiable for the nurse to proceed on the assumption that Mr. Dine's behavior is PROBABLY related to a

    23. _B_

    A. fear of becoming dependent
    B. feeling of loss
    C. reaction to physical pain
    D. response to muscle reconditioning

24. Mr. Dine is now receiving a daily dose of a long-acting insulin preparation that he will continue to take at home.
    Which of these bedtime snacks would be BEST for him?

    24. _A_

    A. Cheese and crackers   B. An apple and diet cola
    C. Orange juice and toast   D. Canned peaches and tea

25. Before Mr. Dine is discharged, he should have which of these understandings about his own care?

    25. _C_

    A. Less insulin will be required since the diseased tissue has been removed.
    B. Social activities must be limited to conserve energy.
    C. The stump should be examined daily.
    D. Tissue breakdown will be prevented if foods high in vitamin C are taken daily.

KEY(CORRECT ANSWERS)

1.	C	11.	C
2.	B	12.	D
3.	A	13.	B
4.	C	14.	C
5.	D	15.	D
6.	A	16.	A
7.	A	17.	A
8.	A	18.	A
9.	A	19.	A
10.	A	20.	B

21.	C
22.	D
23.	B
24.	A
25.	C

TEST 3

DIRECTIONS: Each question or incomplete statement is followed by several suggested answers or completions. Select the one that BEST answers the question or completes the statement. *PRINT THE LETTER OF THE CORRECT ANSWER IN THE SPACE AT THE RIGHT.*

1. A physician orders the following pre-operative medications for a child: Demerol hydro-chloride 8 mg.; Atropine sulfate 0.06 mg. On hand are the following vials: Meperidine (Demerol) hydrochloride 50 mg. in 1 cc.; Atropine sulfate 0.40 mg. in 1 cc. In order to administer the prescribed doses, the nurse should give _____ of meperi-dine and _____ of atropine.

    A. 0.16 cc.; 0.15 cc.
    B. 0.26 cc.; 0.20 cc.
    C. 1 minim; 3 minims
    D. 2 minims; 4 minims

1.___A___

2. To provide care to a patient who has lost a body part or valued function, which of these measures is ESSENTIAL to include in the care plan?

    A. Inviting the assistance of a person who has a similar handicap
    B. Encouraging an immediate independence in self-care
    C. Providing information to the patient about available prosthetic devices
    D. Allowing adequate time for the patient to work through his grief

2.___D___

Questions 3-9.

DIRECTIONS: Questions 3 through 9 are to be answered on the basis of the following infor-mation.

Ms. Gloria Goldstein, 40 years old, visits a physician because of pain in her left leg. The physician determines that Ms. Goldstein has thrombophlebitis in her left leg and hospital admission is arranged. Her orders include bed rest and bishydroxycoumarin (Dicumarol).

3. Bed rest is prescribed for Ms. Goldstein in order to

    A. promote fluctuations in the venous pressure of both extremities
    B. improve the capacity of the venous circulation in both extremities
    C. minimize the potential for release of a thrombus in the affected extremity
    D. prevent thrombus formation in the unaffected extremity

3.___C___

4. The expected action of Dicumarol is to

    A. dissolve a thrombus
    B. prevent extension of a thrombus
    C. promote healing of the infarction
    D. reduce vascular necrosis

4.___B___

5. To detect a common untoward effect of Dicumarol, the nurse should assess Ms. Gold-stein for the possible development of

    A. generalized dermatitis
    B. hematuria
    C. urinary retention
    D. vitamin K deficiency

5.___B___

6. While Ms. Goldstein is receiving Dicumarol, she should be monitored by which of these laboratory tests?   6.__A__

    A. Prothrombin time   B. Clotting time
    C. Red cell fragility   D. Platelet count

7. An order for which of these medications should be questioned because it is usually contraindicated for a patient receiving Dicumarol?   7.__B__

    A. Cortisone
    B. Aspirin
    C. Chlorpromazine hydrochloride (Thorazine)
    D. Isoproterenol (Isuprel) hydrochloride

8. The nurse is talking with Ms. Goldstein on the third day of her hospitalization. Suddenly, Ms. Goldstein, who is in bed, complains of a sharp pain in the left side of her chest. The physician establishes a diagnosis of pulmonary embolus. Ms. Goldstein's orders include absolute bed rest and heparin.   8.__B__
Which of these medications should be readily available while Ms. Goldstein is receiving heparin therapy?

    A. Procainamide (Pronestyl) hydrochloride
    B. Protamine sulfate
    C. Papaverine hydrochloride
    D. Calcium gluconate

9. At lunchtime one day, Ms. Goldstein, who is on a regular diet, states that she does not feel hungry.   9.__D__
The nurse should

    A. encourage her to eat the full meal
    B. emphasize her need for protein
    C. limit her snacks
    D. allow her to eat as she likes

10. The BEST beginning point in offering support to a patient in time of crisis is to   10.__B__

    A. tell the client what to do to solve the problem
    B. imply that the client is a competent person
    C. find a person or agency to take care of the problem
    D. remind the client that everyone has to cope with crises

Questions 11-16.

DIRECTIONS: Questions 11 through 16 are to be answered on the basis of the following information.

    Ms. Sylvia Capp, 53 years old, has a physical examination, and it is determined that she is hypertensive. She attends the medical clinic and is receiving health instruction and supervision. Ms. Capp is to receive a thiazide drug and a diet low in fat, sodium, and triglycerides.

11. The finding that would constitute a significant index of hypertension is a   11.___D___

    A. pulse deficit of 10 beats per minute
    B. regular pulse of 90 beats per minute
    C. systolic pressure fluctuating between 150 and 160 mm. Hg.
    D. sustained diastolic pressure greater than 90 mm. Hg.

12. The nurse asks Ms. Capp to select foods that best meet her diet prescription.   12.___C___
Ms. Capp's knowledge of goods lowest in both fat and sodium would be ACCURATE if
she selected

    A. tossed salad with blue cheese dressing, cold cuts, and vanilla cookies
    B. split pea soup, cheese sandwich, and a banana
    C. cold baked chicken, lettuce with sliced tomatoes, and applesauce
    D. beans and frankfurters, carrot and celery sticks, and a plain cupcake

13. When teaching Ms. Capp about her diet, the nurse should include which of these instruc-   13.___B___
tions?

    A. Avoid eating canned fruits
    B. Season your meat with lemon juice or vinegar
    C. Restrict your intake of green vegetables
    D. Drink diet soda instead of decaffeinated coffee

14. To assist Ms. Capp to comply with a low-fat diet, the information about fats that would be   14.___B___
MOST useful to her is the

    A. amount of fat in processed meats
    B. method of preparing foods to limit the fat content
    C. comparison of hydrogenated fats to emulsified fats
    D. caloric differences of foods containing fats and carbohydrates

15. Because Ms. Capp is receiving a thiazide drug, her diet should include foods that are   15.___B___
high in

    A. calcium   B. potassium
    C. iron   D. magnesium

16. Ms. Capp tells the nurse that she smokes two packs of cigarettes a day.   16.___A___
To initiate a plan that will assist Ms. Capp in overcoming her smoking habit, which of
these actions by the nurse would probably be MOST effective?

    A. Have her identify those times when she feels that she must have a cigarette
    B. Ask her to describe what she knows about the deleterious effects of smoking on
       her condition
    C. Explain to her how smoking contributes to environmental pollution
    D. Impress on her the realization that smoking is a form of addiction that is no longer
       socially acceptable

Questions 17-25.

DIRECTIONS: Questions 17 through 25 are to be answered on the basis of the following information.

Mr. Ethan Allen, 46 years old, is admitted to a center for the treatment of persons who
abuse alcohol. He had been drinking a quart or more of liquor a day for 10 to 15 years. He
was drinking up to the time of his admission. His wife is with him.

17.   Mr. Allen's immediate treatment is MOST likely to include orders for   17. C

    A.   oral fluids, ascorbic acid, and a narcotic
    B.   a cool bath, a barbiturate, and blood lithium level
    C.   full diet as tolerated, thiamine, and a tranquilizer
    D.   a spinal tap, bromides, and restraints

18.   If Mr. Allen develops delirium tremens, which of these environmental factors is likely to be   18. B
MOST disturbing?

    A.   Strangers   B.   Shadows
    C.   Unfamiliar procedures   D.   Medicinal odors

19.   Ms. Allen says to the nurse, *I'd do anything to help my husband stop drinking.*   19. A
The PRIMARY goal of the nurse's response should be to

    A.   get Ms. Allen to clarify the problem as she sees it
    B.   have Ms. Allen join Al-Anon
    C.   tell Ms. Allen that she has done all she could to help her husband
    D.   have Ms. Allen understand that alcoholism is a problem that only her husband can
solve

20.   In giving care to Mr. Allen, the nurse should be alert for complications of withdrawal,   20. D
which include

    A.   aphasia   B.   hypotension
    C.   diarrhea   D.   convulsions

21.   After several weeks of group therapy, Mr. Allen says to the nurse, *I've never been able to*   21. D
face life without alcohol.
Which of the responses would initially be MOST appropriate?

    A.   I know how you feel, Mr. Allen. We all have difficulty in meeting some problems.
    B.   But now you know where to go for help.
    C.   Perhaps you can manage if you join Alcoholics Anonymous, Mr. Allen.
    D.   That has been the way you have dealt with your problems.

22.   Mr. Allen's success in abstaining from drinking is thought to depend on his   22. B

    A.   admission that his behavior is detrimental to himself and his family
    B.   conviction that he must change and has some capacity for change
    C.   ability to express remorse
    D.   having taken a pledge witnessed by fellow alcoholics

23. Mr. Allen is started on disulfiram (Antabuse), which he will continue to take after discharge from the hospital. It should be emphasized to Mr. Allen that while he is on Antabuse, he must NEVER take

    A. elixir of terpin hydrate
    B. aspirin
    C. bicarbonate of soda
    D. antihistamines

23._A_

24. Patients such as Mr. Allen may develop Korsakoff's psychosis. Which of these symptoms is associated with this condition?

    A. Fantastic delusions and fear
    B. Sullenness and suspiciousness
    C. Amnesia and confabulation
    D. Nihilistic ideas and tearfulness

24._C_

25. The nurse explains Alcoholics Anonymous to Mr. Allen. An understanding implemented by Alcoholics Anonymous is that people

    A. feel less alone when they feel understood
    B. are more likely to be able to handle problems when they are alerted to them ahead of time
    C. are dependent upon their environment for cues that keep them oriented
    D. resort to defense mechanisms as a means of coping with anxiety

25._A_

KEY (CORRECT ANSWERS}

1.	A		11.	D
2.	D		12.	C
3.	C		13.	B
4.	B		14.	B
5.	B		15.	B
6.	A		16.	A
7.	B		17.	C
8.	B		18.	B
9.	D		19.	A
10.	B		20.	D

21. D
22. B
23. A
24. C
25. A

EXAMINATION SECTION
TEST 1

DIRECTIONS: Each question or incomplete statement is followed by several suggested answers or completions. Select the one that BEST answers the question or completes the statement. *PRINT THE LETTER OF THE CORRECT ANSWER IN THE SPACE AT THE RIGHT.*

1. The abbreviation *EEG* refers to a(n)   1. _D_

   A. examination of the eyes and ears
   B. inflammatory disease of the urinogenital tract
   C. disease of the esophageal structure
   D. examination of the brain

2. The complete destruction of all forms of living microorganisms is called   2. _C_

   A. decontamination   B. sterilization
   C. fumigation   D. germination

3. A rectal thermometer differs from other fever thermometers in that it has a   3. _C_

   A. longer stem   B. thinner stem
   C. stubby bulb at one end   D. slender bulb at one end

4. The one of the following pieces of equipment which is USUALLY used together with a sphygmometer is a   4. _A_

   A. stethoscope   B. watch
   C. fever thermometer   D. hypodermic syringe

5. A curette is a   5. _D_

   A. healing drug   B. curved scalpel
   C. long hypodermic needle   D. scraping instrument

6. The otoscope is used to examine the patient's   6. _B_

   A. eyes   B. ears   C. mouth   D. lungs

7. A catheter is used   7. _B_

   A. to close wounds
   B. for withdrawing fluid from a body cavity
   C. to remove cataracts
   D. as a cathartic

8. Of the following pieces of equipment, the one that is required for making a scratch test is a   8. _A_

   A. needle   B. scalpel   C. capillary tube   D. tourniquet

9. A hemostat is an instrument which is used to   9. _B_

   A. hold a sterile needle
   B. clamp off a blood vessel
   C. regulate the temperature of a sterilizer
   D. measure oxygen intake

10. Of the following medical supplies, the one that MUST be stored in a tightly sealed bottle is

    A. sodium fluoride   B. alum
    C. oil of cloves   D. aromatic spirits of ammonia

10. D

11. A person who has been exposed to an infectious disease is called

    A. a contact   B. an incubator
    C. diseased   D. infected

11. A

12. A myocardial infarct would occur in the

    A. heart   B. kidneys   C. lungs   D. spleen

12. A

13. The abbreviations *WBC* and *RBC* refer to the results of tests of the

    A. basal metabolism   B. blood
    C. blood pressure   D. bony structure

13. B

14. When a person's blood pressure is noted as 120/80, it means that his

    A. pulse blood pressure is 120
    B. pulse blood pressure is 80
    C. systolic blood pressure is 120
    D. systolic blood pressure is 80

14. C

15. The anatomical structure that contains the tonsils and adenoids is the

    A. pharynx   B. larynx   C. trachea   D. sinuses

15. A

16. An abscess can BEST be described as a

    A. loss of sensation
    B. painful tooth
    C. ruptured membrane
    D. localized formation of pus

16. D

17. Nephritis is a disease affecting the

    A. gall bladder   B. larynx
    C. kidney   D. large intestine

17. C

18. Hemoglobin is contained in the

    A. white blood cells   B. lymph fluids
    C. platelets   D. red blood cells

18. D

19. Bile is a body fluid that is MOST directly concerned with

    A. digestion   B. excretion
    C. reproduction   D. metabolism

19. A

20. Of the following bones, the one which is located BELOW the waist is the

    A. sternum   B. clavicle   C. tibia   D. humerus

20. C

21. The one of the following which is NOT part of the digestive canal is the

21. _B_

    A. esophagus   B. larynx   C. duodenum   D. colon

22. The thyroid and the pituitary are part of the _____ system.

22. _B_

    A. digestive   B. endocrine
    C. respiratory   D. excretory

23. The one of the following which would be included in a *GU* examination is the

23. _C_

    A. rectum   B. trachea   C. kidneys   D. pancreas

24. Of the following, the one which would be included in the x-ray examination known as a *GI series* is the

24. _A_

    A. colon   B. skull   C. lungs   D. uterus

25. A person who, while not ill himself, may transmit a disease to another person is known as a(n)

25. _C_

    A. breeder   B. incubator
    C. carrier   D. inhibitor

KEY (CORRECT ANSWERS)

1.	D	11.	A
2.	C	12.	A
3.	C	13.	B
4.	A	14.	C
5.	D	15.	A
6.	B	16.	D
7.	B	17.	C
8.	A	18.	D
9.	B	19.	A
10.	D	20.	C

21.	B
22.	B
23.	C
24.	A
25.	C

TEST 2

DIRECTIONS: Each question or incomplete statement is followed by several suggested answers or completions. Select the one that BEST answers the question or completes the statement. *PRINT THE LETTER OF THE CORRECT ANSWER IN THE SPACE AT THE RIGHT.*

1. Thorough washing of the hands for two minutes with soap and warm water will leave the hands

    A. sterile
    B. aseptic
    C. decontaminated
    D. partially disinfected

    1. D

2. The one of the following which is BEST for preparing the skin for an injection is

    A. green soap and water
    B. alcohol
    C. phenol
    D. formalin

    2. B

3. A fever thermometer should be cleansed after use by washing it with

    A. soap and cool water
    B. warm water only
    C. soap and hot water
    D. running cold tap water

    3. A

4. The FIRST step in cleaning an instrument which has fresh blood on it is to

    A. wash it in hot soapy water
    B. wash it under cool running water
    C. soak it in a boric acid bath
    D. soak it in 70% alcohol

    4. B

5. If a contaminated nasal speculum cannot be sterilized immediately after use, then the BEST procedure to follow until sterilization is possible is to place it

    A. under a piece of dry *gauze*
    B. in warm water
    C. in alcohol
    D. in a green soap solution

    5. D

6. A hypodermic needle should ALWAYS be checked to see whether it has a good sharp point

    A. when it is being washed
    B. when it is removed from the sterilizer
    C. just before it is sterilized
    D. immediately before an injection

    6. C

7. Of the following, the LOWEST temperature at which cotton goods will be sterilized if placed in an autoclave for 30 minutes is

    A. 130° F   B. 170° F   C. 200° F   D. 250° F

    7. D

8. Of the following procedures, the one which is BEST for sterilizing an ear speculum which is contaminated with wax is to   8. __C__

    A. scrub it with cold soapy water, rinse in ether, and place in boiling water for 20 minutes

    B. soak it in warm water, scrub in cold soapy water, rinse with water, and autoclave at 275° F for 10 minutes

    C. wash it in alcohol, scrub in hot soapy water, rinse with water, and place in boiling water for 20 minutes

    D. wash it in 1% Lysol solution, rinse, and autoclave at 275° F for 15 minutes

9. Assume that clean water accidentally spilled on the outside of a package of cloth-wrapped hypodermic syringes which has been sterilized.
Of the following, the BEST action to take is to   9. __B__

    A. leave the package to dry in a sunny, clean place

    B. sterilize the package again

    C. remove the wet cloth and wrap the package in a dry sterile cloth

    D. wipe off the package with a clean dry towel and later ask the nurse-in-charge what to do

10. Hypodermic needles should be sterilized by placing them in   10. __B__

    A. boiling water for 5 minutes

    B. an autoclave at 15 lbs. pressure for 15 minutes

    C. oil heated to 220° F for 10 minutes

    D. a 1:40 Lysol solution for 10 minutes

11. A cutting instrument should be sterilized by placing it in   11. __A__

    A. a chemical germicide

    B. an autoclave at 15 lbs. pressure for 20 minutes

    C. boiling water for 20 minutes

    D. a hot air oven at 320° F for 1 hour

12. A fever thermometer used by a patient who has tuberculosis should be washed and then placed in   12. __C__

    A. boiling water for 10 minutes

    B. a hot air oven for 20 minutes

    C. a 1:1000 solution of bichloride of mercury for one minute

    D. an autoclave at 15 lbs. pressure for 15 minutes

13. The MOST reliable method of sterilizing a glass syringe is to place it in   13. __D__

    A. Zephiran chloride 1:1000 solution for 40 minutes

    B. oil heated to 250° F for 12 minutes

    C. boiling water for 20 minutes

    D. an autoclave at 15 lbs. pressure for 20 minutes

14. The insides of sterilizers should be cleaned daily with a mild abrasive PRIMARILY to 14. A

    A. remove scale
    B. prevent the growth of bacteria
    C. remove blood and other organic matter
    D. prevent acids from damaging the sterilizer

15. Of the following, the BEST reason for giving a patient a jar in which to bring a urine spec- 15. C
imen on his next visit to the clinic is that the

    A. patient may not have a jar at home
    B. patient may bring the specimen in a jar which is too large
    C. patient may bring the specimen in a jar which has not been cleaned properly
    D. jar may be misplaced if it is not a jar in which urine specimens are usually collected

16. Of the following, the MOST important reason why you should remain with a 4-year-old 16. B
child when his temperature is being taken by mouth is that otherwise the child might

    A. fall off the chair and fracture an arm or leg
    B. break the thermometer while it is in his mouth
    C. remove the thermometer from his mouth and misplace it
    D. leave the examining room and return to his mother

17. The BEST way to take the temperature of an infant is by 17. D

    A. feeling his forehead
    B. using an oral thermometer
    C. placing a thermometer under his armpit
    D. using a rectal thermometer

18. When the temperature of an adult is taken rectally, it is LEAST accurate to say that the 18. C

    A. temperature reading will be higher than if it were taken orally
    B. thermometer should be lubricated before use
    C. thermometer should be in place for at least ten minutes
    D. temperature reading is likely to be more accurate than if it were taken orally

19. When the temperature of an adult is taken orally, it is LEAST accurate to say that the 19. C

    A. thermometer should be washed with alcohol before it is used
    B. thermometer should be taken down below 96° F before it is used
    C. patient's temperature may be taken immediately after he has smoked a cigarette
    D. patient should be inactive just before his temperature is taken

20. The nurse described the test to the patient before bringing him to the examining room for 20. A
a basal metabolism test. Her action may BEST be described as

    A. *correct;* the patient will be more cooperative if he knows what to expect
    B. *wrong;* the nurse does not know how the test will affect the patient
    C. *correct;* the nurse can judge whether the patient is too upset by this information to take the test
    D. *wrong;* explaining the test beforehand will only make the patient nervous

21. When a patient's sputum test is *positive,* it means that the   21. _D_

    A. patient's sputum is plentiful
    B. doctor has made an accurate diagnosis
    C. patient has recovered and is now in good health
    D. laboratory reports that the patient's sputum contains certain disease germs

22. A biopsy can BEST be described as a(n)   22. _B_

    A. pre-cancerous condition   B. examination of tissues
    C. living organism   D. germicidal solution

23. The *scratch* or *patch* test is USUALLY given when testing for   23. _A_

    A. allergies   B. rheumatic fever
    C. blood poisoning   D. diabetes

24. Gamma globulin is frequently given to children after exposure to and before the appear-   24. _A_
ance of symptoms of

    A. measles   B. smallpox
    C. tetanus   D. chicken pox

25. Of the following, the one which is NOT a respiratory disease is   25. _C_

    A. bronchitis   B. pneumonia
    C. nephritis   D. croup

KEY (CORRECT ANSWERS)

1.	D		11.	A
2.	B		12.	C
3.	A		13.	D
4.	B		14.	A
5.	D		15.	C
6.	C		16.	B
7.	D		17.	D
8.	C		18.	C
9.	B		19.	C
10.	B		20.	A

21.	D
22.	B
23.	A
24.	A
25.	C

TEST 3

DIRECTIONS: Each question or incomplete statement is followed by several suggested answers or completions. Select the one that BEST answers the question or completes the statement. *PRINT THE LETTER OF THE CORRECT ANSWER IN THE SPACE AT THE RIGHT.*

1. A physician who specializes in the treatment of conditions affecting the skin is known as a(n)

    A. urologist   B. dermatologist
    C. toxicologist   D. ophthalmologist

1. B

2. The branch of medicine which deals with diseases peculiar to women is

    A. pathology   B. orthopedics
    C. neurology   D. gynecology

2. D

3. The branch of medicine which deals with diseases of old age is called

    A. pediatrics   B. geriatrics
    C. serology   D. histology

3. B

4. *Petit mal* is a form of

    A. epilepsy   B. syphilis   C. diabetes   D. malaria

4. A

5. Glaucoma is a disease of the

    A. thyroid gland   B. liver
    C. bladder   D. eye

5. D

6. A patient who has edema has

    A. not enough red blood cells
    B. too much water in the body tissues
    C. blood in the urine
    D. a swollen gland

6. B

7. The thoracic area of the body is located in the

    A. abdomen   B. lower back
    C. chest   D. neck

7. C

8. An electrocardiograph is MOST usually used in the examination of the

    A. brain   B. heart
    C. kidney   D. gall bladder

8. B

9. The word *coagulate* means MOST NEARLY to

    A. bleed excessively   B. break up
    C. work together   D. form a clot

9. D

10. A stethoscope is used to examine the patient's

    A. heart   B. patellar reflex
    C. blood cells   D. spinal fluid

10. A

11. A pelvimeter is MOST usually used in the examination of a patient in the _____ clinic.   11.___C___

    A. chest   B. cancer   C. prenatal   D. eye

12. Tuberculin may BEST be described as a   12.___B___

    A. virus infection of the lungs
    B. preparation used in the diagnosis of tuberculosis
    C. sanitarium for tuberculous patients
    D. form of cancer of the lung

13. An autoclave is a(n)   13.___C___

    A. automatic dispenser of instruments needed for clinic examinations
    B. sterile place for storing clinic supplies until they are needed
    C. apparatus for sterilizing equipment under steam pressure
    D. portable self-operating general anesthesia unit

14. Radiation therapy is   14.___C___

    A. the recording of electrical impulses of the body on a graph
    B. a study of the effects of radiation fall-out on the human body
    C. a form of treatment used for certain diseases
    D. the filming of internal parts of the body through the use of x-rays

15. Diathermy is the treatment of patients by   15.___D___

    A. scientific use of baths and mineral waters
    B. insertion of radium into diseased tissues
    C. intravenous feedings of vitamins and minerals
    D. electrical generation of heat in the body tissues

16. The measurement of blood pressure involves two readings, which are known as   16.___B___

    A. metabolic and diastolic
    B. systolic and diastolic
    C. metabolic and hyperbolic
    D. hyperbolic and systolic

17. The Snellen chart is used in examinations of the   17.___A___

    A. eyes   B. blood   C. urine   D. bile

18. An enema is MOST generally used to   18.___C___

    A. induce vomiting
    B. irrigate the stomach
    C. clear the bowels
    D. drain the urinary bladder

19. A bronchoscope is USUALLY used in examinations of the   19.___D___

    A. kidneys   B. heart   C. stomach   D. lungs

20. The Wassermann test is used to find out whether a patient has   20._D___

    A. diphtheria   B. leukemia
    C. scarlet fever   D. syphilis

21. If a boiling water sterilizer is used, the minimum time necessary to sterilize instruments is   21._A___
MOST NEARLY _____ hour(s).

    A. 1/2   B. 1   C. 1 1/2   D. 2

22. To sterilize towels and dry gauze dressings in the health clinic, it is MOST advisable to   22._D___

    A. dip them in a sterilizing solution
    B. wash them with a strong detergent
    C. boil them in the sterilizer
    D. steam them under pressure

23. Sterilization by use of chemicals rather than by boiling water is indicated when the instru-   23._B___
ment

    A. is made of soft rubber
    B. has a sharp cutting edge
    C. has pus or blood on it
    D. was used more than 24 hours before sterilization

24. When dusting the furniture in the clinic, it is advisable to use a silicone-treated dustcloth   24._A___
CHIEFLY because the treated cloth will

    A. collect the dust more efficiently
    B. disinfect as well as dust the furniture
    C. not remove the wax from the furniture
    D. make it unnecessary to polish the furniture in the future

25. Assume that the clinic in which you work has issued instructions that all supplies contain-   25._D___
ing poison are to have blue labels with the word *poison* clearly marked on the label, and
that these supplies are to be kept in a storage cabinet separate from other supplies. You
notice that a bottle with no label is on a shelf in the *poison* storage cabinet.
Of the following, the BEST action for you to take is to

    A. place the unlabeled bottle in the back of the regular storage cabinet
    B. put a blue label on the bottle and write *poison* on the label
    C. ask another public health employee to help you decide if the bottle contains poison
    D. pour the contents of the bottle into the slop sink and destroy the bottle

KEY (CORRECT ANSWERS)

1.	B		11.	C
2.	D		12.	B
3.	B		13.	C
4.	A		14.	C
5.	D		15.	D
6.	B		16.	B
7.	C		17.	A
8.	B		18.	C
9.	D		19.	D
10.	A		20.	D

21.	A
22.	D
23.	B
24.	A
25.	D

TEST 4

DIRECTIONS: Each question or incomplete statement is followed by several suggested answers or completions. Select the one that BEST answers the question or completes the statement. *PRINT THE LETTER OF THE CORRECT ANSWER IN THE SPACE AT THE RIGHT.*

1. When storing medical supplies, it is important to remember that liquids should be labeled   1. C

    A. only if the liquids are poisonous and there is the slightest chance that they will not be recognized
    B. whenever there is the slightest chance that they will not be recognized
    C. at all times and discarded if labels have become detached
    D. only in those cases where the liquids will be given to patients

2. When dusting metal counter tops in the clinic, it is BEST to use a clean cloth which is   2. D

    A. medicated   B. wet   C. dry   D. damp

3. Of the following statements concerning a hypodermic syringe, the one that is MOST correct is that a plunger   3. C

    A. used for taking blood specimens can be used with any syringe barrel
    B. can be used for any syringe barrel as long as it goes in easily
    C. can be used only with the syringe barrel that was made for it
    D. must be used with the syringe barrel that was made for it only if it is to be used for injections

4. The one of the following which should NOT be done when using a thermometer is to   4. C

    A. shake down the thermometer to 95° F before taking the patient's temperature
    B. ask the patient to keep his lips closed when taking the temperature orally
    C. wash the thermometer in hot soapy water after use
    D. keep the thermometer in a container of alcohol when not in use

5. The temperature of an adult when taken by rectum is USUALLY   5. A

    A. *higher* than if taken either by mouth or under the armpit
    B. *higher* than if taken by mouth and lower than if taken under the armpit
    C. *lower* than if taken either by mouth or under the armpit
    D. *lower* than if taken by mouth and higher than if taken under the armpit

6. Of the following tests, the one which is associated with tuberculosis is the _____ test.   6. B

    A. Schick   B. Mantoux   C. Dick   D. Kahn

7. A needle that has been used to draw blood should be rinsed immediately after use in   7. C

    A. a disinfectant solution   B. hot water
    C. cold water   D. hot, soapy water

8. Of the following, the statement that is MOST correct is that a hypodermic needle should   8. __B__
   be checked for burrs, hooks, and sharpness

   A. once a week
   B. before it is sterilized
   C. after it has been sterilized
   D. after it has been used three or four times

9. The MOST accurate of the following statements is that when a syringe and needle are   9. __A__
   being sterilized by boiling, the

   A. plunger must be completely out of the barrel
   B. needle should be left attached to the barrel as when in use
   C. plunger may be completely inside the barrel
   D. needle should be boiled at least twice as long as the syringe

10. Of the following, the MOST important reason for washing an instrument in hot, soapy   10. __D__
    water is to

    A. sterilize the instrument
    B. destroy germs by heat
    C. destroy germs by coagulation
    D. remove foreign matter and bacteria

11. Assume that a hypodermic needle which is to be used for injection is accidentally   11. __D__
    brushed at the tip by your hand. Of the following, the action which should be taken before
    this needle is used is that it be

    A. washed under the hot water tap
    B. wiped with a sterile piece of gauze
    C. washed in hot, soapy water, then rinsed in sterile water
    D. boiled for ten minutes

12. The CORRECT way to sterilize a scalpel is to   12. __A__

    A. place it in a chemical germicide
    B. boil it for 10 minutes
    C. put it in the autoclave
    D. pass it through a bright flame

13. Assume that a tray of instruments has been accidentally left uncovered for five minutes   13. __B__
    after it had been sterilized.
    Of the following, the action you should take to ensure that the instruments are sterile
    for use is to

    A. dip them in boiling water
    B. boil them for 10 minutes
    C. replace the cover on the tray
    D. wipe each instrument with sterile gauze

14. An intramuscular injection is MOST likely to be used in the administration of   14. __B__

    A. smallpox vaccine   B. streptomycin
    C. glucose   D. blood

31

15. The one of the following which is NOT a normal element of blood is   15. C

    A. hemoglobin   B. a leucocyte
    C. marrow   D. a platelet

16. Of the following statements regarding the Salk vaccine, the MOST accurate one is that it   16. A

    A. immunizes children and adults against paralytic poliomyelit is
    B. is a test to determine the presence of poliomyelitis virus in the blood
    C. is a test to determine whether a child is immune to poliomyelitis
    D. is used in the treatment of patients suffering from paralytic poliomyelitis

17. The GREATEST success in the treatment of cancer has been in cancer of the   17. D

    A. blood   B. stomach   C. liver   D. skin

18. An autopsy is a(n)   18. C

    A. type of blood test
    B. examination of tissue removed from a living organism
    C. examination of a human body after death
    D. test to determine the acidity of body fluids

19. The word *vascular* is MOST closely associated with   19. A

    A. the circulatory system   B. respiration
    C. digestion   D. the nervous system

20. The word *diagnosis* means MOST NEARLY   20. B

    A. preparation of a diagram
    B. determination of an illness
    C. medical examination of a patient
    D. written prescription

21. A tendon connects   21. B

    A. bone to bone   B. muscle to bone
    C. muscle to muscle   D. muscle to ligament

22. Blood takes on oxygen as it passes through the   22. D

    A. liver   B. heart   C. spleen   D. lungs

23. The fatty substance in the blood which is deposited in the artery walls and which is   23. C
    believed to cause hardening of the arteries is called

    A. amino acid   B. phenol
    C. cholesterol   D. pectin

24. The digestive canal includes the   24. A

    A. stomach, small intestine, large intestine, and rectum
    B. stomach, larynx, large intestine, and rectum
    C. trachea, small intestine, large intestine, and rectum
    D. stomach, small intestine, large intestine, and abdominal cavity

25. When giving artificial respiration, it should be kept in mind that air is drawn into the lungs   25.____
    by the

    A. expansion of the chest cavity
    B. contraction of the chest cavity
    C. expansion of the lungs
    D. contraction of the lungs

———

KEY (CORRECT ANSWERS)

1.	C	11.	D
2.	D	12.	A
3.	C	13.	B
4.	C	14.	B
5.	A	15.	C
6.	B	16.	A
7.	C	17.	D
8.	B	18.	C
9.	A	19.	A
10.	D	20.	B

21.	B
22.	D
23.	C
24.	A
25.	A

———

EXAMINATION SECTION
TEST 1

DIRECTIONS: Each question or incomplete statement is followed by several suggested answers or completions. Select the one that BEST answers the question or completes the statement. *PRINT THE LETTER OF THE CORRECT ANSWER IN THE SPACE AT THE RIGHT.*

1. The *preferred* method of controlling hemorrhage is by

    A.   applying pressure at the pressure points
    B.   using a wide elastic tourniquet
    C.   applying pressure over the wound with a clean cloth
    D.   applying a large gauze dressing to absorb and clot the blood

1. _C_

2. For general use, the BEST method of artificial respiration is

    A.   back pressure - arm lift
    B.   breathe into mouth of the victim
    C.   prone - pressure
    D.   compression - release

2. _B_

3. For an adult with a normal skin, the temperature of the hot water bottle should be *between*

    A.   120°-130° F.   B.   100°-110° F.
    C.   140°-150° F.   D.   160°-170° F.

3. _A_

4. Penicillin was discovered by

    A.   Jonas Salk   B.   Alexander Fleming
    C.   R. J. Diebos   D.   Selman A. Waksman

4. _B_

5. Underweight is the PRIMARY contributory factor in

    A.   still birth   B.   premature labor
    C.   anomalies in the birth process   D.   abnormal deliveries

5. _B_

6. The part of the brain that is associated with memory is the

    A.   cerebellum   B.   pons varolii
    C.   medulla oblongata   D.   cerebrum

6. _A_

7. To restore the markings on a mouth thermometer,

    A.   dip the thermometer in melted wax
    B.   apply sealing wax and scrape off excess
    C.   apply dark red nail polish and wife off at once
    D.   dip in eosin solution and wipe off

7. _C_

8. The compound which is NOT a constituent of normal urine is

    A.   ammonia   B.   creatinine
    C.   hippuric acid   D.   indican

8. _D_

9. A water solution of ammonia is a(n)   9. _C_

    A. acid   B. basic salt   C. base   D. acid salt

10. The substance that is NOT used in testing for sugar is   10. _B_

    A. clinitest   B. phenolsulphonephthalein
    C. Fehling's solution   D. Benedict's solution

11. The substances that are NOT miscible are   11. _A_

    A. olive oil and acetic acid
    B. glycerine and alcohol
    C. soap and water
    D. linseed oil and lime-water

12. The downward pressure of the water in an enema can depend upon the   12. _D_

    A. speed of flow
    B. size of the tube opening
    C. quantity of fluid used
    D. the height of the surface of the water above the patient

13. The administration of vaccine should   13. _A_

    A. precede exposure to the disease
    B. reduce the duration of the disease
    C. follow after the disease has run its course
    D. prevent further spread of the infection

14. The SAFEST way of dusting a sick room is with a   14. _C_

    A. vacuum machine   B. feather duster
    C. damp cloth   D. dry cloth

15. *Before* disposing of food that is left over on a tray of a patient with a communicable dis-   15. _B_
ease, it should be

    A. wrapped in newspaper   B. boiled for 5 minutes
    C. boiled for 10 minutes   D. boiled for 15 minutes

16. A sheet which is stained by body discharges should FIRST be   16. _D_

    A. bleached   B. washed with warm water and soap
    C. boiled   D. rinsed in cold water

17. The ill person should be kept warm because in this way the blood   17. _B_

    A. *increases* in viscosity   B. *decreases* in viscosity
    C. *decreases* in fluidity   D. *increases* in saline cotent

18. Longer-acting penicillin has been an *effective* influence in the control of   18. _A_

    A. gonorrhea   B. tuberculosis   C. meningitis   D. measles

19. A stimulant for the respiratory center is   19. _A_

    A. carbon dioxide   B. ethyl chloride
    C. oxygen   D. nitrous oxide

20. The parts of the nervous system stimulated by strychnine are the　　　　　　　　　　20. _B_

    A. hepatic and renal nerves
    B. brain and spinal cord
    C. autonomic ganglia and sciatic nerves
    D. coronary and pulmonary nerves

21. The GREATEST disease threat to the newborn in the United States is　　　　　　21. _B_

    A. scarlet fever　　　　　　　　　B. diarrhea
    C. whooping cough　　　　　　　　D. measles

22. To keep MOST cut flowers fresh,　　　　　　　　　　　　　　　　　　　　　22. _A_

    A. cut the end slantwise with a sharp knife
    B. cut the stems when they wilt, using scissors
    C. change the water every day
    D. use very cold water

23. Solutions are absorbed MORE rapidly when　　　　　　　　　　　　　　　　　23. _C_

    A. they are in concentrated form
    B. they are slightly diluted
    C. spread over a large surface
    D. spread over a limited area

24. Natural resistance to infection is *lowered* by　　　　　　　　　　　　　　　24. _A_

    A. fatigue　　　　　　　　　　　　B. reducing diets
    C. cold weather　　　　　　　　　　D. lack of immunization

25. Diphtheria can be prevented through the use of　　　　　　　　　　　　　　　25. _B_

    A. the Schick test　　　　　　　　　B. diphtheria toxoid
    C. therapeutic antiserum　　　　　　D. antibiotics

KEY (CORRECT ANSWERS)

1.	C	11.	A
2.	B	12.	D
3.	A	13.	A
4.	B	14.	C
5.	B	15.	B
6.	D	16.	D
7.	C	17.	B
8.	D	18.	A
9.	C	19.	A
10.	B	20.	B

21.	B
22.	A
23.	C
24.	A
25.	B

———

TEST 2

DIRECTIONS: Each question or incomplete statement is followed by several suggested answers or completions. Select the one that BEST answers the question or completes the statement. *PRINT THE LETTER OF THE CORRECT ANSWER IN THE SPACE AT THE RIGHT.*

1.   Audible sound is measured in terms of

    A.   farads   B.   decibels   C.   ohms   D.   rels

1. _B_

2.   Reduction in incidental nausea during pregnancy has been effected by an increase in the intake of

    A.   ascorbic acid   B.   vitamin D
    C.   vitamin B-complex   D.   minerals

2. _C_

3.   Diet therapy is concerned *principally* with

    A.   stimulation of impaired tissues
    B.   maintaining health
    C.   modification of customary diet
    D.   reducing caloric intake

3. _C_

4.   *Most* economic for protein re-enforcement of the diet is

    A.   egg yolk   B.   ice cream
    C.   cream cheese   D.   skim-milk powder

4. _D_

5.   When putting drops in the eyes, place them

    A.   under the upper eyelid
    B.   on the inside of lower eyelid
    C.   in the aqueous chamber
    D.   on the iris

5. _B_

6.   The MOST effective control of the spread of tuberculosis relies on

    A.   vaccine   B.   case finding
    C.   Mantoux test   D.   diet and rest

6. _B_

7.   The effect of below-freezing temperatures on microbes is to

    A.   destroy the pathogens   B.   kill them
    C.   stimulate sporification   D.   check growth and multiplication

7. _D_

8.   An anodyne

    A.   is an antidote
    B.   is an antiseptic
    C.   prolongs the life of red blood corpuscles
    D.   relieves pain

8. _D_

9.   Boiling an article in water for 10 minutes will destroy

    A.   pathogens   B.   non-spore-forming microbes
    C.   spore-forming microbes   D.   spore-forming patgens

9. _B_

10. An *inexpensive* disinfectant is 10.__C__

    A. bichloride of mercury
    B. potassium permanganate
    C. creosote
    D. alcohol

11. The source of infection MOST difficult to control is 11.__D__

    A. water   B. insects   C. food   D. air

12. Pasteurization of milk 12.__A__

    A. kills pathogenic bacteria
    B. destroys bacteria of all kinds
    C. controls the growth of bacteria   D. sterilizes milk

13. The COMMONEST cause of apoplexy is 13.__B__

    A. coronary thrombosis and arterial dilation
    B. hardening of the arteries and hypertension
    C. emotional shock and low blood pressure
    D. uremia and aphasia

14. Poor diet influences MOST the occurrence of 14.__A__

    A. metabolic diseases   B. cancer
    C. nephritis   D. hypertension

15. In proper handwashing, be sure to use 15.__B__

    A. cold water   B. soap, water and adequate friction
    C. liquid soap   D. very hot water

16. At present, antibiotics are recognized to be 16.__A__

    A. a factor in altering the natural germ balance in the body
    B. ineffective in developing toxic reactions
    C. ineffective in developing allergic reactions
    D. most desirable in fixed antibiotic combinaations

17. The study of pathogenic organisms in relation to disease is the science of 17.__A__

    A. microbiology   B. blocking therapy
    C. chemotherapy   D. replacement therapy

18. Atoms of an element that differ in atomic weight are called 18.__C__

    A. molecules   B. neutrons   C. isotopes   D. particles

19. The *danger* of strontium 90 lies in the fact that it 19.__A__

    A. is absorbed and concentrated in bone tissue
    B. causes tumors in smooth muscles
    C. falls back and is absorbed by the soil near the explosion
    D. renders the atmosphere unfit for breathing

20. A vaccine is introduced into the body to
    20. _B_

    A. kill the causative organism
    B. stimulate growth of specific antibodies
    C. inhibit growth of the causative organism
    D. produce bacteriostasis

21. The *preventive* treatment for diphtheria consists of injections of
    21. _C_

    A. gamma globulin
    B. pertussis
    C. toxoid
    D. convalescent serum

22. Gamma globulin *usually* gives temporary immunity after exposure to
    22. _C_

    A. whooping cough
    B. mumps
    C. measles
    D. chicken pox

23. The substance among the following which is an *immunizing* serum is
    23. _B_

    A. diphtheria antitoxin
    B. tubercle bacilli
    C. gamma globulin
    D. BCG (bacillus Calmette-Guerin)

24. The "confection" for pre-school children approved by the American Dental Society is
    24. _C_

    A. non-sweet soft drinks
    B. hard candies
    C. raw fruit
    D. crisp cookies and crackers

25. The effect of morphine which MOST encourages to addiction is
    25. _A_

    A. sensing an exaggerated feeling of well being
    B. the dulling of perception
    C. drowsiness, sleep and dreams
    D. relief from pain

KEY (CORRECT ANSWERS)

1.	B		11.	D
2.	C		12.	A
3.	C		13.	B
4.	D		14.	A
5.	B		15.	B
6.	B		16.	A
7.	D		17.	A
8.	D		18.	C
9.	B		19.	A
10.	C		20.	B

21.	C
22.	C
23.	B
24.	C
25.	A

———

TEST 3

DIRECTIONS: Each question or incomplete statement is followed by several suggested answers or completions. Select the one that BEST answers the question or completes the statement. *PRINT THE LETTER OF THE CORRECT ANSWER IN THE SPACE AT THE RIGHT.*

1. In preparing a patient for hospital care, it would be MOST advisable for the nurse to tell the patient

    A. the length of time he will probably have to stay for complete recovery
    B. that the term "bed rest" means that he will have bathroom privileges
    C. that the best form of therapy for him may be bed rest without medication or surgery
    D. that the hospital is a very fine place, that the food is excellent and that he will enjoy the routine

1. C

2. Of the following symptoms, the one which would be *least likely* to cause a person to consult a physician for chest examination is

    A. continuous loss of weight
    B. a cough lasting longer than three weeks
    C. a slight elevation of temperature in the afternoon
    D. fresh blood in the stools

2. D

3. The PRIMARY purpose of a cancer detection center is to

    A. examine, for diagnosis, persons who are suspected of having cancer
    B. examine people who are presumably healthy
    C. treat people who have a diagnosis of cancer
    D. follow-up patients who have had cancer and are apparently cured

3. B

4. Addition of fluorine to drinking water which has a low fluorine level has PRIMARILY the effect of aiding in the

    A. strengthening of bones
    B. improving of skin texture
    C. preventing of dental caries
    D. preventing of scurvy

4. C

5. The LEADING cause of death in the 5- to 14-year age group is

    A. pneumonia   B. accidents
    C. rheumatic fever   D. scarlet fever

5. B

6. The drug which has given new hope to victims of arthritis is

    A. ACTH   B. histamine   C. penicillin   D. chloromycetin

6. A

7. The one of the following which is the leading cause of death is

    A. tuberculosis   B. diseases of the heart
    C. cancer   D. accidents

7. B

8. Robert Koch is known for his identification of

    A. tubercle bacilli   B. diphtheria bacilli
    C. treponema-pallidum organism   D. Neisseria gonorrhoeae

8. A

9. The BEST definition for *myopia* is   9. A

    A. near-sightedness   B. far-sightedness
    C. cross eyes   D. blocking of the lacrimal duct

10. Of the following, the one which represents *normal* vision is   10. C

    A. 20/200   B. 20/30   C. 20/20   D. 15/30

11. Of the following statements, the one which is MOST accurate is that   11. C

    A. to prevent trichinosis, it is necessary to roast beef and lamb until well done
    B. brucellosis is developed in humans only when they drink milk containing the bru-cellosis organism
    C. because of the possibility of infection by the rabies organism it is necessary that all breaks in the skin caused by the bite of a dog receive immediate medical attention and be reported to the police
    D. because the staphylococcus organisms multiply most readily in a temperature below 50° Fahrenheit, it is safe to keep custard-filled pastry indefinitely at room temperature of 68° Fahrenheit

12. Of the following definitions, the one which is CORRECT is that the   12. A

    A. infant mortality rate is the number of deaths of infants under one year of age per 1000 live births
    B. maternal mortality rate is the number of deaths from puerperal causes per 10,000 population
    C. morbidity rate is the number of deaths per 1000 population
    D. neonatal mortality rate is the number of deaths of infants under one week of age

13. Of the following, the one which is NOT a sign of pregnancy in the first trimester is   13. D

    A. absence of menses   B. marked changes in breasts
    C. nausea in the morning   D. feeling of fetal movements

14. The hazards of childbearing vary with the health or disease of the individual.   14. D
Of the following conditions, the one which is NOT usually considered a childbearing hazard is

    A. tuberculosis
    B. nephritis
    C. diseases of the heart
    D. poliomyelitis involving lower extremities only

15. Of the following statements concerning poliomyelitis, the one that is CORRECT is that   15. B

    A. poliomyelitis is a disease with initial symptoms of an upper respiratory infection and cough
    B. in the care of the acute poliomyelitis case it is important to handle the affected limb at the insertion and origin of the muscle only
    C. poliomyelitis, in the acute stages, may affect the spine. It is important, therefore, that the patient be kept on a soft mattress
    D. if the poliomyelitis victim has a marked weakness of certain muscles two months after onset, there is no hope for further improvement

16. A nurse working with children should know that,of the following statements, the only   16. _A_
CORRECT one is that

    A. Koplik spots in the mucous membrane of the mouth are an early symptom of mea-sles

    B. a strawberry tongue is found in chicken-pox

    C. enlargement of and pain in the parotid glands are early manifestations of scarlet fever

    D. large blisters, first appearing on exposed surfaces, are characteristic of German measles

17. Of the following types of growths, the one which is a *benign* tumor is   17. _A_

    A. adenoma   B. carcinoma   C. sarcoma   D. neuroblastoma

18. A nurse should know that,of the following statements ,the CORRECT one is that   18. _B_

    A. one average serving of dark cereal furnishes the necessary requirement of iron for an adolescent girl for one day

    B. one quart of milk furnishes the necessary calcium requirement of a pregnant woman for one day

    C. bananas are a very rich source of vitamin A

    D. glandular meats, sugars, and cereals are good sources of vitamin C

19. Of the following foods, the one RICHEST in thiamine is   19. _B_

    A. oranges   B. liver

    C. yellow vegetables   D. eggs

20. Of the following diseases, the one NOT caused by a lack of essential food elements is   20. _D_

    A. rickets   B. scurvy   C. beriberi   D. tetanus

21. Of the following explanations, the BEST one that a nurse can give to a mother who com-   21. _A_
plains that her 15-year-old adolescent boy has a huge appetite is that the

    A. boy may gain 20 pounds in a year and 4 to 6 inches in height; also, that if he is active in sports, he may need up to 4000 calories daily

    B. boy is under a great deal of nervous tension, and that,therefore,he eats huge amounts to satisfy this desire to be "doing something"

    C. boy is in danger of becoming excessively heavy, and that,therefore ,his diet should be restricted by limiting milk and meats

    D. boy's diet should be restricted by reducing amounts of all food taken until his weight is 10% below the average

22. With respect to obesity and diet, the LEAST acceptable statement of the following is that   22. _D_

    A. obesity constitutes a public health problem of importance, since obese persons are more apt to develop diabetes and degenerative diseases

    B. obesity usually results from an habitual intake of more food than the energy output requires

    C. the treatment of obesity should involve re-education of the appetite

    D. the recommended intake for an obese person is 3000 calories daily, since the diet should be adequate in respect to all essential nutrients

23. Diseases associated with the aged are assuming increasing importance.   23. C
One of these chronic conditions, the nurse frequently finds, is acute cerebral thrombo-
sis with resulting hemiplegia. To bring about *maximum* rehabilitation, the nurse should
assist in a program in which

    A. the patient is encouraged to help himself only when, and if, he feels he is able to do
so

    B. the patient is immobilized until the acute phase is over and the patient is able to
start to help himself

    C. any portion of the body is prevented from remaining in a position of flexion long
enough to permit muscle shortening to occur

    D. the use of the affected muscles and the opposing muscles is discouraged for at
least four weeks following the onset of illness

24. The nurse should know that the age period during which there is the LARGEST inci-   24. B
dence of rheumatic fever is from

    A. birth to five years   B. six to twelve years
    C. fourteen to twenty years
    D. twenty-one to twenty-six years

25. A lateral curvature of the spine is known as   25. A

    A. scoliosis   B. lordosis   C. kyphosis   D. trichinosis

---

KEYS (CORRECT ANSWERS)

1.	C	11.	C
2.	D	12.	A
3.	B	13.	D
4.	C	14.	D
5.	B	15.	B
6.	A	16.	A
7.	B	17.	A
8.	A	18.	B
9.	A	19.	B
10.	C	20.	D

21.	A
22.	D
23.	C
24.	B
25.	A

TEST 4

DIRECTIONS: Each question or incomplete statement is followed by several suggested answers or completions. Select the one that BEST answers the question or completes the statement. *PRINT THE LETTER OF THE CORRECT ANSWER IN THE SPACE AT THE RIGHT.*

1. Cerebral palsy can BEST be described as a   1. _C_

    A. nerve infection which causes the incoordination of the muscles
    B. muscular deformity chiefly affecting the upper extremities
    C. neuro-muscular disability caused by injury to the motor centers of the brain
    D. muscular disfunction caused by injury to the spinal column

2. Of the following statements, the one which would be the MOST *inadvisable* for a nurse to   2. _D_
    tell diabetic patients is that

    A. it is advisable to see a doctor at regular intervals
    B. extreme cleanliness is very important. Feet should be washed daily and skin kept
        soft
    C. as gangrene may develop in older diabetics from simple bruises or breaks in the
        skin, all injuries should be treated immediately
    D. in giving foot care, the nails should be cut as short as possible and the cuticle
        removed by cutting

3. Of the following definitions, the one which is BEST is that   3. _D_

    A. pneumoperitoneum is the incision and drainage of the pleural space
    B. pneumolysis is an operation in which the infected lobe is removed
    C. pneumothorax is the introduction of air into the potential peritoneal cavity
    D. thoracoplasty is an operation in which parts of several ribs are removed to give a
        permanent collapse of the lung

4. With reference to tuberculosis, the one of the following statements which is INCORRECT   4. _B_
    is that

    A. the death rate from tuberculosis among men is approximately 50% higher than
        among women
    B. from birth until six months of age infants have an immunity to tuberculosis
    C. mortality from tuberculosis reaches its highest peak in men between the ages of 50
        and 60
    D. the mortality rate for tuberculosis is very much lower in the elementary school age
        group than in all other groups

5. In counseling a person who has had tuberculosis, a nurse should suggest to him that, of   5. _A_
    the following types of work, the one which would be the MOST advisable for him to avoid
    is

    A. a job which requires rapid prolonged motions of the arms
    B. light assembly work in which the worker fits small parts together
    C. work in which the worker's value depends on delicacy of touch and close attention
    D. work which involves clerical, stenographic, or bookkeeping tasks

6. The age at which the average baby starts to creep is, *approximately,*   6. _B_

    A. 5 months   B. 9 months   C. 12 months   D. 14 months

7. Of the following statements, the one which is the MOST accurate is that   7. _A_

    A. a young baby begins to suck his thumb because he has not had enough sucking at breast or bottle to satisfy his sucking instinct
    B. diarrhea is a more frequent occurrence than constipation among very young babies that are bottle fed
    C. a baby weighing 6 to 8 pounds must be kept at a room temperature of 75 to 80° F ahrenheit, as his system for regulating body temperature has not been well developed
    D. a normal baby does not recognize a human face and does not respond to it until 4 to 5 months of age

8. In counseling a young mother of pre-school children, the one of the following which represents the MOST accurate statement is that   8. _B_

    A. by the age of two, a child is quite a social being; he is very easily satisfied and,in his emotional development , identifies himself with his parents
    B. between the ages of one and three years, an occasional temper tantrum merely means some frustrations that are normal; more frequent tantrums may indicate that the mother has not learned to handle the child tactfully
    C. at two and one half years of age, the frequent hitting of a playmate for taking toys, instead of asking for them, is abnormal and needs psychiatric guidance
    D. a two-year-old dresses himself, with the exception of tying shoe laces; he is toilet trained, and, if day wetting occurs, medical advice should be sought

9. On physical inspection of the young infant, the nurse looks for symptoms of brachial birth palsy.   9. _A_
Of the following, the one which MOST accurately describes these symptoms is that

    A. the arm is limp at the side, the elbow is straight, and the forearm is pronated; inability to abduct, raise, and outwardly rotate the upper arm is noted
    B. the foot is twisted into a position of plantar flexion and inversion; this position raises the height of the longitudinal arch, causing a deformity
    C. there is a shortening of the leg, as the femoral head slides up along the sides of the ilium; abduction of the hip is limited
    D. the head is tipped to the side and twisted so that the chin points in the opposite direction

10. A nurse asked to appraise a home preparatory to discharge from the hospital of a premature baby, present weight 5 pounds, would NOT recommend that the baby be sent to this home at this time if   10. _C_

    A. the father has an income of $50 a week, and there are three young children
    B. the apartment is on the fourth floor, walk up; there are four rooms, of which two can be used as bedrooms
    C. one of the children was exposed to pertussis two weeks ago; he apparently has no symptoms
    D. the mother is under medical care for the treatment of nutritional anemia

11. A nurse should know that, of the following conditions, the one which is NOT a congenital deformity is   11.___D

    A.   wryneck   B.   club foot   C.   spine bifida   D.   kyphosis

12. A nurse should know that, with reference to the care of the premature infant, the one of the following which is NOT indicated is   12.___D

    A.   the maintenance of normal body temperature
    B.   proper feeding
    C.   protection of the infant from exposure to infection
    D.   removal from the incubator at least once a day for exercise

13. The term, "rooming in" program, refers to the program where the   13.___C

    A.   patient in labor is allowed to have her husband with her
    B.   parents are advised to keep the infant in the sleeping room with them the first month of its life
    C.   newborn is kept in the hospital room with the mother
    D.   patient comes to the hospital five days prior to the expected delivery to become acquainted with the institution

14. The BEST advice you can give parents disturbed by their five-year-old child's habit of nailbiting is to tell them to   14.___A

    A.   find out what some of the pressures on the child are and try to relieve them
    B.   paint the child's fingers with the product "bitter aloes"
    C.   point out to the child that this is a baby habit and not desirable in a school child
    D.   punish the child by not allowing him to watch television or go to the movies

15. In certain periods of development, anti-social behavior in young children is considered normal.
However, of the following situations, the one which merits referral to a mental hygiene clinic is where a   15.___D

    A.   two-year-old persists in hitting his four-year-old brother
    B.   three-year-old develops enuresis when a new baby is brought into the home
    C.   four-year-old runs away from home at every opportunity
    D.   six-year-old is not friendly, has no "pals" after six months in school, and participates in activities only when compelled to

16. Of the following, the one which is NOT in accord with accepted theories in child psychology is that a young child should be   16.___C

    A.   comforted when he cries
    B.   fed when he is hungry
    C.   toilet trained when the mother feels it is necessary
    D.   accepted as he is

17. With reference to syphilis, the one of the following statements which is CORRECT is that   17.___A

    A.   the incubation period is 10 to 90 days; average is 3 weeks
    B.   the period of communicability is 2 weeks
    C.   the mode of transmission is usually through indirect contact, as through towels and clothing
    D.   methods of control include routine taking of blood pressure

18. Of the following statements concerning syphilis, the one which is MOST accurate is that   18.___

    A. a positive blood test for syphilis always indicates that the patient is in an infectious state of the disease

    B. when a pregnant woman with syphilis reports for treatment early in pregnancy and follows the doctor's orders throughout, there is very little danger of the baby being born with congenital syphilis

    C. if the prescribed number of penicillin injections have been received by the patient with secondary syphilis, he will not be re-infected if exposed

    D. the period between exposure and appearance of the first symptoms of syphilis is usually two to six days

19. The stage in which syphilis is usually NOT considered contagious is   19.___

    A. primary   B. secondary   C. tertiary   D. chancre

20. The incubation period of scarlet fever is   20.___

    A. two to seven days   B. seven to fourteen days
    C. seven to twenty-one days   D. fourteen to eighteendays

21. As a nurse you are frequently asked how to protect children against poliomyelitis. According to present teaching, the one of the following which you should NOT recommend is   21.___

    A. avoiding groups and places of general assemblage where new contacts would be made

    B. maintaining good personal and environment hygiene

    C. avoiding chilling which lowers body resistance

    D. exercising as much as possible, even to the point of tiring, in order to strengthen the body

22. Of the following diseases, the one characterized by "strawberry tongue" is   22.___

    A. meningococcus meningitis   B. poliomyelitis
    C. German measles   D. scarlet fever

23. Of the following statements concerning the transfer of communicable diseases from animal to man, the one which is CORRECT is that   23.___

    A. tetanus is confined to persons who have eaten raw or insufficiently cooked meat, usually pork or pork product containing viable larvae

    B. brucellosis is usually transmitted by house pets, such as parrots, canaries and pigeons

    C. psittacosis is usually transmitted by cows, hogs, or goats

    D. rickettsial pox is transmitted by common house mice, probably from mouse to man by a rodent mite

24. Of the following statements, the one which is CORRECT is that   24.___

    A. Pasteur treatment is instituted to prevent the development of rabies

    B. a smallpox epidemic may be prevented by rigid inspection of milk

    C. hydrophobia is a synonym for tetanus

    D. the feces and urine in cases of Vincent's agina should be disinfected

25. With reference to serum hepatitis (jaundice), the one of the following statements which is   25.____A____
CORRECT is that

    A.   the virus causing it may be transmitted through parenteral inoculations of infected blood
    B.   it has an incubation period of one to two months
    C.   it is characterized by severe paroxysms of coughing, with little or no fever, and general muscle pains
    D.   the victims do not receive immunizing agents or convalescent serum early enough

---

KEY (CORRECT ANSWERS)

1.	C		11.	D
2.	D		12.	D
3.	D		13.	C
4.	B		14.	A
5.	A		15.	D
6.	B		16.	C
7.	A		17.	A
8.	B		18.	B
9.	A		19.	C
10.	C		20.	A

21.	D
22.	D
23.	D
24.	A
25.	A

TEST 5

DIRECTIONS: Each question or incomplete statement is followed by several suggested answers or completions. Select the one that BEST answers the question or completes the statement. *PRINT THE LETTER OF THE CORRECT ANSWER IN THE SPACE AT THE RIGHT.*

1. Vitamin A is stored in the

   A. skeletal muscles   B. liver
   C. thyroid   D. brain

   1._B_

2. The MOST important single item of the diet is

   A. carbohydrates   B. water   C. milk   D. protein

   2._B_

3. The control of diabetes in children is

   A. more difficult than in adults   B. impossible
   C. relatively simple   D. not necessary

   3._A_

4. Obesity may be caused by

   A. lack of vitamins   B. excessive calorie intake
   C. gastronomy   D. high protein diet

   4._B_

5. Beriberi is caused by

   A. lack of thiamine   B. heredity
   C. faulty hygiene   D. a virus

   5._A_

6. Emotional disturbances

   A. hasten digestion   B. delay digestion
   C. cause uremia   D. result in loss of Vitamin B

   6._B_

7. Calorie is a

   A. unit of measurement   B. term used for digestibility
   C. need for nutrients   D. catalytic agent

   7._A_

8. A *substantial* source of iron is found in

   A. apricots   B. almonds   C. potatoes   D. cheese

   8._A_

9. Pasteurized milk is *valuable* in the diet because it is a good source of

   A. Vitamin K   B. amino acid   C. Vitamin B   D. rutin

   9._B_

10. Vitamin A helps to prevent

    A. night blindness   B. hemorrhage in newborn infant
    C. scurvy   D. destruction of connective tissue

    10._A_

11. In diarrhea, feed

    A. orange juice   B. boiled milk
    C. chopped spinach   D. stewed prunes

    11._B_

12. Swelling, heat and redness occur in an inflamed area because the capillaries become   12. _B_

    A. constricted   B. dilated
    C. ruptured   D. fenestrated

13. Bone owes its hardness CHIEFLY to the mineral salt   13. _A_

    A. calcium phosphorus   B. potassium iodide
    C. sodium carbonate   D. stearic acid

14. The number of vertebrae of the spinal column of a human is   14. _A_

    A. 33   B. 42   C. 28   D. 21

15. Sebaceous glands   15. _B_

    A. aid digestion   B. have ducts
    C. are attached to the muscles of the eye
    D. increase blood pressure

16. The audiometer is an instrument for measuring   16. _A_

    A. hearing acuity   B. vision accuracy
    C. temperature   D. pressure

17. Tic is a(n)   17. _D_

    A. poisonous product   B. insect
    C. connective tissue   D. twitching

18. Ringworm is caused by   18. _A_

    A. fungi   B. pediculi
    C. infection of the intestines   D. impetigo

19. Mastoid is   19. _C_

    A. a woman who practices massage   B. marasmus
    C. part of the temporal bone   D. inflammation of the breast

20. Morphology is a study of   20. _A_

    A. form   B. trench mouth   C. death   D. the fetus

21. The Rh factors are   21. _C_

    A. negative   B. positive
    C. negative and positive   D. none of these

22. Insomnia refers to   22. _B_

    A. unconsciousness   B. sleeplessness
    C. sleep walking   D. insensibility

23. Mortality refers to   23. _B_

    A. pulverization   B. death   C. motion   D. illness

24. Fungus is a   24. A___

    A. form of plant life   B. division of a nucleus
    C. medication for inducing sleep   D. vitamin deficiency

25. The incubation period of the common cold is   25. A___

    A. 27-36 hours   B. 7 days   C. 14 days   D. 21 days

KEY (CORRECT ANSWERS)

1.	B		11.	B
2.	B		12.	B
3.	A		13.	A
4.	B		14.	A
5.	A		15.	B
6.	B		16.	A
7.	A		17.	D
8.	A		18.	A
9.	B		19.	C
10.	A		20.	A

21. C
22. B
23. B
24. A
25. A

TEST 6

DIRECTIONS: Each question or incomplete statement is followed by several suggested answers or completions. Select the one that BEST answers the question or completes the statement. *PRINT THE LETTER OF THE CORRECT ANSWER IN THE SPACE AT THE RIGHT.*

1. Morphine addiction causes

   A. constriction of the pupil of the eye
   B. increase in heart rate   C. dilation of the cervix
   D. difficulty in hearing

   1.___A___

2. Pigmentation

   A. depends upon the hemoglobin   B. reduces body heat
   C. protects tissues of the skin   D. produces color

   2.___D___

3. In respiration,

   A. expiration is slower than inspiration
   B. receptors of the skin respond
   C. the hypothalmus is expanded
   D. enzymes are rendered inert

   3.___A___

4. The permanent teeth in human adults should number

   A. 27   B. 32   C. 26   D. 34

   4.___D___

5. The Newburgh-Kingston fluoridation experiment dealt with

   A. vitamin B in nutrition   B. anemia
   C. dental caries   D. malnutrition

   5.___C___

6. The brain

   A. is dependent upon glucose for its energy
   B. functions in the final destruction of the red blood
   C. appears biconcave, is elastic and pliable
   D. separates the high pressure system of the arterial tree from the lower pressure system of the venous tree

   6.___A___

7. Taste buds are located on the tongue *and*

   A. on the soft palate   B. at the Eustachian tube
   C. on posterior descending branch of the coronary
   D. in the atrium

   7.___A___

8. Color blindness *sometimes* means

   A. hues of green and red are indistinguishable
   B. continuous winking when colors are dull
   C. disturbed equilibrium   D. irritated conjunctiva

   8.___A___

9. Metabolism

   A. expresses the fact that nerve fibres give only one kind of reaction
   B. summarizes the activities each living cell must carry on

   9.___B___

C. possesses the properties of irritability and conductivity
D. describes the membrane theory

10. The heat of the body is maintained by

    A. oxidation   B. vertigo   C. gravity   D. hyperpnea

10. A

11. All cells

    A. exist proximal to liquid environment
    B. secrete a hormone which helps maintain the normal calcium level of the blood
    C. differ in origin and function
    D. are cone-shaped

11. A

12. Anoxia is

    A. a colloidal solution that exerts pressure
    B. plasma volume
    C. body proteins
    D. lack of oxygen

12. D

13. The heart rate

    A. varies in individuals
    B. increases from birth to old age
    C. increases during first hours of sleep
    D. decreases in hemorrhage

13. A

14. The heart begins to "beat"

    A. immediately preceding birth
    B. in the fetus at about the fourth week of fetal life
    C. in the fetus during seventh month of fetal life
    D. with the first cry after birth

14. B

15. A neuron consists of

    A. fluid in the semicircular canals
    B. conjugated protein which yields globin and hemin
    C. a cell body and processes
    D. a band of spectrum colors ranging from red to violet

15. C

16. The process of swallowing is called

    A. delactation   B. diastasis   C. deglutition   D. emission

16. C

17. Histology

    A. dissolves essential constituents in water
    B. connects arterial and venous circulation
    C. describes microscopic structure
    D. reduces diseased structures

17. C

18. Prevent noise for the sick patient by

18. _C_

    A. removing the door hinges
    B. keeping the window shades rolled up
    C. padding the door latches
    D. repairing faucets

19. For the patient, select a room that is

19. _A_

    A. near the bathroom
    B. large enough for necessary furniture
    C. equipped with screened windows
    D. exposed to sunshine

20. Devices for elevating the patient's bed may be

20. _C_

    A. large books   B. kitchen chairs
    C. wooden bed-blocks   D. foot stools

21. A substitute for the rubber draw sheet is a(n)

21. _D_

    A. average sizedplastic dressercover
    B. old raincoat
    C. Sunday newspaper
    D. shower curtain

22. Prevent accidents due to poisons by

22. _A_

    A. labeling properly   B. storing outside of home
    C. substituting non-poisons   D. destroying poisons

23. Most prone to accidents in the home is the

23. _D_

    A. young adult   B. middle-aged individual
    C. adolescent   D. aged individual

24. Mortality due to tuberculosis is rapidly declining through the use of

24. _C_

    A. tuberculin tests   B. preventive measures
    C. chemicals   D. statistics

25. A drug used in the treatment of mental illness is

25. _C_

    A. streptomycin   B. paramino-salicylic acid
    C. reserpine   D. cortisone

KEY (CORRECT ANSWERS)

1.	A	11.	A
2.	D	12.	D
3.	A	13.	A
4.	B	14.	B
5.	C	15.	C
6.	A	16.	C
7.	A	17.	C
8.	A	18.	C
9.	B	19.	A
10.	A	20.	C
21.	D		
22.	A		
23.	D		
24.	C		
25.	C		

TEST 7

DIRECTIONS: Each question or incomplete statement is followed by several suggested answers or completions. Select the one that BEST answers the question or completes the statement. *PRINT THE LETTER OF THE CORRECT ANSWER IN THE SPACE AT THE RIGHT.*

1. As a substitute for an emesis basin, use a(n)   1. _A_

    A. metal coffee can   B. small pyrex bowl
    C. old kitchen dish   D. small enamel sauce pan

2. To keep the feet of the patient in normal position,   2. _C_

    A. soak the feet   B. lubricate the feet
    C. use bed cradle   D. flex the ankles and toes

3. When using an aerosol bomb in the sick room,   3. _B_

    A. close the windows   B. remove the patient
    C. keep all food covered   D. follow-up with chlordane

4. When in doubt about the nature of a stain,   4. _C_

    A. swab with water   B. apply carbon tetrachloride
    C. consult professional cleaner   D. saturate with kerosene

5. Flammable chemicals, if used in stain removal, should be used   5. _B_

    A. in a room   B. out-of-doors
    C. sparingly   D. with lint-free cloths

6. Paper supplies are used freely in the sick room since they are   6. _A_

    A. helpful in prevention   B. inexpensive
    C. clean   D. bright and colorful

7. Keep house pets out of the sickroom because they may   7. _C_

    A. be noisy   B. tire the patient
    C. carry disease elsewhere   D. jar furniture

8. Protect the top edge of the bed blanket from being soiled by   8. _C_

    A. folding the spread over it
    B. folding paper towels over it
    C. sewing a strip of muslin over it
    D. pinning a table napkin over it

9. Some nurses never become good housekeepers because they lack   9. _D_

    A. observation   B. interest   C. sensitivity   D. ability

10. When water is added to dry mustard, the reaction is   10. _B_

    A. polymerization   B. hydrolysis
    C. dehydration   D. neutralization

11. The efficacy of saline cathartics depends upon the   11. _B_

    A. selective action   B. osmotic pressure
    C. relaxation of smooth muscle   D. retarding of peristis

12. The chemical which stimulates the respiratory center is   12. _B_

    A. oxygen   B. carbon dioxide   C. calcium   D. nitrogen

13. Carbon dioxide and oxygen are exchanged in the air sacs by   13. _B_

    A. infusion   B. diffusion   C. reaction   D. filtration

14. The absorption of water through the intestinal wall is by   14. _B_

    A. filtration   B. osmosis   C. infiltration   D. fusion

15. Oils and water do not mix readily because of the difference in   15. _B_

    A. heat of fusion   B. surface tension
    C. heat of sublimation   D. freezing point

16. The lowering of the head, when a person feels faint, will increase the blood supply to the head by   16. _B_

    A. suction   B. gravity   C. siphonage   D. centripetalforce

17. The ventricles of the heart act like a   17. _B_

    A. lever   B. pump   C. siphon   D. barometer

18. Radon is radioactive gas which results when radium emits a(n)   18. _B_

    A. beta particle   B. alpha particle
    C. gamma ray   D. neutron

19. A rubber hot water bottle transfers heat to the skin CHIEFLY by   19. _A_

    A. conduction   B. convection   C. radiation   D. oxidation

20. A clinical thermometer is a(n)   20. _B_

    A. thermograph   B. maximum thermometer
    C. minimum thermometer   D. absolute thermometer

KEY (CORRECT ANSWERS)

1.	A	11.	B
2.	C	12.	B
3.	B	13.	B
4.	C	14.	B
5.	B	15.	B
6.	A	16.	B
7.	C	17.	B
8.	C	18.	B
9.	D	19.	A
10.	B	20.	B

EXAMINATION SECTION
TEST 1

DIRECTIONS: Each question or incomplete statement is followed by several suggested answers or completions. Select the one that BEST answers the question or completes the statement. *PRINT THE LETTER OF THE CORRECT ANSWER IN THE SPACE AT THE RIGHT.*

1. A nurse instructing a family in the home should emphasize that of the following the MOST effective way of controlling tuberculosis infection is to

    A. soak all the patient's linen in soap and water solution for 6 hours before laundering
    B. admit no one to the room except the attendant
    C. have the patient cover his mouth and nose with disposable tissues when coughing or expectorating
    D. remove all rugs, curtains, and unnecessary furniture from the room

1. _C_

2. When a post-operative patient complains of pain in the calf of the leg, aggravated by dorsiflexion of the foot, the BEST course of action for the nurse to take is to recommend

    A. hot soakings
    B. walking about to relieve pain
    C. massaging locally
    D. remaining in bed and calling the doctor

2. _D_

3. Morbidity rates are statistics relative to

    A. births   B. deaths
    C. sickness and disease   D. marriages

3. _C_

4. The Snellen test is a

    A. visual screening test   B. diagnostic test for syphilis
    C. blood test for anemia   D. hearing test

4. _A_

5. The nurse should instruct families that the temperature of water for hot water bottles should be between

    A. 95° and 110° F   B. 115° and 130° F
    C. 135° and 150° F   D. 155° and 170° F

5. _B_

6. When planning a feeding schedule for a premature infant, it is of PRIMARY importance to

    A. feed the baby regularly every two hours
    B. establish a food tolerance since the intestinal tract is undeveloped
    C. include Vitamins A, B, C, D and K in the feeding
    D. provide for additional carbohydrates

6. _B_

7. B.C.G. vaccine is being given at the present time

    A. to all children with a positive tuberculin test
    B. to all children exposed to tuberculosis

7. _D_

C. to all children with minimal tuberculosis lesions
D. experimentally to non-reactors to the tuberculin test who are subject to frequent exposure to tuberculosis

8. When teaching a colostomy patient self-care at home, the MOST important point for the nurse to emphasize is that

8._C_

A. a colostomy bag is essential to assure safety from leakage
B. the irrigation can should hang five feet above hip level
C. the irrigation should be done at the same time each day
D. the irrigation should be followed by one hour of bed-rest

9. The destruction of all organisms, including spores, is known as

9._D_

A. disinfection
B. sterilization
C. antiseptic action
D. germicidal action

10. The MOST frequent and serious complication likely to arise after a patient has undergone surgery is

10._C_

A. wound infection
B. blood poisoning
C. respiratory infection
D. decubitus ulcers

11. A disarrangement of the normal relation of the bones entering into the formation of a joint BEST defines

11._A_

A. a dislocation
B. a fracture
C. a sprain
D. ankylosis

12. The Non-Protein Nitrogen (N.P.N.) test is a

12._A_

A. blood test to determine renal function
B. blood test to determine liver function
C. urine test to determine concentration
D. patency test of the Fallopian tubes

13. When eating pork, a person may AVOID trichinosis by

13._D_

A. not eating it in warm weather
B. soaking it in salt water two hours before cooking
C. buying pork which has a government inspection stamp
D. thoroughly cooking it

14. Beriberi is a nutritional disease caused by lack of a sufficient amount of vitamin

14._B_

A. A
B. B_1
C. B_{12}
D. K

15. The one of the following groups of foods which is the BEST source of thiamine is

15._D_

A. milk, egg yolks, cheese, lettuce
B. green peas, broccoli, kale, cabbage
C. escarole, carrots, cream cheese
D. whole grain bread and cereals, pork, organ meats

16. The vitamin believed to be of GREATEST aid in the healing of wounds is vitamin   16. __C__

    A. B_2 B. B_{12} C. C   D. D

17. Following the ingestion of contaminated food, acute food poisoning USUALLY occurs   17. __B__
after the elapse of from _____ hours.

    A. 2 to 6   B. 7 to 12
    C. 13 to 24   D. 25 to 36

18. A slowly progressive degenerative disease of the nervous system usually occurring in or   18. __B__
after middle life, and characterized by tremors and rigidity of the skeletal muscles, BEST
defines the condition known as

    A. arthritis   B. Parkinson's disease
    C. Jacksonian epilepsy   D. multiple sclerosis

19. Of the following, the PREFERRED site for intramuscular injections is   19. __D__

    A. the deltoid muscle
    B. the quadriceps muscle
    C. any section of the buttocks
    D. the upper outer quadrant of the buttock near its inner angle

20. Of the following, the one which is MALIGNANT is   20. __C__

    A. papilloma   B. lipoma
    C. lymphosarcoma   D. myoma

21. Of the following organisms, the one which causes MORE THAN HALF of all kidney infec-   21. __A__
tions is

    A. bacterium coli   B. staphylocoecus
    C. streptococcus   D. escherichia coli

22. Of the following antibiotics, the one which produces a TOXIC effect on the auditory nerve   22. __C__
is

    A. chloromycetin   B. aureomycin
    C. streptomycin   D. penicillin

23. Antibiotics are UNIFORMLY excreted through the   23. __B__

    A. skin   B. urine   C. stool   D. lungs

24. Isonicotinic acid hydrazide is used CHIEFLY in the treatment of   24. __D__

    A. rheumatic fever   B. arthritis
    C. cancer   D. tuberculosis

25. The one of the following which attacks the enamel of the teeth is   25. __B__

    A. gingivitis   B. dental caries
    C. pyorrhea alveolaris   D. vitamin C deficiency

KEY (CORRECT ANSWERS)

1.	C		11.	A
2.	D		12.	A
3.	C		13.	D
4.	A		14.	B
5.	B		15.	D
6.	B		16.	C
7.	D		17.	B
8.	C		18.	B
9.	D		19.	D
10.	C		20.	C

21.	A
22.	C
23.	B
24.	D
25.	B

TEST 2

DIRECTIONS: Each question or incomplete statement is followed by several suggested answers or completions. Select the one that BEST answers the question or completes the statement. *PRINT THE LETTER OF THE CORRECT ANSWER IN THE SPACE AT THE RIGHT.*

1. Failure of muscle coordination to bring the image of an object upon the fovea centralis retinae at the same time in each eye BEST defines the condition known as

    A. glaucoma   B. optic neuritis
    C. retrobulbar neuritis   D. strabismus

1. _D_

2. ANOTHER term for farsightedness is

    A. hyperopia   B. myopia
    C. ophthalmia   D. astigmatism

2. _A_

3. A condition which in its advanced stages is characterized by symptoms of halos or rainbows around light is known as

    A. cataracts   B. detached retina
    C. glaucoma   D. corneal ulcers

3. _C_

4. Blocking of the eustachian tube in children is caused MOST often by

    A. adenoid growth around the nasal end of the tube
    B. deterioration in the inner ear
    C. ear wax
    D. perforation of the eardrum

4. _A_

5. It is generally agreed among authorities that a child should have training in lip reading when successive audiometric tests indicate that the better ear shows a LOSS of _____ decibels.

    A. 5   B. 10   C. 15   D. 25

5. _D_

6. The MOST satisfactory way to measure a patient for crutches is to have him

    A. stand against a wall, with his arms straight at side
    B. lie on his back, with his arms straight at side
    C. lie on his back, with his arms elevated over his head
    D. stand against a wall, with his arms extended over his head

6. _B_

7. In crutch walking, the weight is placed on the

    A. quadriceps muscle
    B. trapezius muscle
    C. deltoid muscle
    D. palms of the hands with wrists in hyperextension

7. _D_

8. If a nurse sees that a newborn holds his head to one side with his chin rotated in the opposite direction, she SHOULD recognize the condition as

    A. facial paralysis   B. cerebral palsy
    C. torticollis   D. cephalhematoma

8. _C_

9. Of the following types of cerebral palsy, the one which is characterized by tense con-   9. A
tracted muscles is

   A. spastic   B. athetoid
   C. ataxic   D. dystonic

10. Of the following communicable diseases, the one that is characterized by the eruption of   10. A
successive crops of rose pink spots which change into vesicles and finally into crusts is

   A. chicken pox   B. German measles
   C. scarlet fever   D. measles

11. The remarkable reduction in the incidence of typhoid fever is due PRIMARILY to   11. B

   A. immunization
   B. control of human environment
   C. the use of antibiotics
   D. isolation of typhoid carriers

12. Antibodies which neutralize toxins are called   12. C

   A. lysins   B. agglutinins
   C. antitoxins   D. opsonins

13. Brucellosis is USUALLY acquired in man by   13. C

   A. direct contact with a human being having the disease
   B. direct contact with infected cattle
   C. ingestion of raw milk or milk products
   D. inhaling bacteria from the air

14. Immunity following successful vaccination against smallpox is now believed to last   14. D

   A. for the lifetime of the individual
   B. at least seven years
   C. from one to three years
   D. a varying length of time from individual to individual

15. The gamma globulin fraction of pooled human plasma is an EFFECTIVE agent for pre-   15. B
venting or modifying

   A. chicken pox   B. measles
   C. scarlet fever   D. diphtheria

16. Of the following, the one which is capable of ALTERING the course of tuberculosis is   16. A

   A. streptomycin   B. B.C.G. vaccine
   C. the tuberculin test   D. the Schick test

17. Of the following, the FIRST symptom of spontaneous pneumothorax is   17. A

   A. tightening of the chest with or without dyspnea
   B. acute dyspnea
   C. anxious expression of the face
   D. restlessness plus anxiety

18. To function effectively in the follow-up of a venereal disease patient, the one MOST important thing for the nurse to know is the

    18. _B_

    A. number of contacts the patient has had
    B. correct medical diagnosis of the patient concerned
    C. structure of the family
    D. economic status of the family

19. The incubation period of neisseria gonorrhea is GENERALLY from _____ days.

    19. _A_

    A. 3 to 6   B. 7 to 10
    C. 11 to 14   D. 15 to 18

20. Of the following, the one which prenatal syphilis SELDOM affects is the

    20. _D_

    A. nervous system   B. spleen
    C. liver   D. heart

21. Even without treatment, a person infected with non-congenital syphilis is NOT dangerous to others after he has had the disease _____ months.

    21. _D_

    A. 6   B. 12   C. 18   D. 2

22. In the treatment of syphilis, the antibiotic which has proven the MOST effective, with the LEAST toxic results, as well as the MOST economical, is

    22. _C_

    A. streptomycin   B. aureomycin
    C. penicillin   D. chloromycetin

23. Of the following communicable diseases that may be contracted in the first trimester of pregnancy, the one which is BELIEVED to produce malformation in the newborn is

    23. _B_

    A. scarlet fever   B. German measles
    C. diphtheria   D. measles

24. In the normal course of pregnancy, the total blood volume

    24. _D_

    A. decreases
    B. increases and decreases at various times
    C. remains normal
    D. increases

25. In fetal growth, the period characterized by membranous nails and tooth buds occurs at the end of the _____ lunar month.

    25. _B_

    A. 1st   B. 3rd   C. 5th   D. 7th

KEY (CORRECT ANSWERS)

1.	D		11.	B
2.	A		12.	C
3.	C		13.	C
4.	A		14.	D
5.	D		15.	B
6.	B		16.	A
7.	D		17.	A
8.	C		18.	B
9.	A		19.	A
10.	A		20.	D

21.	D
22.	C
23.	B
24.	D
25.	B

TEST 3

DIRECTIONS: Each question or incomplete statement is followed by several suggested answers or completions. Select the one that BEST answers the question or completes the statement. *PRINT THE LETTER OF THE CORRECT ANSWER IN THE SPACE AT THE RIGHT.*

1. The exercises included in the program of "natural childbirth" are PRIMARILY aimed at

    A. making the waiting time more interesting to the patient
    B. assuring the patient of a painless labor period
    C. relaxing the patient
    D. eliminating the use of anesthesia during labor

1.__C__

2. The UNDERLYING principle of "rooming in" for newborn infants and their mothers is that it

    A. prevents nursery infections in the baby
    B. requires less nursing time
    C. provides an opportunity for the mother to know and care for her baby while in the hospital
    D. encourages breast feeding

2.__C__

3. Erythroblastosis due to the RH factor in newborn infants MOST frequently results from

    A. transfusing an RH negative woman with RH positive blood
    B. the mating of an RH positive father and an RH negative mother
    C. the failure to determine the RH status of pregnant women
    D. transfusing the mother during pregnancy

3.__B__

4. A premature baby is BEST defined as an infant who

    A. is less than 9 months in gestation
    B. weighs 6 pounds at birth
    C. was born in the 7th month of gestation
    D. weighs 2500 grams or less at birth

4.__D__

5. Retrolental fibroplasia occurs in

    A. premature infants   B. pre-school children
    C. adolescents   D. old age

5.__A__

6. When advising a mother regarding infant feeding, the nurse should know that MOST pediatricians recommend that

    A. babies be fed when they cry
    B. mothers plan a three or four hour schedule and adhere to it without variation
    C. mothers need not adhere to a strict feeding schedule since each child has an individual feeding pattern which should be used as a guide
    D. infants never be fed more often than once every four hours

6.__C__

7. An average normal infant may FIRST be expected to sit alone at the age of _____ months.

    A. 5   B. 7   C. 9   D. 11

7.__C__

8. Of the following, the GREATEST single cause of infant and neonatal mortality is   8. B

    A. accidents   B. prematurity
    C. congenital malformation   D. pneumonia

9. Of the following statements relating to epilepsy, the one which is MOST correct is that   9. C

    A. epilepsy indicates feeblemindedness
    B. children with epilepsy should be treated as invalids
    C. seizures in about 50% of children with epilepsy can best be controlled with medicines now in use
    D. children with epilepsy should have permanent home teaching

10. The MOST rapid period of biological growth is during the _____ period.   10. A

    A. prenatal   B. pre-adolescent
    C. adolescent   D. post-adolescent

11. A nurse should advise a mother that bowel training is ORDINARILY successful   11. B

    A. at the same time as bladder training
    B. earlier than bladder training
    C. later than bladder training
    D. when the child is four months old

12. When cautioning about carbon monoxide poisoning, the nurse should recommend that the family   12. C

    A. keep a fire extinguisher handy at all times
    B. inspect gas, appliances daily
    C. keep a window open at least two inches in any room where there is a gas appliance
    D. do not inspect gas appliances with wet hands

13. In the treatment of severe burns, the FIRST consideration should be given to   13. B

    A. dressing the burned area
    B. treating for shock
    C. estimating the extent of the burned area
    D. giving large amounts of fluids

14. The FIRST step recommended in first aid treatment for an animal bite is   14. A

    A. cleansing the wound thoroughly with soap under running water
    B. application of any antiseptic solution
    C. application of tincture of iodine
    D. application of tincture of iodine followed by a band-aid

Questions 15-19.

DIRECTIONS: Next to Numbers 15 through 19, write the letter preceding the disease or condition mentioned in Column II which is most closely connected with the test mentioned in Column I, Numbers 15 through 19.

Column I		Column II			
15.	Aschheim-Zondek	A.	tuberculosis	15.	D
16.	Dick	B.	syphilis	16.	C
17.	Kline	C.	scarlet fever	17.	B
18.	Mantoux	D.	pregnancy	18.	A
19.	Papanicolaou	E.	diphtheria	19.	G
		F.	diabetes		
		G.	cancer		

Questions 20-25.

DIRECTIONS: Next to Numbers 20 through 25, write the letter preceding the term mentioned in Column II which is most closely connected with the definition given in Column I, Numbers 20 through 25.

Column I		Column II			
20.	Inflammation of the kidneys	A.	cretinism	20.	E
21.	Alzeimer's disease	B.	enuresis	21.	C
22.	Involuntary passage of urine	C.	geriatrics	22.	B
23.	White blood corpuscle	D.	leucocyte	23.	D
24.	A form of idiocy and dwarfism	E.	nephritis	24.	A
25.	Lateral curvature of the spine	F.	paraphasia	25.	G
		G.	scoliosis		
		H.	silicosis		

KEY (CORRECT ANSWERS)

1.	C		11.	B
2.	C		12.	C
3.	B		13.	B
4.	D		14.	A
5.	A		15.	D
6.	C		16.	C
7.	C		17.	B
8.	B		18.	A
9.	C		19.	G
10.	A		20.	E

21.	C
22.	B
23.	D
24.	A
25.	G

———

TEST 4

DIRECTIONS: Each question or incomplete statement is followed by several suggested answers or completions. Select the one that BEST answers the question or completes the statement. *PRINT THE LETTER OF THE CORRECT ANSWER IN THE SPACE AT THE RIGHT.*

1. The victim of a neck fracture should be transported

    A. face downward on a rigid support
    B. face upward on a rigid support
    C. lying on the left side of a rigid support
    D. sitting upright on a chair

1. B

2. Of the following, the PRIMARY cause of acne in adolescents is

    A. too much carbohydrate in the diet
    B. the inability of the fat gland ducts and outlets to allow passage of increased secretions of sebum
    C. lack of vitamin A in the diet
    D. lack of good personal hygiene

2. B

3. The nutritional needs of older people differ from those of young adults in that older people require MORE

    A. protein   B. minerals   C. calcium   D. calories

3. C

4. Planning for aging should be the responsibility CHIEFLY of

    A. the individual   B. the family
    C. industry   D. the total community

4. D

5. Prophylaxis against the diseases of old age is USUALLY directed toward

    A. preventing the onset of a disease
    B. preventing or minimizing the disability disease produces
    C. prohibiting all physical exercise
    D. providing for early retirement

5. B

6. Of the following, the MOST accurate statement with regard to the life expectancy of the diabetic today is that

    A. his life span is 1/3 that of the non-diabetic
    B. his life span approximates that of the non-diabetic, provided proper precautions are taken
    C. the diabetic seldom lives beyond age 60 because of complications which shorten life
    D. if diabetes occurs in childhood, the prognosis is good for a normal life span

6. B

7. N.P.H. insulin is generally considered the MOST valuable of the different types of insulin because it

    A. has a low protamine content as compared with protamine zinc insulin
    B. reaches its peak in eight hours, thus providing safety for the patient during the night

7. D

C.   is well-adapted to the mild cases
D.   meets the requirements of the greatest number of patients

8.   When caring for elderly people with diabetes, it is MOST important for the nurse to   8. _B___

A.   know that all diabetics must have insulin daily
B.   understand their individual personalities and habits
C.   teach them how to do urinalysis and give their own insulin
D.   know that their diets require major adjustments

9.   The GREATEST social problem affecting health which has increased in the past few   9. _B___
years is

A.   juvenile delinquency
B.   juvenile narcotic addiction
C.   crowding of children in housing projects
D.   migration of industrial workers

10.   The MOST important reason for the nurse to keep records of patients is to   10. _A___

A.   provide better service to the patients
B.   give information to other agencies in the community
C.   compile information for legal documents
D.   keep *data* for tabulating vital statistics

11.   The function of the nurse on a school health council is to   11. _A___

A.   act in an advisory capacity to the principal and teaching staff in matters pertaining
to health
B.   secure needed facilities for treatment of children with defects
C.   plan the health education program for the school
D.   organize the entire facilities of the school for the promotion of health

12.   With regard to health services, the recommendation for enactment into law that was car-   12. _C___
ried out was that

A.   the Children's Bureau be abolished
B.   compulsory health insurance be inaugurated for all people in the United States
C.   the Federal Security Agency be reorganized into a Department of Health, Educa-
tion and Welfare
D.   the Children's Bureau and the United States Health Service be combined

13.   If a nurse has been assigned the following four visits, all within a radius of a few blocks,   13. _D___
she should visit FIRST the case in which a(n)

A.   anxious prenatal patient is going to be evicted from her home
B.   school child was sent home from school because of Koplik spots
C.   newborn baby is regurgitating every other feeding
D.   newborn baby was discharged against the advice of the hospital to a home in
which the father has a positive sputum for tuberculosis

14. A nurse is assigned four visits. Of the following, the FIRST visit she should make is to a   14. _C_

    A. cardiac patient who receives mercuhydrin regularly twice a week
    B. patient receiving 20U. of N.P.H. insulin
    C. mother delivered of a baby by a non-nurse midwife at 4 A.M. that morning
    D. child sent home from school the previous day with a rash resembling scarlet fever

15. Assume that a mother expresses concern over her one-year-old baby's feeding habits.   15. _B_
As a nurse, you can BEST advise this mother by telling her that

    A. she should feed her baby, although he refuses to eat
    B. appetites of children begin to diminish at the end of the first year and continue to be
       small for a year or two
    C. poor eating habits in children are often a result of emotional problems between
       parents
    D. she should feed her child every two hours whether he is hungry or not

16. Assume that a nine-year-old boy comes to you for help. He has a splinter in his finger   16. _D_
which has been embedded for 24 hours and around which there is a reddened *area*.
The BEST course of action for you to take is to

    A. remove the splinter and apply an antiseptic solution
    B. wash the area with tincture of green soap, express gently, and apply an antiseptic
       solution
    C. have the boy soak his finger in hot water and instruct him to have his mother con-
       tinue the soakings at home in order to loosen the splinter
    D. cover the area with a sterile dressing and call the mother to instruct her to take the
       child to a physician for treatment

17. A city of 100,000 reported 30 maternal deaths last year. Of the following, the statement   17. _C_
regarding the maternal death rate which is CORRECT is that it

    A. is 30%
    B. cannot be computed because we do not know the general death rate
    C. cannot be computed because we do not know the number of live births
    D. cannot be computed because we do not know the infant death rate

18. The agency which has as its objective "the attainment of the highest possible level of   18. _B_
health of all the people" is the

    A. American Red Cross
    B. World Health Organization
    C. United States Public Health Service
    D. The Children's Bureau

19. In the event of an atom bomb attack, civil defense authorities state that the one of the fol-   19. _A_
lowing which will cause the GREATEST number of deaths is

    A. radioactivity   B. injuries
    C. infections   D. hemorrhage

20. Insulin was isolated from other products of the pancreas by   20. _B_

    A. Louis Pasteur   B. Frederick Banting
    C. George Baker   D. Anton Von Leeuwenhoek

21. Recent studies indicate that the MOST economical and practical public health control method for dental caries is to

    A. promote a community-wide nutrition program
    B. provide community dental services for bi-yearly examination of school children
    C. provide individual daily fluoride supplements
    D. fluoridate the domestic water supply

21. D

22. During a poliomyelitis epidemic, of the following, the one precaution NOT recommended by the National Foundation for Infantile Paralysis is to

    A. keep clean
    B. avoid new groups
    C. avoid getting chilled
    D. keep children home from school

22. D

23. The LEADING cause of all deaths in the United States is

    A. cancer   B. diseases of infancy
    C. accidents   D. heart disease

23. D

24. The LEADING cause of school absences in the United States is

    A. accidents   B. skin diseases
    C. digestive disorders   D. respiratory infections

24. D

25. The National Cancer Institute established in the U.S. Public Health Service in 1937 has as its MAJOR goal

    A. research and dissemination of knowledge concerning the causes and treatment of cancer
    B. improving standards for the care of the cancer patient in both the home and hospital
    C. training of medical personnel in the treatment of cancer
    D. granting financial aid to states in the development of cancer control programs

25. D

KEY (CORRECT ANSWERS)

1.	B		11.	A
2.	B		12.	C
3.	C		13.	D
4.	D		14.	C
5.	B		15.	B
6.	B		16.	D
7.	D		17.	C
8.	B		18.	B
9.	B		19.	A
10.	A		20.	B

21.	D
22.	D
23.	D
24.	D
25.	D

EXAMINATION SECTION
TEST 1

DIRECTIONS: Each question or incomplete statement is followed by several suggested answers or completions. Select the one that BEST answers the question or completes the statement. *PRINT THE LETTER OF THE CORRECT ANSWER IN THE SPACE AT THE RIGHT.*

1. A nurse arrives in a home immediately after the birth of a premature baby for whom no preparation has been made. The MOST important factor to be considered in the immediate care of the baby is

    A. maintenance of body temperature
    B. removal to a hospital
    C. feeding with breastmilk
    D. demonstration of the infant's bath to the mother
    E. securing someone to give full-time care to the baby

1.__A__

2. The CHIEF cause of infant mortality is

    A. gastroenteritis   B. pneumonia
    C. prematurity   D. suffocation
    E. birth injuries

2.__C__

3. A child who carries the RH positive factor when his mother is an RH negative may develop a condition known as

    A. hypopituitarism   B. erythroblastosis
    C. autosomal genes   D. mongolism
    E. acromegaly

3.__B__

4. According to studies of child development, the one of the following behavior characteristics which you would expect to find in a normal two-year-old child is

    A. bladder control day and night
    B. ability to play well with a group
    C. ability to feed himself without help
    D. ability to converse in sentences
    E. ability to ride a tricycle

4.__C__

5. Authorities are agreed that the BEST time to begin training a child for bladder control is

    A. as soon as the mother observes a definite rhythm in urination
    B. when the child begins to walk
    C. not until the child can indicate verbally a desire to void
    D. at one year of age
    E. at nine months of age

5.__A__

6. In the age group 15 to 30, the one of the following diseases which is the CHIEF cause of death is

    A. puerperal sepsis   B. heart disease
    C. tuberculosis   D. syphilis
    E. appendicitis

6.__C__

7. In the age group 55 to 64, the one of the following diseases which is the CHIEF cause of death is

    A. circulatory disease   B. pneumonia
    C. tuberculosis   D. hemiplegia
    E. cancer

7. A

8. In 1976, the expectancy of life at birth had increased to about 61.5. This was a 20-year saving since 1900.
Of the following factors, the one to which MOST of this saving in life has been attributed is the

    A. improved living conditions, as a result of higher incomes
    B. effects of the discovery of bacteria
    C. increase in recreational facilities which has lowered nervous tension
    D. curtailment of arduous physical labor due to mechanical inventions
    E. federal, state, and municipal assistance to the indigent and the handicapped

8. B

9. The term *acquired immunity,* when used in connection with communicable disease, means the

    A. specific immunity developed as a result of a natural selection in a group of people living in any particular area
    B. immunity existing in an area where people have never contracted the disease
    C. immunity existing for a few months after birth given physiologically to the newborn baby by the mother
    D. specific immunity resulting from an attack of the disease or from artificial means
    E. immunity human beings have against certain diseases of lower animals

9. D

10. Children who have had rheumatic fever and, as a result, exhibit symptoms of heart disease, must be given special protection against

    A. exposure to acute communicable diseases
    B. cathartics which contain kidney irritants
    C. dietary fads to control weight
    D. sight and sounds which frighten them
    E. living in an enervating warm climate

10. A

11. A twenty-one-year-old man is found by x-ray to have minimal tuberculosis. The physician orders sanitorium care. Temporarily no beds are available.
The BEST advice the nurse can give in this instance until he can be admitted to the sanitorium is to

    A. encourage the man to visit a friend in Arizona.
    B. plan bed rest and isolation of the patient at home where his mother can care for him
    C. advise that he may continue work in his office position since the work is light and the lesion minimal
    D. encourage a seashore vacation where he may lie for hours in the sun
    E. advise an outdoor mountain vacation

11. B

12. The time of a well-prepared nurse in a busy syphilis clinic can BEST be used in

12. C

A. acting as receptionist to put patients at ease
B. giving intravenous treatments, thereby releasing the physicians to do physical examinations
C. taking histories and interpreting the disease and its treatment to patients
D. assisting the physician and taking notes on his physical examinations
E. managing the clinic smoothly so patients need not wait

13. The effect of syphilitic involvement of the eighth nerve in individuals with congenital syphilis is that it   13. _E_

A. usually causes facial paralysis, if the patient is not treated promptly
B. manifests itself very slowly and, therefore, may be easily controlled
C. is a relatively unimportant complication of the disease and responds readily to treatment
D. may be disregarded as a probable complication of the disease if the patient is over 6 years old
E. usually causes total deafness and is not readily responsive to treatment

14. The only way in which syphilis can be detected with CERTAINTY in pregnant women is by   14. _D_

A. actual discovery of active lesions, since in a new case the serology will remain negative until after parturition
B. a vaginal smear and dark-field examination, since in pregnancy the spirochetes migrate to the vagina mucosa
C. a careful case history, since recent discoveries indicate that serologic tests are non-specific in pregnancy
D. routine serologic tests, since the primary and secondary signs and symptoms are often repressed in pregnancy
E. the Rorschach test

15. The method which is GENERALLY recommended for preventing premature infant deaths resulting from inter-cranial hemorrhage is to   15. _A_

A. administer vitamin K to the mother before delivery and to the baby after birth
B. give the mother massive doses of calcium by hypodermic injection
C. increase the amount of codliver oil given to the mother so that the calcium is better utilized by the baby
D. give the infant parathyroid hormone in order to utilize available calcium
E. give the baby transfusions of gum tragacanth in normal saline

16. The MOST important factor in the control of breast cancer is   16. _D_

A. application of radium as soon as a lump appears in the breast
B. deep x-ray therapy of all suspected lipomas
C. biopsy of the glands in the axilla
D. operative intervention early in the disease
E. breastfeeding of infants as a preventive measure

17. Although there are still many unknown factors in the complete etiology of cancer, there is one to which authorities agree cancer can usually be validly attributed. This factor is   17. _C_

A. the tendency to cancerous growths passed on in the chromosomes and genes
B. the mechanical action of finely divided airborne proteins
C. chronic irritation in various forms
D. degeneration of cells in the older age groups
E. the implantation, in some way yet unknown, of malignant growths

18. The type of tuberculosis that has been generalized as a result of the bacilli having been seeded into the bloodstream from a tuberculosis infection is

    18. A

    A. miliary tuberculosis   B. tuberculosis meningitis
    C. tuberculosis enteritis   D. silicotic tuberculosis
    E. tuberculosis scrofula

19. The MOST common immediate cause of unsuccessful collapse of the lung by artificial pneumothorax is

    19. E

    A. hemoptysis   B. cavitation
    C. pleurisy with effusion   D. caseous lesion
    E. pleural adhesions

20. A child is given the Mantoux test to detect the existence of tuberculosis infection. After three days, a raised edematous reddened area appears at the site of the test.
    The CORRECT interpretation of the test result is:

    20. B

    A. A primary infection is present which makes the child completely resistant to further exogenous infections
    B. The test shows evidence of infection, but does not indicate whether the process is active or quiescent
    C. The test shows evidence of active pulmonary tuberculosis
    D. The reaction may be due to protein sensitivity and a control test is required to eliminate this factor
    E. The child has been exposed to active tuberculosis, but has not acquired an infection

21. Of the following, the one which should receive the MOST emphasis by the school nurse in order to achieve the best results in improving school health education is

    21. C

    A. classroom teaching in hygiene
    B. home visits to expand parent education
    C. assisting teachers to integrate health education in classroom teaching
    D. active participation in the health education programs of Parent-Teacher Associations
    E. parent education through group instruction at the time of the school health examination

22. A high school student is found to have a heart condition which warrants bed rest at home. Because only six weeks of the school term remain, the student wishes to complete the term, and is inclined to disregard the school physician's advice until the school term closes.
    The BEST method the school nurse can take in handling this situation is to

    22. A

A.   visit the home to enlist the parents' cooperation and assist them in planning the necessary care, and encourage the student to follow the doctor's advice
B.   discuss it with the school doctor and get his suggestions for adjustment in the school schedule to allow the student to complete the school term
C.   refer the student to the Visiting Nurse Association for follow-up and instruction
D.   advise the student that if she does remain in school to go to bed every day as soon as she gets home from school
E.   advise the student to see her pharmacist for confirmation of the school physician's diagnosis

23.   The one of the following criteria which is the BEST method for evaluating the success of the school health program is   23. _A_

A.   improved health behavior as evidenced by the application of health knowledge in daily habits of living
B.   an increased number of health classes in the school curriculum
C.   the number of defects discovered and corrected in school children
D.   the number of school children examined annually by their family physicians
E.   an increased number of children entering school each year without defects

24.   A kindgergarten school child is found by a visual acuity test to have 20/30 vision. The action the school nurse should take in this situation is to   24. _E_

A.   send the child to an oculist for a complete eye examination
B.   send a note to the child's parents advising that the child should wear glasses
C.   do nothing since farsightedness is normal in young children
D.   advise the teacher to reduce the amount of class work required of the child until the condition is corrected
E.   enlist the cooperation of parents and teacher in teaching the child good eye hygiene

25.   A nurse should know that blepharitis is a(n)   25. _C_

A.   skin disease which is highly communicable
B.   infection of the bladder
C.   inflammation of the eyelids
D.   disease caused by a fungus
E.   nutritional deficiency disease

KEY (CORRECT ANSWERS)

1.	A		11.	B
2.	C		12.	C
3.	B		13.	E
4.	C		14.	D
5.	A		15.	A
6.	C		16.	D
7.	A		17.	C
8.	B		18.	A
9.	D		19.	E
10.	A		20.	B

21.	C
22.	A
23.	A
24.	E
25.	C

EXAMINATION SECTION
TEST 1

DIRECTIONS: Each question or incomplete statement is followed by several suggested answers or completions. Select the one that BEST answers the question or completes the statement. *PRINT THE LETTER OF THE CORRECT ANSWER IN THE SPACE AT THE RIGHT.*

1. Which of these occurrences in a postpartal woman would be MOST indicative of an abnormality?   1.____

   A. A chill shortly after delivery
   B. A pulse rate of 60 the morning after delivery
   C. Urinary output of 3,000 ml. on the second day after delivery
   D. An oral temperature of 101° F. (38.3° C.) on the third day after delivery

2. While discussing nutrition with the nurse, a woman who is a primigravida says that she eats an egg for breakfast every day.   2.____
   The woman should be informed that the absorption of iron from the egg would be BEST facilitated by the woman's also eating _____ at the same meal.

   A. toast
   C. orange juice
   B. butter
   D. bacon

Questions 3-8.

DIRECTIONS: Questions 3 through 8 are to be answered on the basis of the following information.

Ms. Judy Lee, 28 years old and gravida I, is attending the antepartal clinic regularly. Ms. Lee is carrying twins. In the 38th week of gestation, she is admitted to the hospital in labor. Her membranes have ruptured.

3. Since Ms. Lee's admission, the nurse has been able to hear and count the heartbeats of both twins. Suppose that at a later time during Ms. Lee's labor, the nurse can hear only one heartbeat, even after several attempts. Which of these interpretations of this finding would be ACCURATE?   3.____

   A. Inaudibility of one of the heartbeats can result from a change in the position of the twins, but it could also be due to fetal distress; prompt evaluation of the situation by the physician is mandatory.
   B. Muffled fetal heartbeats are common when uterine contractions are strong and frequent, as they are in a multiple pregnancy; more frequent evaluation of the fetal heartbeats is advisable.
   C. Inability to hear one heartbeat in a twin pregnancy can normally be expected at intervals throughout labor; no action is indicated.
   D. Inability to hear fetal heartbeats in a twin pregnancy does not indicate fetal difficulty unless accompanied by additional symptoms; amniotic fluid should be examined for meconium staining.

4. Ms. Lee's labor progresses, and she delivers spontaneously two girls - one weighs 4 lbs. (1,814 gm.) and the other weighs 4 lb. 8 oz. (2,041 gm.). The twins are transferred to the premature nursery, and Ms. Lee is transferred to the postpartum unit.
Which of these concepts should be MOST basic to planning care for the Lee twins?   4.____

   A. Circulatory function is enhanced by frequent change of position.
   B. A well-lubricated skin is resistant to excoriation and damage.
   C. A premature infant's rectal temperature reflects the infant's ability to conserve heat.
   D. Optimal environmental temperature results in minimal oxygen consumption in the premature infant.

5. The method used for a premature infant's first formula feeding and the time at which it is begun will be based CHIEFLY upon the infant's   5.__C__

   A. birth weight
   B. degree of hydration
   C. level of physiologic maturity
   D. total body surface

6. The smaller of the Lee twins is to be gavaged.
In determining the location of the catheter after its insertion into the infant, it would be MOST desirable to insert   6.__C__

   A. the tip of a large syringe into the catheter and withdraw an amount of air equal to the amount of feeding
   B. a few drops of sterile water into the catheter, hold the end of the catheter below the level of the infant's stomach, and observe it for drainage of gastric contents
   C. about 0.5 to 1 ml. of air into the catheter and listen to the infant's abdomen with a stethoscope
   D. about 5 ml. of sterile water into the catheter and observe the infant's respirations

7. On her second postpartum day, Ms. Lee says to the nurse,
I've been to the bathroom four times in the past hour to urinate. The funny thing about it is that I only pass a small amount of urine each time.
Which of these initial actions by the nurse would demonstrate the BEST judgment?   7.__A__

   A. Palpate Ms. Lee's abdomen for bladder distention.
   B. Explain to Ms. Lee that frequent voiding is expected during the first few days after delivery.
   C. Advise Ms. Lee to use a bedpan for her next voiding.
   D. Discuss with Ms. Lee the relationship between trauma during delivery and signs of bladder irritation during the postpartum period.

8. On the third postpartum day, Ms. Lee is discharged. The twins are to remain until they have reached an appropriate weight. When the twins are to be discharged, Mr. and Ms. Lee come to the hospital to take them home.
Which of these statements, if made by Ms. Lee, would indicate the BEST understanding of her babies' needs?   8.__D__

   A. Our babies' needs are different from those of full-term infants, and we will do all we can to protect them.
   B. We are going to try very hard to counteract the effects of our babies' having been born prematurely.

C. For a while the smaller baby will need special attention, and then we will be able to treat both of our babies similarly.

D. We expect to enjoy our babies and will give them the kind of care babies need.

Questions 9-18.

DIRECTIONS: Questions 9 through 18 are to be answered on the basis of the following information.

Ms. Angela Dobbs, 32 years old and gravida I, is now in her third trimester of pregnancy. She has had diabetes mellitus since the age of 16 and has been attending the antepartal clinic regularly for the past 5 months.

9. Compared with Ms. Dobbs' insulin requirements when she was not pregnant, it can be expected that the insulin dosage during her third trimester will

9.___B

A. remain the same
B. be increased
C. be decreased
D. be increased or decreased, depending upon fetal activity

10. At 30 weeks' gestation, Ms. Dobbs has an ultrasonic examination. The results of this examination disclose information about the fetus'

10.___B

A. circulatory function
C. presence of surfactant
B. gestational age
D. presence of congenital defects

11. Because the incidence of fetal death is higher in women who have diabetes mellitus, indications of placental insufficiency should be suspected if Ms. Dobbs has a(n)

11.___A

A. sustained drop in her blood glucose level
B. urinary output of more than 1500 ml. a day
C. increase in the secretion of gonadotropin
D. albumin content in her urine of +1

12. At 35 weeks' gestation, Ms. Dobbs is admitted to the hospital for evaluation of her pregnancy and diabetic status. Ms. Dobbs is to have a urinary estriol level determination. Which of these instructions should be among those given to her about collecting the urine for this procedure? Collect

12.___C

A. the first morning specimen before eating breakfast
B. a specimen about an hour after the evening meal
C. a twenty-four hour specimen
D. a clean-voided specimen

13. Ms. Dobbs is to have an amniocentesis done to determine the lecithin/sphingomyelin (L/S) ratio.
The purpose of this study is to

13.___D

A. assess placental functioning
B. assess the amount of fetal body fat
C. determine fetal kidney functioning
D. determine fetal pulmonary maturity

14. Ms. Dobbs has a cesarean section and is delivered of a boy who weighs 8 lb. 4 oz.   14. C
(3,742 gm.). He is transferred to the intensive care nursery. Ms. Dobbs is transferred to
the postpartum unit from the recovery room.
Postpartum orders for Ms. Dobbs include an estrogen preparation to

   A. promote sodium excretion
   B. suppress the production of chorionic gonadotropin
   C. inhibit secretion of the lactogenic hormone
   D. diminish lochial flow

15. Two hours after delivery, the nurse observes that Baby Boy Dobbs is lethargic and has   15. A
developed mild generalized cyanosis and twitching.
In view of the fact that his mother has diabetes mellitus, the infant is PROBABLY exhib-
iting symptoms of a

   A. low blood sugar level   B. high CO_2 level
   C. subnormal temperature   D. withdrawal from insulin

16. Because Ms. Dobbs has diabetes mellitus, her infant should be assessed for the pres-   16. D
ence of

   A. a blood group incompatibility
   B. meconium ileus
   C. phenylketonuria
   D. a congenital abnormality

17. Ms. Dobbs is bottle-feeding her baby. Ms. Dobbs, who has previously observed a demon-   17. C
stration of diapering, is changing her baby's diaper for the first time, under the supervision of the registered nurse. Ms. Dobbs is holding the baby's feet correctly, but when she
starts to raise his legs to remove the diaper, the feet slip from her grasp, and the baby's
legs drop back onto the mattress of the bassinet. The baby whimpers briefly, and Ms.
Dobbs looks dismayed.
Which of these responses by the nurse would be BEST?

   A. I'll show you again how to change the baby's diaper, Ms. Dobbs.
   B. I'll diaper the baby for you this time, Ms. Dobbs.
   C. You've almost got it, Ms. Dobbs. Try again?
   D. Why are you so nervous, Ms. Dobbs?

18. Some time after discharge, Ms. Dobbs calls the hospital to report the loss of her baby's   18. B
birth certificate. Where would it be BEST for her to apply for a duplicate? The

   A. record room of the hospital where the baby was born
   B. agency that records vital statistics for the community in which the baby was born
   C. Census Bureau
   D. National Office of Vital Statistics

Questions 19-25.

DIRECTIONS: Questions 19 through 25 are to be answered on the basis of the following information.

Ms. Linda Young, a 17-year-old high school student, attends the antepartal clinic on a regular basis. This is Linda's first pregnancy.

19.   Linda is now 7 months pregnant.   19._A_
In assessing whether Linda is retaining abnormal amounts of fluid, it would be ESPE-
CIALLY significant that she has gained

    A.   3 lb. (1,361 gm.) during the past week
    B.   4 1/2 lb. (2,041 gm.) since her last clinic visit a month ago
    C.   11 lb. (4,990 gm.) in the second trimester of pregnancy
    D.   14 lb. (6,350 gm.) since the onset of pregnancy

20.   Which of these measures will contribute MOST to the prevention of postpartal uterine   20._C_
infections?

    A.   Routine use of serologic tests for syphilis early in the antepartal period
    B.   Limitation of sexual intercourse during the last six weeks of pregnancy
    C.   Maintenance of cleanliness of the perineal area during labor
    D.   Taking showers or sponge baths exclusively during the last six weeks of pregnancy

21.   At term, Linda is admitted to the hospital in active labor. Linda's cervix is 2 cm. dilated   21._D_
and 80% effaced. Which of these interpretations of these findings is CORRECT?
The

    A.   cervix is 2 cm. short of complete dilatation, and it is 80% thinner than it was before
labor started
    B.   cervix is still 2 cm. long, and 80% of the thinning of the cervix is completed
    C.   walls of the cervix are 2 cm. thick, and 80% of the widening of the cervical opening
has been achieved
    D.   opening of the cervix is 2 cm. wide, and the cervical canal is 80% shorter than nor-
mal

22.   Linda has an episiotomy and delivers a 7 lb. (3,175 gm.) boy. Baby Boy Young is trans-   22._B_
ferred to the nursery and Linda is transferred to the postpartum unit. Linda plans to bottle-feed her baby. The nurse is assessing Baby Boy Young.
Which of these observations, if made, would be considered characteristics of a newborn?

    A.   Branlike desquamation of the hands and fee; alternating limpness and stiffness of
the body; and pink, moist skin
    B.   Cool, mottled hands and feet; quivering lower jaw; and flexion of body parts
    C.   Clenched fists; arching of the back when recumbent; and frequent crying
    D.   Butterfly-shaped area of pigmentation at the base of the spine; extension of the
arms and legs when the head is turned to the side; and diaphragmatic breathing

23. When Linda has been admitted to the postpartum unit, she says to the nurse, *I'm so glad my baby is a boy. Maybe Jack will marry me now because he'll be so proud to have a son.*
It is probably MOST justifiable to say that Linda

    A.   wants to get married in order to gain her independence from her family
    B.   is capable of subordinating her personal needs to the needs of others
    C.   is showing a beginning awareness of the problems associated with having a baby out of wedlock
    D.   lacks insight into the factors that contribute to a successful marriage

23. D

24. When Baby Boy Young is brought to his mother for the first time to be fed, Linda asks the nurse, *What's wrong with my baby's eyes? He looks cross-eyed.*
Which of these initial responses by the nurse would probably be MOST helpful?

    A.   Babies seem to be cross-eyed for a while after birth because the muscles in their eyes aren't able to work together.
    B.   You feel that your baby's eyes are abnormal?
    C.   I can see that you're upset about this. It would be advisable for you to talk with the doctor about it.
    D.   Your baby will appear cross-eyed for some time because his eyes won't be completely developed until he is about six months old.

24. A

25. When Linda is talking with the nurse about feeding her baby, she says, *I've heard that if I breastfed him, he'd* develop a close feeling toward me more quickly. I had planned to bottle-feed him.
The nurse's initial reply should convey which of these understandings about the development of a mother-child relationship?

    A.   A satisfactory mother-child relationship will develop more readily through breast-feeding than bottle-feeding.
    B.   Holding the baby during bottle-feeding will help to promote a good mother-child relationship.
    C.   The times at which the baby is fed by the mother will affect the quality of the mother-child relationship more than the feeding method.
    D.   Since bottle-feeding is less complicated than breastfeeding, the mother will be able to focus more attention on mothering functions such as cuddling and talking while the baby is eating.

25. B

KEY (CORRECT ANSWERS)

1.	D		11.	A
2.	C		12.	C
3.	A		13.	D
4.	D		14.	C
5.	C		15.	A
6.	C		16.	D
7.	A		17.	C
8.	D		18.	B
9.	B		19.	A
10.	B		20.	C

21. D
22. B
23. D
24. A
25. B

———

TEST 2

DIRECTIONS: Each question or incomplete statement is followed by several suggested answers or completions. Select the one that BEST answers the question or completes the statement. *PRINT THE LETTER OF THE CORRECT ANSWER IN THE SPACE AT THE RIGHT.*

1. The instructions that are ESPECIALLY important to give to a pregnant woman who has heart disease are:

   A. Increase protein intake
   B. Take no drugs unless they have been prescribed
   C. Limit high-calorie foods
   D. Avoid fatigue

   1. _D_

Questions 2-9.

DIRECTIONS: Questions 2 through 9 are to be answered on the basis of the following information.

Ms. Mary White, 35 years old, is pregnant for the third time. She is receiving antepartal care from a private physician. Ms. White is in the seventh month of pregnancy and has symptoms of preeclampsia.

2. The physician instructs Ms. White not to eat foods which have a high sodium content. The nurse tells Ms. White about foods containing sodium and then asks her to identify foods lowest in sodium.
   Which of these foods, if selected by Ms. White, would be CORRECT?

   A. Creamed chipped beef on dry toast
   B. Cheese sandwich on whole wheat toast
   C. Frankfurter on a roll
   D. Tomato stuffed with diced chicken

   2. _D_

3. In Ms. White's 39th week of gestation, her physician recommends that she be hospitalized. When the physician leaves after examining Ms. White, Ms. White says to the nurse, *It's easy for you people to say, "Go to the hospital," but it's not so easy for me to do it. I can't go just like that!*
   After acknowledging her feeling, which of these approaches by the nurse would probably be BEST?

   A. Stress to Ms. White that her husband would want her to do what is best for her health.
   B. Explore with Ms. White ways that immediate hospitali-zation could be arranged.
   C. Repeat the physician's reasons for advising immediate hospitalization for Ms. White.
   D. Explain to Ms. White that she is ultimately responsible for her own welfare and that of her baby.

   3. _B_

4. Ms. White is admitted to the hospital.
   Because of the possibility of convulsive seizures, which of these articles should be readily available for Ms. White's care?

   4. _A_

A. Oxygen and suction machine
B. Suction machine and mouth care tray
C. Mouth care tray and venous cutdown set
D. Venous cutdown set and oxygen

5. The next morning, Ms. White tells the nurse that she thinks she is beginning to have contractions.
For the timing of uterine contractions, it is recommended that she place

5.____ C

A. her hands on the upper part of the abdomen, on opposite sides, and curve them somewhat around the uterine fundus
B. the heel of the hand on the abdomen, just above the umbilicus, and press firmly
C. her hand flat on the abdomen over the uterine fundus, with the fingers apart, and press lightly
D. her hand in the middle of the upper part of the abdomen and then move the hand several times to different parts of the upper abdomen during each contraction

6. Ms. White goes into labor.
If Ms. White were to complain of a severe headache while she is in labor, the nurse should INITIALLY

6.____ B

A. put Ms. White flat in bed with one pillow under her head
B. take Ms. White's blood pressure
C. check Ms. White's chart to determine whether she has recently received an analgesic
D. count the fetal heart rate

7. Ms. White delivers a girl. Baby White's Apgar score at 1 minute is 8.
The CHIEF purpose of the first Apgar scoring of a newborn is to

7.____ B

A. obtain a baseline for comparison with the infant's future development
B. evaluate the efficiency of the infant's vital functions
C. assess the effectiveness of the initial care given to the infant
D. determine the presence of gross malformations in the infant

8. Ms. White is transferred to the postpartum unit, and Baby Girl White is transferred to the newborn nursery. Ms. White had a normal vaginal delivery, but is having difficulty voiding in the early postpartum.
The cause of her difficulty is MOST likely due to

8.____ A

A. decreased abdominal pressure and trauma to the trigone of the bladder
B. decreased blood volume and increased production of estrogen and progesterone
C. increased bladder tone and emotional stress
D. constriction of the kidney pelves and ureters

9. Ms. White is bottle-feeding her baby.
Which of these manifestations developing in her nipples or breasts on the third day after delivery would be NORMAL?

9.____ B

A. Decrease in secretion from the breasts
B. Engorgement of the breasts
C. Inversion of the nipples
D. Tenderness and redness of the nipples

Questions 10-11.

DIRECTIONS: Questions 10 and 11 are to be answered on the basis of the following information.

Ms. Ellen Stone, an 18-year-old primigravida, is brought to the hospital in early active
labor. She has received no antepartal care during her pregnancy.

10.   Which of these observations of Ms. Stone would be the MOST reliable indication that she   10.___
is in true labor?

   A.   Strong, intermittent uterine contractions
   B.   Progressive cervical effacement and dilatation
   C.   Rupture of the membranes
   D.   Engagement of the presenting part

11.   During the first stage of Ms. Stone's labor, which of these measures by the nurse would   11.___
be MOST supportive of her?

   A.   Administering sufficient analgesia to minimize pain from uterine contractions and
        encouraging her to remain on her back
   B.   Keeping her informed about the progress of her labor and helping her to relax
        between contractions
   C.   Having her hold on to the nurse's hand during the height of contractions and
        reminding her to breathe rapidly with her mouth open
   D.   Telling her to bear down with her contractions and instructing her to sleep between
        contractions

Questions 12-21.

DIRECTIONS: Questions 12 through 21 are to be answered on the basis of the following information.

Ms. Karen Newman, a 26-year-old multipara, is pregnant. Her obstetric history includes 2
full-term pregnancies terminating in normal deliveries and, prior to her present pregnancy, a
spontaneous abortion at 14 weeks' gestation. She is receiving antepartal care from a private
physician.

12.   On the basis of Ms. Newman's obstetric history, she is designated as a gravida _____,   12.___
para _____.

   A.   III; II   B.   III; IV   C.   IV; II   D.   IV; III

13.   Ms. Newman weighs 152 lb. (68.95 kg.) at the end of the fourth month of gestation. Her   13.___
weight before she became pregnant was 135 lb. (61.23 kg.), which was normal for her
age and body build.
It is justifiable to say that Ms. Newman's 17-lb. (7.72 kg.) weight gain for her stage of
pregnancy is

   A.   below average   B.   average
   C.   somewhat above average   D.   excessive

14. Ms. Newman tells the nurse that her 2 1/2-year-old son, Danny, tends to be jealous and   14.___C___
that she is worried about how he may react to the new baby.
The nurse's reply should indicate that jealousy in a 2 1/2-year-old

    A. can be lessened by providing a mother-substitute for the child when the mother
        first returns home from the hospital
    B. can be suppressed if the child's contact with the new baby is restricted
    C. cannot be handled by reasoning with the child
    D. cannot be dealt with therapeutically

15. Ms. Newman is 2 weeks past term. She is admitted to the hospital for induction of labor   15.___C___
with an oxytocic drug. Upon admission, Ms. Newman is permitted to have liquids by
mouth.
Which of these foods would probably be CONTRAINDICATED for her?

    A. Tea with lemon   B. Ginger ale
    C. Milk   D. Gelatin dessert

16. Which of these findings, if present in Ms. Newman, would it be ESSENTIAL for the regis-   16.___D___
tered nurse to report to the physician before the oxytocic infusion is started?

    A. Low backache
    B. A rise in blood pressure from 122/80 to 130/84
    C. An increase in pulse rate from 88 to 98
    D. Regular contractions of 60 seconds' duration

17. Ms. Newman has an intravenous infusion running, to which oxytocin injection (Pitocin)   17.___C___
has been added.
Which of these conditions would warrant IMMEDIATE discontinuation of Ms. Newman's intravenous infusion of Pitocin?

    A. Increase in show
    B. Rupture of the membranes
    C. A sustained uterine contraction
    D. A fetal heart rate of 120 during a contraction

18. Ms. Newman has an order for 100 mg. of meperidine (Demerol) hydrochloride.   18.___C___
Which of these groups of signs in Ms. Newman would MOST clearly indicate that a
dose of Demerol could be given to her with safety?
Cervical dilatation, _____ cm.; presenting part at _____ station; uterine contractions
q._____ minutes, lasting _____ seconds; fetal heart rate, _____ beats per minute.

    A. 3; 0; 10; 45; 100   B. 4; 0; 3; 50; 172
    C. 5; -1; 5; 40; 144   D. 7; -1; 2; 60; 120

19. In view of the fact that Ms. Newman had general anesthesia, it would be safe to start giv-   19.___B___
ing her oral fluids

    A. after she voids for the first time
    B. after she has coughed voluntarily
    C. when her pulse rate is 70 beats per minute
    D. when she has rested for about an hour after admission to the postpartum unit

20. Penicillin ointment rather than silver nitrate is used in the prophylactic eye care of Baby Boy Newman to   20. __D__

    A.   promote a more lasting bacteriostatic effect
    B.   gain a more rapid systemic effect
    C.   administer therapeutic amounts with greater ease
    D.   cause less irritation of the conjunctivae

21. Six weeks after the birth of her baby, Ms. Newman returns to the clinic for a routine follow-up visit. At the clinic, Ms. Newman says to the nurse, *Having so many children makes it very hard for us to manage, but my husband won't do anything to prevent me from getting pregnant. He gets angry when I even mention the idea.* Which of these approaches by the nurse is LIKELY to be MOST useful?   21. __D__

    A.   Give Ms. Newman a pamphlet for her husband that describes various contraceptive methods.
    B.   Ask Ms. Newman to have her husband accompany her to the clinic to talk with the nurse about contraception.
    C.   Refer Ms. Newman to an agency that provides family planning services.
    D.   Find out from Ms. Newman if her husband would be willing to accept a method of contraception that would not involve him directly.

Questions 22-30.

DIRECTIONS: Questions 22 through 30 are to be answered on the basis of the following information.

    Ms. Barbara Wing, 21 years old, attends the antepartal clinic for the first time when she has missed two menstrual periods. The physician determines that she is pregnant and finds her to be in good health. This is her first pregnancy.

22. During Ms. Wing's initial conference with the registered nurse, she mentions that although she usually feels well, there are times when she feels tired.
Which of these responses by the nurse would be BEST?   22. __A__

    A.   Fatigue is normal when the body is adjusting to the pregnant state. Let's talk about your daily schedule so we can plan extra rest for you.
    B.   It will be necessary for you to cut down on your usual activities and try to get more rest. About how many hours of sleep do you get at night?
    C.   Your fatigue is probably due to hormonal changes that occur in early pregnancy. As your body adapts to the demands of your developing baby, this feeling will pass.
    D.   Your fatigue at this time indicates that you probably will have to give special consideration to rest, and possibly even to diet, throughout your pregnancy.

23. Ms. Wing is to include extra amounts of vitamin C in her diet.
She should be instructed that the juice that has the
LEAST vitamin C per average serving is   23. __D__

    A.   canned apple   B.   canned tomato
    C.   fresh grapefruit   D.   frozen orange

24. Ms. Wing's pregnancy progresses normally.   24. _D_
    In the latter part of the third trimester, Ms. Wing should be advised to take which of
    these precautions relative to bathing?

    A. Take sponge baths exclusively
    B. Avoid using bath salts
    C. Bathe only in tepid water
    D. Place nonskid material at the bottom of the bathtub

25. Ms. Wing is at term and in early active labor when she is brought to the hospital by her   25. _A_
    husband. Mr. and Ms. Wing attended a series of preparation for childbirth classes.
    Such a program is MOST likely to be successful if the

    A. parents and the medical and nursing staff have accepted the philosophy, princi-
       ples, and techniques of the classes
    B. physician is present during labor and gives support to the mother
    C. nurse who is to stay with the mother during labor and delivery is prepared to assist
       the father in coaching his wife
    D. mother and father are truly prepared for their roles during labor and delivery

26. The nurse makes all of the following observations of Ms. Wing during the second stage   26. _B_
    of her labor.
    Which one would be of GREATEST significance in terms of her welfare and that of her
    baby?
    A(n)

    A. sudden increase in blood-tinged show
    B. change in the baseline blood pressure from 110/80 to 90/60
    C. fetal heart rate of 152 to 160 beats per minute between contractions
    D. increase in maternal pulse rate from 90 to 95 beats per minute during contractions

27. Ms. Wing has an episiotomy and delivers a girl weighing 7 lb. 5 oz. (3,317 gm.).   27. _D_
    Which of these observations of Ms. Wing would indicate that normal placental separa-
    tion is occurring? She has

    A. hardening and thickening of the exposed portion of the umbilical cord, softening of
       the uterine fundus, and a steady stream of blood from the vagina
    B. strong uterine contractions, recession of the uterine fundus below the symphysis
       pubis, and temporary absence of vaginal bleeding
    C. gaping of the vulva in conjunction with strong uterine contractions, rapid enlarge-
       ment of the uterus, and oozing of blood from the vagina
    D. increased protrusion of the umbilical cord from the vagina, the uterus' becoming
       globular-shaped, and a sudden spurting of blood from the vagina

28. Ms. Wing is transferred to the postpartum unit, and Baby Girl Wing is transferred to the   28. _C_
    newborn nursery.
    In examining Ms. Wing's episiotomy incision, which of these positions would be appro-
    priate for the patient and would BEST help to minimize strain on the sutures?

    A. Prone   B. Knee-chest
    C. Sim's   D. Trendelenburg

29. Which of these measures, if carried out before Baby Girl Wing's discharge, will PROBA-   29. _B_
BLY contribute to Ms. Wing's confidence in her ability to care for her baby?

   A. Having Ms. Wing observe demonstrations of infant care in which equipment commonly found in the home is used
   B. Having Ms. Wing take care of the baby in the hospital under the guidance of the
registered nurse
   C. Arranging for Mr. Wing to learn how to assist Ms. Wing with caring for the baby
   D. Arranging to have the community health nurse visit with Ms. Wing and discuss
areas that are of concern to Ms. Wing

30. Mr. and Ms. Wing discuss birth control with the nurse. In selecting a method of birth con-   30. _C_
trol, the Wings should give priority to

   A. Ms. Wing's age
   B. the length of their marriage
   C. the technique they find most acceptable
   D. the success rate of a particular method

KEY (CORRECT ANSWERS)

1.	D		16.	D
2.	D		17.	C
3.	B		18.	C
4.	A		19.	B
5.	C		20.	D
6.	B		21.	D
7.	B		22.	A
8.	A		23.	A
9.	B		24.	D
10.	B		25.	A
11.	B		26.	B
12.	C		27.	D
13.	D		28.	C
14.	C		29.	B
15.	C		30.	C

EXAMINATION SECTION
TEST 1

DIRECTIONS: Each question or incomplete statement is followed by several suggested answers or completions. Select the one that BEST answers the question or completes the statement. *PRINT THE LETTER OF THE CORRECT ANSWER IN THE SPACE AT THE RIGHT.*

1. Symptoms characteristic of severe preeclampsia include

    A. ringing in the ears and rapid pulse
    B. elevated temperature and excitability
    C. vomiting and excessive urination
    D. persistent headache and blurred vision

1.__D__

2. In the care of a newborn with hydrocephalus, which of these measures is *especially* important?

    A. Keeping the baby dry
    B. Changing the baby's position at regular intervals
    C. Feeding the baby small amounts of formula frequently
    D. Placing the baby so that his head is lower than the rest of his body

2.__B__

3. A newborn who has a cleft palate is to be bottle-fed.
Which of these measures would it be MOST important to take when feeding this infant?

    A. Apply elbow restraints to the infant prior to each feeding
    B. Hold the infant in an upright position during feedings
    C. Give the infant a small amount of sterile water after each feeding
    D. Feed the infant small amounts frequently

3.__B__

QUESTIONS 4-12.

Mrs. Connie Tong, 21 years old, attends the antepartal clinic. The physician examines Mrs. Tong and finds her to be about 3 months pregnant.

4. The licensed practical nurse is talking with Mrs. Tong about her nutritional needs. The nurse should advise Mrs. Tong that she will get the HIGHEST amount of vitamins and minerals from the vegetables in her diet if she

    A. eats them raw
    B. stores them in the refrigerator
    C. cooks them in unsalted water
    D. boils them in a covered pot

4.__A__

5. Mrs. Tong says to the licensed practical nurse, "I try to drink as much milk as I'm sup-posed to, but it's hard to do because I don't like milk."
Which of these responses by the nurse would be BEST?

    A. Ask Mrs. Tong what foods she likes that contain milk
    B. Ask Mrs. Tong if she understands why milk is important for the development of her baby

5.__A__

C. Suggest that Mrs. Tong substitute one whole egg for every glass of milk that she omits from her diet
D. Suggest that Mrs. Tong talk with her physician about taking calcium tablets as a substitute for milk

6. During Mrs. Tong's clinic visit when she is 4 months pregnant, which of these procedures will be carried out for her? 6.___

A. Vaginal smear and pelvic measurements
B. Vaginal examination and Rh factor determination
C. Blood test for syphilis and rectal examination
D. Blood pressure determination and weighing

7. Which of these understandings regarding activity for pregnant women would it be BEST for the licensed practical nurse to have? 7.___

A. Activities that require stretching and bending should be avoided
B. Usual activities should be continued in moderation
C. Emphasis should be given to active participation in outdoor activities
D. Each new activity should be preceded by a short period of rest

Mrs. Tong's pregnancy progresses normally. She is admitted to the hospital at term in early active labor.

8. Which of these occurences is the MOST reliable indication of the onset of true labor? 8.___

A. The woman's report of a burst of energy
B. Regular progression of uterine contractions
C. Increased vaginal discharge
D. Rupture of the membranes

Mrs. Tong has a normal spontaneous delivery of a girl. Mrs. Tong plans to breast-feed her infant.

9. When Mrs. Tong is 6 hours postpartum, she is placed on a bedpan to void. After trying for a period of time, Mrs. Tong states that she is unable to void. Her bladder is distended. Which of these measures would it be BEST for the licensed practical nurse to use to help Mrs. Tong to void? 9.___

A. Pour warm water over her vulva
B. Apply gentle manual pressure over her bladder
C. Encourage her to drink fluids freely
D. Explain to her that she will have to be catheterized if she does not void

10. When Baby Girl Tong is brought to Mrs. Tong for the first breast-feeding, Mrs. Tong asks the licensed practical nurse, "How much of the nipple should the baby be given?" Which of these replies is it CORRECT for the nurse to give Mrs. Tong? 10.___

A. "The baby should have the nipple and some of the dark area around the nipple well into her mouth."
B. "Since she's had some water from a bottle in the nursery, she has already learned the amount of nipple she needs to nurse adequately."

C. "Babies' mouths are of different sizes, and the baby will take the correct amount of nipple for her."

D. "Babies nurse best when only the nipple is in the mouth."

11. On Mrs. Tong's third postpartum day, the licensed practical nurse finds her crying. When asked what seems to be wrong, Mrs. Tong says, "I really don't know. I have so much to be grateful for – a healthy baby, a good husband – I really should be happy."
Which of these actions by the nurse would demonstrate the BEST judgment in this situation?

11.___D___

A. Provide privacy for Mrs. Tong
B. Ask Mrs. Tong if her relationship with her husband will permit her to discuss her feelings with him.
C. Explain to Mrs. Tong that her reaction is an unusual one
D. Remain with Mrs. Tong for a while

12. Because Mrs. Tong is breast-feeding her baby, the diet recommended for her is likely to differ from that recommended for a mother who is NOT nursing by it being

12.___C___

A. lower in roughage, and higher in carbohydrates
B. lower in sodium, and higher in iron
C. higher in calcium and protein
D. higher in fat and cellulose

QUESTIONS 13-19.

Mrs. Merrilee Stone, 31 years old, comes to the antepartal clinic because she has missed 2 menstrual periods. She is found to be about 10 weeks pregnant. This is Mrs. Stone's third pregnancy. The Stones have 2 children.

13. Mrs. Stone has been advised by the physician to increase her intake of iron.
Which of these sandwiches, as *ordinarily* prepared, is HIGHEST in iron?

13.___A___

A. Egg salad
B. Peanut butter
C. Cream cheese and jelly
D. Lettuce and tomato

Mrs. Stone attends the clinic when she is 8 months pregnant.

14. Three of the following symptoms are common at this stage of pregnancy.
Which one is NOT?

14.___B___

A. Frequent urination
B. Nausea and vomiting
C. Edema of the ankles
D. Dyspnea when lying flat in bed

15. Mrs. Stone says to the licensed practical nurse, "Sometimes I think about what would happen if I died during childbirth." Which of these approaches by the nurse would be BEST?

15.___C___

A. Explain to her that such thoughts are common at her stage of pregnancy
B. Tell her that maternal deaths are extremely rare
C. Find out what prompted these feelings in her
D. Ask her if she has discussed these feelings with her husband

At term Mrs. Stone is admitted to the hospital in active labor. Mrs. Stone's labor is being electronically monitored.

16. Which of these findings, if observed in Mrs. Stone, should be reported to the nurse in charge IMMEDIATELY?   16. ____

    A. A decrease in the fetal heart rate from 144 to 132 during a contraction
    B. A decrease in the interval between contractions from 6 to 7 minutes to 4 to 5 minutes
    C. A sudden increase in the amount of blood in the vaginal show
    D. An increase in blood pressure from 120/76 to 132/80 at the beginning of a contraction

17. The duration of Mrs. Stone's contractions should be timed from the   17. ____

    A. beginning of a contraction to the beginning of the next contraction
    B. beginning of a contraction to the end of that contraction
    C. end of a contraction to the beginning of the next contraction
    D. end of a contraction to the end of the next contraction

Mrs. Stone's labor progresses normally. She delivers a boy.

18. A few hours after Mrs. Stone's delivery, the licensed practical nurse notes that Mrs. Stone has saturated two perineal pads with blood within a 20-minute period. Which of these actions should the nurse take FIRST?   18. ____

    A. Check the consistency of Mrs. Stone's uterine fundus
    B. Encourage Mrs. Stone to void
    C. Take Mrs. Stone's blood pressure
    D. Notify the nurse in charge

Mrs. Stone is transferred to the postpartum unit.

19. Mrs. Stone says to the licensed practical nurse, "I guess I really want some help. I don't need any more children. Three are enough."
Which of these approaches by the nurse would be *best* FIRST?   19. ____

    A. Find out what Mrs. Stone knows about the availability of family planning services
    B. Ask Mrs. Stone if her husband is interested in conception control
    C. Discuss with Mrs. Stone the effectiveness of various contraceptive methods
    D. Commend Mrs. Stone for her determination to limit her family size

QUESTIONS 20-26.

Mrs. Ulule Braxton, 32 years old, has 6 children, aged 1, 2, 3, 5, 7, and 9 years. Mrs. Braxton is visiting the physician because she has not menstruated for several months.

20. In the waiting room, Mrs. Braxton says to another patient, "Here I am again. I kind of hope that I'm not pregnant." When the licensed practical nurse is helping Mrs. Braxton to prepare for her examination, the nurse says to Mrs. Braxton, "I overheard your comments to the other patient in the waiting room."
Which of these additional remarks by the nurse would be MOST appropriate to follow this initial comment?   20. ____

A. "You may feel negative about another pregnancy now. These feelings are bound to change."
B. "It's healthy to express your feelings. Let's talk about them."
C. "You ought to discuss these feelings with the doctor, since they may affect the outcome of your pregnancy."
D. "The doctor may advise you to seek professional counseling. Such feelings often precede emotional problems in the postpartum period."

Mrs. Braxton is about 3 months pregnant.

21. A presumptive diagnosis of pregnancy can be made at 3 months' gestation by   21. _B_

    A. hearing fetal heart tones via a fetoscope
    B. the presence of chorionic gonadotropin in the mother's urine
    C. seeing the fetal skeleton on an x-ray
    D. the mother's confirmation of quickening

22. Why is it especially IMPORTANT for Mrs. Braxton to be under medical supervision during   22. _D_
her pregnancy?

    A. Premature labor is a common occurence in women such as Mrs. Braxton who are extremely active and over 25 years of age
    B. Fetal anoxia results from placental aging, which is common in women of Mrs. Braxton's age group
    C. Multigravidas are especially susceptible to infectious diseases
    D. Grand multiparas have a higher incidence of complications

At term Mrs. Braxton is admitted to the hospital and delivers a 9-lb., 4-oz. (4,196-gm.) boy. Mrs. Braxton is planning to breast-feed her baby.

23. At 5 minutes of life, Baby Boy Braxton's Apgar score is 9. Which of these findings is NOT   23. _C_
present in babies with such a score?

    A. Pulse rate of 120
    B. Regular abdominal breathing
    C. Flaccidity of the lower extremities
    D. Crying in response to being physically stimulated

24. Three of the following drugs may be administered to Mrs. Braxton while she is in the   24. _D_
delivery room.
Which one would NOT be given to her since she is planning to breast-feed her infant?

    A. Oxytocin injection (Pitocin)
    B. Ergonovine maleate (Ergotrate)
    C. Methylergonovine (Methergine) maleate
    D. Testosterone enanthate and estradiol valerate (Deladumone)

25. Mrs. Braxton expresses concern about her ability to supply the baby with enough milk   25. _D_
because of his large size.
Which of these ideas should most certainly be included in the licensed practical
nurse's response?

A. Supplemental feedings can be added for babies who weigh more than 9 pounds
B. Eight to ten glasses of fluid per day, half of which should be milk, will insure an adequate milk supply
C. Smoking should be avoided since it interferes with blood circulation in the mammary glands, thus reducing milk production
D. The more the baby sucks, the more milk the breasts will produce to meet the baby's needs

26. Mrs. Braxton asks the licensed practical nurse how effective oral contraceptive drugs are in preventing pregnancy. Which of these replies would be accurate?   26. _C_

A. "They are quite effective in women whose menstrual cycle is regular."
B. "They vary in effectiveness according to the woman's age."
C. "They are very effective when taken exactly as prescribed."
D. "They are highly effective only if used in conjunction with a birth control device such as a diaphragm."

QUESTIONS 27-36.

Mrs. Dolores Garcia is a 24-year-old multigravida who is 8 months pregnant. She comes to the hospital and is admitted to the labor room with bright red vaginal bleeding. The physician suspects that Mrs. Garcia may have placenta previa or abruptio placentae.

27. During the admission process, three of the following measures would be appropriate for Mrs. Garcia. Which one would be *contraindicated* for her?   27. _A_

A. Giving an enema
B. Obtaining a urine specimen
C. Checking for uterine contractions
D. Shaving the perineal area

28. When Mrs. Garcia is admitted, which of the following information should be obtained FIRST?   28. _B_

A. Her temperature and respiratory rate
B. Her blood pressure and pulse rate
C. Her height and weight
D. The date of her last menstrual period and the dates of her previous pregnancies

29. Which of these symptoms is *frequently* found in women with abruptic placentae, but is rare in women with placenta previa?   29. _C_

A. Thirst
B. Projectile vomiting
C. Abdominal pain
D. Small cysts in the vaginal discharge

It is determined that Mrs. Garcia has placenta previa, and a cesarean section is performed under spinal anesthesia. A 4-lb. (1,814-gm.) girl is delivered and is transferred to the premature nursery, where she is placed in an incubator. Mrs. Garcia is transferred from the recovery room to the postpartum unit with an intravenous infusion in her left arm and an indwelling urinary catheter attached to gravity drainage.

30. Identification tags were placed on both Baby Girl Garcia and her mother before they left   30.___D___
the delivery room.
The CHIEF reason this was done at that time is that

    A. it is the recommended hospital policy
    B. it is the most convenient time
    C. the procedure can be done under aseptic conditions
    D. the baby and her mother had not yet been separated

31. Mrs. Garcia is to be kept flat in bed for about 8 hours postoperatively.   31.___A___
The purpose of this measure is to prevent

    A. headache   B. hemorrhage
    C. hypertension   D. pulmonary embolus

32. An hour after Mrs. Garcia is transferred to the postpartum unit, the licensed practical   32.___C___
nurse notes that her blood pressure reading has changed from 120/80 to 96/70 and that
her abdominal dressings are dry.
Which of these actions should the nurse take FIRST?

    A. Massage Mrs. Garcia's uterine fundus
    B. Elevate the foot of Mrs. Garcia bed
    C. Check Mrs. Garcia's perineal pad
    D. Change Mrs. Garcia's position

33. Mrs. Garcia's indwelling urinary catheter is removed at 10 a.m. on the day after delivery.   33.___A___
The time and amount of each of Mrs. Garcia's first three voidings after the catheter is
removed are as follows: 5 p.m., 350 ml.; 11 p.m., 280 ml.; and 6 a.m., 370 ml.
The licensed practical nurse should know about Mrs. Garcia's urinary pattern the
amounts voided

    A. and the intervals between voidings are within normal limits
    B. are normal, but the intervals between voidings are above normal
    C. are above normal, nut the intervals between voidings are normal
    D. and the intervals between voidings are below normal

34. It is important for the mother of a premature infant to to have *early* contact with her   34.___C___
baby because this practice

    A. reduces the mother's dependency needs
    B. stimulates the physical growth rate of the baby
    C. enhances the mother-infant relationship
    D. decreases the likelihood that postpartum blues might occur

35. Which of these statements is correct about breast engorgement and afterpains in Mrs.   35.___A___
Garcia in comparison with multiparas who have delivered vaginally?

    A. She is likely to have breast engorgement and afterpains similar to those of women
       who delivered vaginally
    B. She is likely to have afterpains similar to those of women who delivered vaginally,
       but breast engorgement will be absent

C. Her breast engorgement will be similar to that of women who delivered vaginally, but afterpains will be absent

D. Her breast engorgement and her afterpains will be different from those of women who delivered vaginally

36. On Mrs. Garcia's sixth postpartum day, her lochia is bright red and moderate in amount. Which of these actions should the licensed practical nurse take FIRST?

36.___

A. Encourage Mrs. Garcia to increase her ambulation in order to aid involution

B. Have Mrs. Garcia lie on her abdomen for about an hour in order to apply pressure to the uterus

C. Chart the observation

D. Report the observation to the nurse in charge

QUESTIONS 37-40.

Mrs. Abby Cunningham, 27 years old, is at a ski lodge when she goes into active labor. A severe blizzard has blocked all roads. No physician is available and the nearest hospital is 60 miles away. A licensed practical nurse who is also a guest at the lodge is called to assist Mrs. Cunningham. This is Mrs. Cunningham's second pregnancy.

37. The licensed practical nurse determines that the birth of the baby is imminent. Which of these actions should the nurse take during the delivery of the baby?

37.___

A. Apply gentle pressure to Mrs. Cunningham's abdomen and tell her to push with each contraction

B. Support Mrs. Cunningham's perineum and the baby's head as it emerges

C. Tell Mrs. Cunningham to take slow, deep breaths during each contraction and to push between contractions

D. Place a clean towel under Mrs. Cunningham's buttocks and help her to hold her legs in lithotomy position

Mrs. Cunningham delivers a boy.

38. To promote a patent airway in the baby immediately after delivery, the licensed practical nurse should

38.___

A. place him in a semisitting position

B. stimulate his swallowing reflex

C. hold his tongue forward

D. position his head lower than his body

39. After the delivery of the placenta, it will be ESSENTIAL for the licensed practical nurse to

39.___

A. determine if involution has occured

B. see if pulsations of the umbilical cord have ceased

C. check the firmness of the uterine fundus

D. palpate the bladder area

40. If Mrs. Cunningham were to bleed heavily from perineal laceration, which of these actions would be appropriate?

    A. Place her in Trendelenburg position
    B. Apply pressure to the tear
    C. Massage the uterus
    D. Put the baby to breast

40. _B_

KEY (CORRECT ANSWERS)

1. D	11. D	21. B	31. A
2. B	12. C	22. D	32. C
3. B	13. A	23. C	33. A
4. A	14. B	24. D	34. C
5. A	15. C	25. D	35. A
6. D	16. C	26. C	36. D
7. B	17. B	27. A	37. B
8. B	18. A	28. B	38. D
9. A	19. A	29. C	39. C
10. A	20. B	30. D	40. B

EXAMINATION SECTION
TEST 1

DIRECTIONS: Each question or incomplete statement is followed by several suggested answers or completions. Select the one that BEST answers the question or completes the statement. *PRINT THE LETTER OF THE CORRECT ANSWER IN THE SPACE AT THE RIGHT.*

1.   In order to accomplish toilet training with a minimum of conflict for the child and the parent, which of these methods by the parent would be BEST?   1. _D_

    A.   Put the child on the toilet after breakfast and have him stay there until his bowels move.
    B.   Put the child on the toilet and promise him candy when his bowels move.
    C.   Disapprove of the child each time he soils himself.
    D.   Start toileting the child when he begins fussing about soiling his diapers.

2.   Jennifer, 2 years old, is to receive an antibiotic orally in liquid form.
Before pouring the medication, it is ESSENTIAL for the licensed practical nurse to   2. _D_

    A.   wipe the lip of the container with a sterile cotton ball
    B.   hold the bottle under warm running water for a few seconds
    C.   find out if Jennifer has ever taken a liquid medication
    D.   shake the bottle well if there is a precipitate

3.   An 11-year-old boy who is in a spica cast often eats too much and then complains of discomfort.
Which of these measures is likely to be MOST helpful to him concerning this problem?   3. _A_

    A.   Give him smaller but more frequent meals
    B.   Continue to give him three meals a day, but give him smaller portions
    C.   Restrict his fluid intake
    D.   Encourage him to eat slowly and to alternate liquids with solids

Questions 4-9.

DIRECTIONS: Questions 4 through 9 are to be answered on the basis of the following information.

    Reggie Dabney, 8 years old, has sickle cell anemia. He is admitted to the hospital in sickle cell crisis.

4.   Sickle cell anemia is caused by   4. _A_

    A.   genetic factors
    B.   antigen-antibody reactions
    C.   nutritional deficiencies
    D.   metabolic disorders

5. Reggie complains of pain in his legs and abdomen. Such pain is MOST probably the result of

   5. _B___

   A. bleeding into the cellular spaces
   B. clumping of erythrocytes
   C. a generalized infectious process
   D. a shift of intestinal fluid

6. Reggie is very quiet and lies facing the wall much of the time.
   Which of these measures by the licensed practical nurse would be BEST?

   6. _A___

   A. Spend time with Reggie other than giving him physical care
   B. Provide Reggie with an opportunity to talk with an older child who also has sickle cell anemia
   C. Assure Reggie at frequent intervals that he is improving
   D. Remind Reggie that being upset might make his condition worse

7. Mrs. Dabney says to the licensed practical nurse, *I hope Reggie will stop having these crises.*
   The nurse's response should be based on which of these understandings?

   7. _B___

   A. Sickle cell anemia can be controlled if the disease is diagnosed at birth.
   B. Sickle cell anemia is a chronic disease characterized by periods of crisis through-out life.
   C. If the child with sickle cell anemia is in remission for two years, the disease is considered arrested.
   D. If the child with sickle cell anemia reaches puberty, the crises will no longer occur.

8. The understanding about children of Reggie's age (8 years) that the licensed practical nurse should keep in mind when planning their play activities is that they

   8. _C___

   A. need to have highly structured activities
   B. prefer being with children of the opposite sex
   C. like to be involved with a group of children their own age
   D. usually include an imaginary playmate in their activities

9. Reggie's condition improves, and plans are made with Mr. and Mrs. Dabney for his discharge.
   Mrs. Dabney says to the licensed practical nurse, *We're planning to go camping at a lake for the entire summer. It's about four hundred miles from here.*
   Because Reggie has sickle cell anemia, which of these suggestions would it be APPROPRIATE for the nurse to make to Mrs. Dabney?

   9. _D___

   A. Be sure that Reggie is not exposed to the sun.
   B. Plan to drive for only short periods at a time so that Reggie will have a chance to exercise his legs.
   C. Limit Reggie's fluids while traveling to help prevent him from being carsick.
   D. Ask your physician about the medical facilities that are available where you are going.

Questions 10-13.

DIRECTIONS: Questions 10 through 13 are to be answered on the basis of the following information.

Reijo Sinisalo, 12 years old, is brought to the emergency room by his parents. A diagnosis of acute appendicitis is made, and Reijo is scheduled for surgery.

An appendectomy is performed. Because the appendix had ruptured, a drain is inserted in the incision. Reijo is brought to the pediatric unit with an intravenous infusion running. He has a nasogastric tube connected to intermittent suction.

10. A nasogastric tube may be inserted for three of the following purposes.
    It would NOT be inserted to

    A. relieve distension
    B. re-establish normal peristalsis
    C. facilitate drainage from the stomach
    D. allow for the measurement of stomach contents

10. B

11. An antibiotic has been added to Reijo's intravenous fluids.
    The purpose of the antibiotic for Reijo is to

    A. promote drainage
    B. facilitate rapid healing
    C. treat the existing peritonitis
    D. prevent the development of pneumonia

11. C

12. In the early postoperative period, which of these understandings about administering medication for pain to children such as Reijo is ACCURATE?

    A. Analgesia is usually necessary and is safe if the dosage is calculated for the individual child.
    B. Potential drug addiction should be a major concern in the care of an acutely ill child.
    C. Since children are active earlier in the postoperative period than adults, they will need little or no analgesia.
    D. Children have a higher tolerance for pain than do adults and, therefore, need smaller doses of drugs.

12. A

13. Which of these behaviors is characteristic of MOST normal 12-year-olds?

    A. Rejection of new routines
    B. Shyness when meeting new people
    C. Anxiety caused by separation from parents
    D. Embarrassment associated with elimination

13. D

113

Questions 14-19.

DIRECTIONS: Questions 14 through 19 are to be answered on the basis of the following information.

Bonnie Tansy, a 3-month-old infant with two siblings, is brought by her mother to the clinic for routine health care. Bonnie has some localized scaling and red areas on her cheeks, neck, and elbows, which are diagnosed as eczema.

14. Which of these suggestions regarding Bonnie's care is it MOST important for the licensed practical nurse to give Mrs. Tansy?

   A. Bathe Bonnie daily with a mild soap.
   B. Keep Bonnie's nails cut short.
   C. Use only long-sleeved clothing for Bonnie.
   D. Have the other children in the family avoid contact with Bonnie.

14. B

15. Which of these behaviors should the licensed practical nurse expect to observe a normal 3-month-old infant doing?

   A. Holding the bottle during a feeding
   B. Smiling in response to being talked to
   C. Turning from the back to the abdomen
   D. Crying when a stranger approaches

15. B

16. Bonnie's eczema remains under control until she is 6 months of age. She is then admitted to the hospital because of a severe flare-up of the eczema on her arms and trunk. Bonnie is wearing elbow restraints.
It would be MOST appropriate to remove her restraints when

   A. she is being held
   B. she is sleeping
   C. she is being wheeled in a carriage around the unit
   D. the nurse is in her room

16. A

17. Bonnie is receiving an antihistamine.
The purpose of this medication is to _____ of the lesions.

   A. promote healing   B. reducing itching
   C. limit the spread   D. prevent infection

17. B

18. Bonnie is discharged. When she is 1 year old, she is readmitted to the hospital with another flare-up of the eczema.
Which of these recent changes in Bonnie's life is MOST likely related to the increased severity of her eczema?

   A. A new foam-rubber mattress was placed in her crib.
   B. Eggs were included in her diet for the first time.
   C. Her parents had their home air-conditioned.
   D. She has a new cotton blanket on her bed.

18. B

19. Bonnie has all of the following abilities.
Which one was probably acquired MOST recently?

   A. Sitting for extended periods without support
   B. Transfering a toy from one hand to the other
   C. Sitting down from a standing position without help
   D. Rolling over completely

19. C

Questions 20-26.

DIRECTIONS: Questions 20 through 26 are to be answered on the basis of the following information.

Greta Wade, 4 months old, is admitted to the hospital with severe diarrhea and dehydration. Isolation precautions are instituted. She is to receive nothing by mouth. Mrs. Wade plans to spend each afternoon with Greta.

20.   It would be MOST important to weigh Greta when she is admitted to the unit in order to   20. _D_

    A.   assess the seriousness of her condition
    B.   determine the presence of edema
    C.   compare her weight with the normal range for her age
    D.   calculate her fluid requirements

21.   Greta should received NOTHING by mouth in order to   21. _D_

    A.   reduce the spread of disease-producing organisms
    B.   provide for a more accurate measurement of stool volume
    C.   prevent aspiration
    D.   decrease activity in the gastrointestinal tract

22.   Greta is receiving intravenous fluids.   22. _B_
Greta's intravenous equipment is to be adjusted so that she receives 18 microdrops per minute. The licensed practical nurse notices that only 2 microdrops are being delivered per minute.
Before reporting this observation to the nurse in charge, which of these actions should the nurse take?

    A.   Milk the intraveous tubing
    B.   Check the site of the intravenous infusion
    C.   Open the clamp on the intravenous tubing completely
    D.   Raise the intravenous bottle

23.   If Greta's intravenous infusion were to run too fast, which of these complications would   23. _D_
be MOST likely to occur?

    A.   Severe diarrhea   B.   Thrombus formation
    C.   Renal failure   D.   Circulatory overload

24.   Greta's mother, Mrs. Wade, asks the licensed practical nurse what she could do to be   24. _C_
helpful to Greta. Which of these suggestions should the nurse give to Mrs. Wade?

    A.   Write down the number of stools Greta has.
    B.   Keep track of the fluid in Greta's I.V. bottle.
    C.   Caress Greta frequently when she is awake.
    D.   Remind me when it is time to change Greta's position.

25.   Greta's condition improves, and she is started on oral feedings.   25. _A_
The licensed practical nurse is to feed Greta for the first time.
Which of these measures should be taken in relation to the feeding situation?

    A.   Give Greta a small amount of the feeding at a time.
    B.   Hold Greta in an upright position during the feeding.

C. Bubble Greta each time she has taken a half ounce of the feeding.
D. Position Greta with her head slightly lower than her chest after feeding her.

26. Greta is to be weighed daily.   26. A
    At which of these times would it be BEST to weigh her?

    A. Prior to her first morning feeding
    B. After she has been bathed
    C. After her first bowel movement
    D. Whenever her mother is available to assist with the procedure

Questions 27-32.

DIRECTIONS: Questions 27 through 32 are to be answered on the basis of the following infor-
              mation.

Allen Beam, 20 months old, is to be admitted to the hospital for surgical repair of an
inguinal hernia.

27. A COMMON symptom of inguinal hernia is   27. C

    A. protrusion of the umbilicus
    B. visible peristalsis
    C. a mass in the groin
    D. abdominal distension

28. Allen arrives at the hospital clutching a rather soiled, ragged baby blanket. When his   28. A
    mother attempts to remove the blanket to take it home, Allen cries and holds on to it.
    Which of these comments by the licensed practical nurse would indicate the BEST
    understanding of Allen's needs?

    A. It looks as if that's Allen's favorite blanket. It's all right for him to keep it with him.
    B. Let's wait until Allen is involved in an activity, and then I'll take the blanket and give
       it to you next time you come.
    C. I'll get Allen another blanket. Then he won't mind giving up this one.
    D. Tell Allen that you only want to take the blanket to wash it and that you'll bring it
       back next time you come.

29. Allen is to have a venipuncture to obtain a blood specimen. When the physician is ready   29. B
    to take Allen's blood, which of these approaches by the licensed practical nurse would be
    BEST?

    A. Tell Allen which arm to extend to the physician
    B. Hold Allen's arm in position for the physician
    C. Show Allen how to squeeze his fist tight while the needle is being inserted
    D. Have Allen cover his eyes with one hand while the specimen is being withdrawn

30. Mrs. Beam tells the licensed practical nurse that she has to leave because she has a 6-   30. C
    month-old baby at home.
    Mrs. Beam says, *Allen has never been away from home without me and I think he's
    going to be very upset.*
    Which of these responses by the nurse would be BEST?

A. Maybe if you promise to bring him his favorite toy when you return, he won't cry so much.
B. If we hear Allen crying, we will send someone in to care for him.
C. I'll stay here with Allen and try to comfort him.
D. Most children only cry for a little while after their mothers leave.

31. Allen is scheduled for surgery and is to have nothing by mouth.
While Allen can have nothing by mouth, he is unhappy and cries for something to drink.
Which of these measures would it be APPROPRIATE to include in his care?

31. A

A. Taking Allen for a walk
B. Giving Allen chips of ice to suck
C. Having Allen use a pleasant-flavored mouthwash.
D. Explaining to Allen why he cannot have fluids

32. Allen has surgery. He is to be discharged the next day. Mrs. Beam tells the licensed practical nurse that Allen does not drink enough milk.
Which of these foods is the BEST substitute for milk?

32. C

A. Citrus fruit juice
C. Cheese

B. Cream
D. Root vegetables

Questions 33-40.

DIRECTIONS: Questions 33 through 40 are to be answered on the basis of the following information.

Anna Amorosa, 2 years old, is admitted to the hospital with a diagnosis of laryngotracheobronchitis. She is placed in a Croupette with oxygen.

33. Common symptoms of severe laryngotracheobronchitis include

33. B

A. swelling of the neck and drooling
B. dyspnea and temperature elevation
C. nausea and vomiting
D. shrill cry and head rolling

34. The licensed practical nurse is unable to count Anna's respirations accurately because she is restless and crying.
Which of these actions by the nurse would be BEST?

34. C

A. Ask another staff member to count Anna's respirations
B. Record an approximate respiratory rate
C. Postpone taking Anna's respirations until she becomes quiet
D. Average her respirations per minute after taking them for 3 minutes

35. The evening after Anna's admission, Mrs. Amorosa arrives to visit Anna. Mrs. Amorosa says to the licensed practical nurse, *I just put my hand in the tent. Anna's clothing is damp.*
In addition to changing Anna's clothing, which of these actions should the nurse take in response to Mrs. Amorosa's comment?

35. D

A. Report Mrs. Amorosa's observation to the nurse in charge
B. Encourage Anna to drink fluids to replace those she is losing
C. Take Anna's temperature to compare it with her previous temperature
D. Explain the function of the humidity to Mrs. Amorosa

36. Expected outcomes of oxygen therapy are

36. D

A. increase in the respiratory and pulse rates
B. increase in the respiratory rate and decrease of the pulse rate
C. decrease of the respiratory rate and increase in the pulse rate
D. decrease of the respiratory and pulse rates

37. Anna's condition improves, and she is to be removed from the Croupette for short periods during the day.
Before returning Anna to the Croupette, the licensed practical nurse should take which of these actions?

37. A

A. Close the tent and turn on the oxygen flow meter
B. Wipe the inside of the canopy with a disinfectant solution
C. Give Anna fluids to drink
D. Assist Anna in doing deep-breathing exercises

38. Anna's condition has improved. She is ambulatory and is to be discharged soon. Anna is in the playroom.
Which of these behaviors is typical of a 2-year-old child?

38. D

A. Playing a simple board game with another child of the same age
B. Sitting quietly with a group of children while listening to a story
C. Coloring within the lines of drawings in a coloring book, using the jumbo-size crayons
D. Engaging in activities near other children but not with them

39. Mrs. Amorosa tells the licensed practical nurse that for the past month Anna has not been eating as much as usual and that she is eating less than her 1-year-old brother.
The MOST likely reason for this change in Anna's appetite is

39. B

A. dislike of the food she is being given
B. a decrease in her growth rate
C. jealousy of her brother
D. a reluctance to feed herself

40. When Anna is ready for discharge, Mrs. Amorosa asks the licensed practical nurse what she should do if Anna begins to develop symptoms of croup again.
Which of these questions would it be BEST to ask Mrs. Amorosa INITIALLY?

40. D

A. Has anyone ever showed you how to do postural drainage with Anna?
B. How far from your home is the nearest emergency room?
C. Does rocking Anna or singing to her help to relax her?
D. Does your bathroom steam up easily when you run the hot water?

KEY (CORRECT ANSWERS)

1.	D	11.	C	21.	D	31.	A
2.	D	12.	A	22.	B	32.	C
3.	A	13.	D	23.	D	33.	B
4.	A	14.	B	24.	C	34.	C
5.	B	15.	B	25.	A	35.	D
6.	A	16.	A	26.	A	36.	D
7.	B	17.	B	27.	C	37.	A
8.	C	18.	B	28.	A	38.	D
9.	D	19.	C	29.	B	39.	B
10.	B	20.	D	30.	C	40.	D

EXAMINATION SECTION
TEST 1

DIRECTIONS: Each question or incomplete statement is followed by several suggested answers or completions. Select the one that BEST answers the question or completes the statement. *PRINT THE LETTER OF THE CORRECT ANSWER IN THE SPACE AT THE RIGHT.*

1. Mothers of infants and toddlers should be instructed that diets for their children that include milk at the expense of other foods are MOST likely to result in the development of a deficiency in   1. __A__

   A. iron
   C. vitamin D
   B. carbohydrate
   D. vitamin K

2. A 1-week-old boy, weighing 6 pounds, has just been returned to the pediatric unit after having surgery for an intestinal obstruction. He has nasogastric suction and is receiving intravenous fluids via a venous cutdown. In addition to meeting the infant's special needs, which of these measures would be ESSENTIAL?   2. __D__

   A. Restraining all four of the baby's extremities
   B. Handling the baby as little as possible
   C. Explaining the equipment used in the baby's treatment to his mother so that she can assist the nurse with his care
   D. Spending time stroking the baby

3. A mother makes all of these comments about her infant daughter to the physician. Which one describes a characteristic MORE likely to be observed in an infant with hypothyroidism than in a normal 3-month-old infant?   3. __B__

   A. She smiles a lot.
   B. She's so good and she never cries.
   C. She notices her toys and she knows my voice.
   D. She seems to spend a great deal of time watching her hands.

Questions 4-7.

DIRECTIONS: Questions 4 through 7 are to be answered on the basis of the following information.

   Bruce Alfonse, 9 years old, has an acute asthmatic attack and is admitted to the hospital because he did not respond to treatment in the emergency room. He has had bronchial asthma since early childhood.

4. Bruce is to receive 100 mg. of aminophylline intravenously.
   If the ampules of aminophylline available on Bruce's unit contain aminophylline gr. 7 1/2 in 10 cc. of solution, how much solution from the ampule will contain 100 mg. of aminophylline?   4. __A__

   A. 2 cc.   B. 4 cc.   C. 6 cc.   D. 8 cc.

5. Which of these events in Bruce's life would be MOST likely to cause an increase in the frequency and intensity of his asthmatic attacks?   5. __B__

A. Ms. Alfonse's buying new furniture for Bruce's bedroom
B. The Alfonse's moving to another city
C. Mr. Alfonse's being away from home on business for several days
D. Bruce's favorite grandparent's coming to visit for a week

6. An IMPORTANT objective of the medical and nursing management of Bruce should be to help him to

6. _B_

   A. accept the fact that he cannot be like other children and that he will have to limit his goals
   B. accept his condition and live a productive life
   C. understand the underlying cause of his condition
   D. accept being dependent upon his mother until he is in his middle teens

7. The nurse is planning Bruce's care.
Consideration should be given to the fact that most normal 8-year-olds

7. _A_

   A. prefer to associate with a peer of the same sex
   B. seek opportunities for socializing with older boys
   C. enjoy small heterosexual groups
   D. function best as a member of a large group of somewhat younger boys and girls

Questions 8-13.

DIRECTIONS: Questions 8 through 13 are to be answered on the basis of the following information.

Jeff Green, age 2 1/2, sustained a simple fracture of the shaft of the left femur when he fell down stairs at home. Upon his admission to the hospital, Jeff is placed in Bryant's traction.

8. Among the equipment used in the application of Bryant's traction is

8. _A_

   A. adhesive material on the skin of both limbs
   B. metal calipers in the malleoli of both ankles
   C. a Kirschner wire in the affected femur
   D. a Thomas splint on the fractured extremity

9. During his first two days in the hospital, Jeff lies quietly, sucks his thumb, and does not cry.
It is MOST justifiable to say that he

9. _D_

   A. has made a good adjustment to the traction
   B. is accustomed to being disciplined at home
   C. has confidence in the nurses caring for him
   D. is experiencing anxiety

10. Prior to his admission, Jeff was partially bowel-trained, but now he defecates involuntarily.
The nurse's approach to this problem should be based on which of these assessments?

10. _A_

   A. What is Jeff's reaction to his soiling
   B. How compulsive is Jeff about cleanliness

C. Is Jeff too young for bowel training
D. Is bowel training important for Jeff

11. Ms. Green is upset because when she comes to visit, Jeff turns his head away from her   11.__A__
and holds his arms out to the nurse.
It is probably MOST justifiable to say that Jeff

    A. is angry with his mother for leaving him in the hospital
    B. is testing the relationship between his mother and the nurse
    C. now has a stronger emotional tie with the nurse than with his mother
    D. is consciously trying to make his mother jealous

12. One day when the nurse offers Jeff a cookie, he says *No!* and at the same time holds out   12.__C__
his hand for it.
Which of these interpretations of Jeff's behavior is PROBABLY justifiable?

    A. His mother has forbidden sweets, and he is in conflict about accepting any.
    B. He is confused about the meaning of yes and no.
    C. His negativism is a beginning attempt at independence.
    D. He is unaccustomed to being offered choices.

13. To prevent accidents such as Jeff's among toddlers, which one of the following measures   13.__B__
would probably help MOST?

    A. Having carpeting on stairs
    B. Using adjustable gates on stairways
    C. Providing the toddler with a plentiful supply of play materials in one room
    D. Keeping the toddler in a playpen placed near the mother's work area

Questions 14-19.

DIRECTIONS: Questions 14 through 18 are to be answered on the basis of the following infor-
                 mation.

Adam Crane, 13 years old, is admitted to the hospital for treatment of acute rheumatic
fever. He is placed on bed rest.

14. Adam MOST probably has which of these groups of symptoms that are characteristic of   14.__D__
acute rheumatic fever?

    A. Swelling of the fingers, petechiae, and general malaise
    B. Nodules overlying bony prominences, dependent edema, and elevated blood pres-
       sure
    C. Bleeding gums, dyspnea, and failure to gain weight
    D. Fever, rash, and migratory joint pain

15. Adam is receiving a corticosteroid drug.   15.__D__
He should be observed for common side effects of this type of drug therapy, such as

    A. hypotension   B. weight loss
    C. pallor   D. acne

16. An oral potassium preparation is ordered for Adam. The CHIEF purpose of this drug for   16.__B__
him is to

A. promote excretion of bacterial toxins
B. prevent hypokalemia
C. enhance the action of the corticosteroid drug
D. reduce the electrical potential of the cardiac conduction system

17. Adam's blood tests include all of the following results. Which of these results would be MOST indicative of improvement in his condition?   17. D

    A. Positive C-reactive protein
    B. Hemoglobin, 14.0 Gm. per 100 cc. of blood
    C. White blood cell count, 11,000 per cu. mm. of blood
    D. Decreasing erythrocyte sedimentation rate

18. Permanent functional impairment would MOST likely result if Adam developed   18. C

    A. erythema marginatum   B. polyarthritis
    C. carditis   D. subcutaneous nodules

19. Recurrent attacks of rheumatic fever in Adam can BEST be prevented by   19. A

    A. keeping him on prophylactic drug therapy for an indefinite period
    B. including foods in his diet that are rich in vitamins and minerals
    C. improving his family's socioeconomic condition
    D. providing daily afternoon rest periods for him for about a year after recovery from an acute attack

Questions 20-25.

DIRECTIONS: Questions 20 through 25 are to be answered on the basis of the following information.

Daniel Rich, 6 weeks old, is admitted to the pediatric unit with pyloric stenosis. He is to have a pyloromyotomy.

20. Daniel's parents tell the nurse that they do not quite understand what the doctor has told   20. D
    them about the operation, and they ask for clarification.
    Which of these explanations to the parents would be MOST appropriate?

    A. Daniel's stomach is contracted and its capacity diminished, making it necessary for the doctor to dilate it with instruments.
    B. Nerves have produced contraction of certain muscles in Daniel's stomach called sphincters, and these nerves must be cut in order to produce relaxation.
    C. Constricting bands of tissue in the middle of Daniel's stomach, which are causing vomiting, will be resected.
    D. The doctor will make a cut in a tight muscle at the bottom of Daniel's stomach, which has caused his symptoms.

21. Preoperatively, Daniel is to receive 0.15 mg. (gr. 1/400) of atropine sulfate.   21. C
    If a vial containing 0.4 mg. (gr. 1/150) in 1 cc. of solution is used to prepare Daniel's dose, how much of the stock solution should be given to him?
    _____ cc.

    A. 0.28   B. 0.33   C. 0.38   D. 0.43

22. Daniel should be observed for early symptoms of side effects of atropine, which include   22. _C_

    A.   vomiting and subnormal temperature
    B.   lethargy and bradycardia
    C.   rapid respirations and flushed skin
    D.   muscle spasms and diaphoresis

23. Daniel has a pyloromyotomy.   23. _D_
Assuming that Daniel's operation is successful, his parents should be informed that his convalescence can be expected to be

    A.   *gradual,* with the persistence of mild preoperative symptoms for a few weeks
    B.   *prolonged,* with gradual reduction and eventual disappearance of preoperative symptoms over a period of a few months
    C.   *brief,* but with periodic recurrence of preoperative symptoms during his first 6 months of life
    D.   *rapid,* and characterized by the absence of preoperative symptoms

24. Daniel is now 8 weeks old. He should be expected to   24. _B_

    A.   cry when a stranger approaches
    B.   pay attention to a voice
    C.   laugh aloud
    D.   make sounds such as *ba-ba* and *da-da*

25. In response to Ms. Rich's questions, the nurse discusses with her the introduction of new foods into Daniel's diet.   25. _B_
Which of these suggestions by the nurse would be MOST appropriate?

    A.   Whenever a new food is added to Daniel's diet, decrease the amount of milk offered to him.
    B.   Give Daniel new foods one at a time.
    C.   Allow Daniel to touch each new solid food before he tastes it.
    D.   Mix new foods with a small amount of some food Daniel has previously had.

KEY (CORRECT ANSWERS)

1.	A		11.	A
2.	D		12.	C
3.	B		13.	B
4.	A		14.	D
5.	B		15.	D
6.	B		16.	B
7.	A		17.	D
8.	A		18.	C
9.	D		19.	A
10.	A		20.	D

21. C
22. C
23. D
24. B
25. B

———

TEST 2

DIRECTIONS: Each question or incomplete statement is followed by several suggested answers or completions. Select the one that BEST answers the question or completes the statement. *PRINT THE LETTER OF THE CORRECT ANSWER IN THE SPACE AT THE RIGHT.*

1. Parents are given information relative to the nutrition of normal newborn infants. Which of the following statements is INACCURATE?

    A. Formulas made of modified cow's milk are well absorbed.
    B. A high protein intake assures a rapid growth rate.
    C. The total daily intake of nutrients is more important than the size or frequency of individual feedings.
    D. Infants born of well-nourished mothers are likely to have adequate stores of nutrients at birth.

1. B

2. A 3-year-old has nephrosis and marked ascites. In which position is she likely to be MOST comfortable?

    A. Semi-Fowler's   B. Sims'
    C. Dorsal recumbent   D. Prone

2. A

3. A 5-year-old with leukemia is to be discharged because his condition is in a state of remission.
It will be MOST helpful to the child when he is at home if his parents understand that

    A. the child's condition is terminal, and it will be their responsibility to make him as happy as possible without making demands upon him
    B. they should guide their child, encouraging him and setting limits for him, so that he may develop to his full potential
    C. it will not be necessary for them to control their child's behavior because his condition makes him aware of his own limitations
    D. it will be important for them to develop a carefully planned schedule for the child that will conserve his strength

3. B

Questions 4-7.

DIRECTIONS: Questions 4 through 7 are to be answered on the basis of the following information.

Josh Greene, 9 1/2 months old, is admitted to the hospital. He has a provisional diagnosis of intussusception.

4. Josh MOST probably has which of these symptoms that are characteristic manifestations of the onset of intussusception in an infant?

    A. Abdominal distention and coffee-ground vomitus
    B. Hyperpyrexia and rectal prolapse
    C. Passage of large amount of flatus associated with straining
    D. Paroxysmal abdominal pain accompanied by screaming

4. D

5. When the physician tells Mr. and Ms. Greene that immediate surgery will be necessary if   5. D
   Josh's diagnosis is confirmed, they are reluctant to give permission for the operation.
   If surgery is not performed soon after a diagnosis of intussusception is made, which of
   these conditions is LIKELY to result?

   A. Chronic ulcerative colitis
   B. Megacolon
   C. Meckel's diverticulum
   D. Gangrene of the bowel

6. A barium enema is ordered to help confirm Josh's diagnosis. An additional reason why a   6. D
   barium enema is ordered for Josh at this time is that it may result in

   A. elimination of offending toxins
   B. diminution of microbial flora of the intestine in preparation for surgery
   C. control of bleeding due to the barium's astringent effect on the bowel lining
   D. reduction of the telescoped bowel segment

7. Josh has intussusception, and the condition is corrected by surgery. His recovery is sat-   7. C
   isfactory.
   When Josh begins to feel better, the play material that would probably be MOST
   appropriate for him is a

   A. mobile
   B. beanbag
   C. roly-poly animal with a weighted base
   D. tinker toy with parts securely fastened

Questions 8-15.

DIRECTIONS: Questions 8 through 15 are to be answered on the basis of the following infor-
             mation.

   Amy Simpson, 13 1/2 years old, is in the hospital for treatment of newly diagnosed diabetes mellitus. A teaching program for Amy and her mother has been instituted by the nursing
staff.

8. To plan a teaching program for Amy, the nurse should consider that the factor that will   8. B
   have the GREATEST influence on its success is

   A. the child's age
   B. the child's parents' acceptance of the diagnosis
   C. whether or not teaching is done consistently by the same nurse
   D. whether or not teaching is limited to one-hour periods

9. When teaching Amy and her parents about insulin, it is important to include the fact that   9. D
   insulin

   A. requirements will decrease with age
   B. dosage is determined, primarily, on the basis of daily food intake
   C. dosage, after adolescence, can be adjusted by the person in terms of variations in
      physical activity
   D. will be needed for life

10. One morning when the nurse goes to help Amy with morning care, Amy is argumentative   10. B
    and restless. She makes unkind remarks to the other children.
    It is essential for the nurse to give IMMEDIATE consideration to which of these ques-
    tions?

    A. Does Amy need a more structured plan of care?
    B. When did Amy have her insulin and did she eat her breakfast?
    C. Was there some incident that occurred the previous day that has upset Amy?
    D. Is Amy bored and does she need help in selecting recreational activities that will
       utilize her excess energy?

11. One day Amy asks the nurse, *Will I be able to go with the gang after school to get ice*   11. D
    cream or a hot dog? Which of these responses by the nurse would give Amy accurate
    information?

    A. You can go with the group, but the hot dogs, ice cream, and other foods that they
       eat are prohibited for you. Your friends will learn to be considerate of your special
       needs.
    B. Both hot dogs and ice cream contain valuable nutrients. But if you have a hot dog,
       don't eat the roll.
    C. You can have a hot dog if you omit a corresponding amount of food from your next
       meal. Since sweets are not good for you, avoid foods like ice cream.
    D. Being with your friends is important. You can eat a hot dog or ice cream some-
       times. We'll help you learn how to choose foods.

12. One day Amy tells her mother and the nurse that she does not want to give herself insu-   12. A
    lin. Her mother says to her, *You don't have to give yourself the injection if you don't want*
    to. I'll do it for you.
    Which of these understandings should be the basis of the nurse's response?

    A. The mother must be helped to understand the importance of the girl's participation
       in her own care.
    B. The girl needs to assume responsibility for her treatment; therefore, Amy and her
       mother should be taught separately.
    C. Children with diabetes often rebel against puncturing themselves with needles,
       and teaching should be discontinued until signs of readiness are demonstrated.
    D. The reaction of the mother is normal and should be overlooked.

13. A few days before Amy is discharged, her scout leader visits her. The scout leader stops   13. C
    at the nurses' station before leaving and says, *The troop is going on a four-day camping*
    trip next month. Amy is very eager to go, and I'd like to have her come. But I'm rather
    concerned about having her out in the woods with us.
    Before replying, which of these questions should the nurse consider?

    A. Are such trips contraindicated for children who have diabetes?
    B. Would it be too hazardous for Amy to attempt the trip so soon after her hospitaliza-
       tion?
    C. Will there be an adult accompanying the children who has had experience with
       children who have diabetes?
    D. Does Amy have enough information about her condition so that she is unlikely to
       have any difficulty?

14. Ms. Simpson says to the nurse, *Amy has never been a complainer. I'm afraid that she will not tell me if she doesn't feel well before she goes to school.* Which of these responses by the nurse would be MOST helpful to Amy's mother?   14. A

    A. It will be important to find out how Amy is feeling without stressing symptoms in talking with her.
    B. It is the school nurse's responsibility to help you with problems like this.
    C. Since Amy behaves this way, it will be necessary for you to question her frequently about how she feels.
    D. You don't need to worry about this because when Amy leaves the hospital her diabetes will be controlled.

15. In the management of a child with diabetes mellitus, occasional minimal glycosuria may be allowed.   15. C
The purpose of this management is to

    A. retard degenerative tissue changes
    B. detect early symptoms of impending coma
    C. reduce the incidence of insulin shock
    D. facilitate diet supervision

Questions 16-22.

DIRECTIONS: Questions 16 through 22 are to be answered on the basis of the following information.

Jimmy Brown, 6 years old, is brought to the hospital immediately after sustaining burns that occurred in his home when he pulled a pan of boiling water off the stove. He has severe burns, mostly third degree, of the anterior chest, upper arms, forearms, and hands.

Jimmy is placed in a single room. An intravenous infusion is started, an indwelling urethral (Foley) catheter is inserted, and pressure dressings are applied to his burned areas.

16. Jimmy develops burn shock.   16. D
He can be expected to exhibit

    A. restlessness and bradycardia
    B. air hunger and hyperreflexia
    C. intense pain and convulsions
    D. pale, clammy skin and thirst

17. To plan for Jimmy's fluid replacement needs, it should be noted that the   17. A

    A. younger the child, the greater amount of fluid he needs in proportion to his body weight
    B. proportion of body weight contributed by water is smaller during early childhood than it is during adulthood
    C. fluid needs per kilogram of body weight are variable until the kidneys become functionally mature at adolescence
    D. total volume of extracellular fluid per kilogram of body weight increases gradually from birth to adolescence and then stabilizes at the adult level

18. On admission, Jimmy's rectal temperature was 99° F. (37.2° C.) Twelve hours later, it is   18.___A___
    101.6° F. (38.7° C.). On the basis of the information provided about him, it is MOST justi-
    fied to say that it

    A. is an expected development in injuries such as Jimmy's
    B. is indicative of damage to Jimmy's heat-control center
    C. is a manifestation of rapidly spreading infection
    D. has resulted chiefly from a marked increase in serum potassium

19. Twenty-four hours after his admission, Jimmy complains that his chest dressing feels too   19.___A___
    tight.
    The nurse should FIRST

    A. check Jimmy's respirations
    B. loosen the chest bandage
    C. call the doctor
    D. find out whether Jimmy has a p.r.n. order for an analgesic

20. When selecting a site for the administration of a parenteral drug to Jimmy, it would be   20.___A___
    MOST important for the nurse to consider that

    A. impaired circulation hampers drug absorption
    B. decreased blood volume shortens the period of drug action
    C. drug action is potentiated by increased amounts of circulating epinephrine
    D. concentration of blood plasma in the tissues potentiates the desired effects of
       drugs

21. Which of these meals for Jimmy would be HIGHEST in proteins and calories?   21.___B___

    A. Vegetable soup, cottage cheese on crackers, applesauce, hot chocolate
    B. Cheeseburger, french fried potatoes, carrot sticks, cantaloupe balls, milk
    C. Fresh fruit plate with sherbet, buttered muffin, slice of watermelon, fruit-flavored
       milk drink
    D. Chicken noodle soup, cream cheese and jelly sandwich, buttered whole kernel
       corn, orange sherbet, cola drink

22. Jimmy is scheduled to go to the physical therapy department at 9:30 A.M. every day. One   22.___B___
    morning at 8:30, after Jimmy has had his breakfast, the nurse who goes in to bathe him
    finds him sound asleep.
    Which of these actions by the nurse would demonstrate the BEST judgment?

    A. Allow Jimmy to sleep until necessary equipment for his bath is gathered and then
       wake him for the procedure.
    B. Let Jimmy sleep and postpone his bath until sometime later in the day.
    C. Wake Jimmy gently and bathe him, explaining to him that he can rest when he
       returns from physical therapy
    D. Bathe Jimmy as quickly as possible and then let him sleep until it is time to go for
       physical therapy.

Questions 23-24.

DIRECTIONS: Questions 23 through 24 are to be answered on the basis of the following infor-
                mation.

Ralph Dunn, 15 years old, is admitted to the hospital for treatment of ulcerative colitis.

23. Ralph is receiving methantheline (Banthine) bromide. The CHIEF purpose of this drug for Ralph is to

     23.___

    A. suppress inflammation of the bowel
    B. reduce peristaltic activity
    C. neutralize acid in the gastrointestinal tract
    D. increase bowel tone

24. Ralph is on a low-residue, high-protein, high-calorie diet.
To meet the requirements of Ralph's diet prescription, the nurse should guide Ralph to select as an evening snack

     24.___

    A. a roast beef sandwich
    B. strawberry shortcake with whipped cream
    C. canned peaches
    D. fresh orange juice

25. The nurse is discussing nutrition with the mother of two sons, a preadolescent and an adolescent. The mother should be instructed that in terms of nutritional needs, as compared with most normal preadolescent boys, MOST normal adolescent boys need _____ calories _____ protein.

     25.___

    A. more; but less   B. more; and more
    C. fewer; but more   D. fewer; and less

KEY (CORRECT AHSWERS)

1.	B		11.	D
2.	A		12.	A
3.	B		13.	C
4.	D		14.	A
5.	D		15.	C
6.	D		16.	D
7.	C		17.	A
8.	B		18.	A
9.	D		19.	A
10.	B		20.	A

21.	B
22.	B
23.	B
24.	A
25.	B

EXAMINATION SECTION
TEST 1

DIRECTIONS: Each question or incomplete statement is followed by several suggested answers or completions. Select the one that BEST answers the question or completes the statement. *PRINT THE LETTER OF THE CORRECT ANSWER IN THE SPACE AT THE RIGHT.*

1.   Which approach by the nurse to a newly admitted toddler, who is not acutely ill, and to his mother would probably be MOST reassuring to both?

    A.   Getting acquainted with the toddler before discussing his likes and dislikes with the mother
    B.   Having the mother hold the toddler while questioning her about his habits
    C.   Leaving the toddler with the play lady in the playroom while talking with the mother about his habits and preferences
    D.   Holding the toddler while asking the mother questions about his habits

1. _D_

2.   The nurse is assessing whether a normal 5-year-old is achieving the primary developmental task for children of his age.
If the child is achieving this task, the child's behavior should indicate that he is developing a sense of

    A.   trust   B.   identity   C.   intimacy   D.   initiative

2. _D_

3.   The mother of a 1-year-old and a 3-year-old is talking with the nurse about the eating habits of her children. In comparing the eating habits of most normal children of those ages, which DIFFERENCE is likely to be evident?

    A.   The food intake of a 3-year-old will be about three times greater than that of a 1-year-old.
    B.   A 1-year-old will have stronger food preferences than a 3-year-old.
    C.   A 3-year-old will do more fingering of foods than a 1-year-old.
    D.   The appetite of a 3-year-old is likely to be more capricious than that of a 1-year-old.

3. _D_

Questions 4-7.

DIRECTIONS: Questions 4 through 7 are to be answered on the basis of the following information.

Liz Thomas, 18 months old, is admitted to the hospital with symptoms of a subdural hematoma.

4.   Liz's mother asks about her daughter's diagnosis. She should be told that a subdural hematoma is

    A.   under the outer layer of the meninges
    B.   between the inner layer of the meninges and the brain
    C.   in the soft tissues of the scalp
    D.   under the periosteum and above the meninges

4. _A_

5. Liz has a craniotomy with removal of a hematoma. Her condition is good. Mr. and Ms. Thomas are suspected of physically abusing Liz.
The day after Liz's surgery, a nurse's aide says to the nurse, *Every time I see Ms. Thomas, I see red. How could any adult, least of all a mother, deliberately hurt a little child?*
Which of these initial responses by the nurse would probably be MOST helpful to the aide?

5.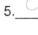

    A. Making judgments about parents' actions is not appropriate for nursing personnel.
    B. You must not let Ms. Thomas know how you feel.
    C. It is an upsetting situation, isn't it?
    D. There is no legal proof that Liz's parents have been abusing her.

6. Which of these measures is MORE important for toddlers who have been battered than for other hospitalized toddlers?

6.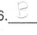

    A. Providing opportunities for physical activity
    B. Arranging to have them cared for consistently by the same personnel
    C. Scheduling specific visiting times for parents
    D. Providing opportunities for play with other toddlers

7. A staff nurse asks the nurse in charge, *Suppose I report to the appropriate agency that a child in my community has sustained a multiplicity of unexplained injuries and may have been abused by the parents. What could happen to me for reporting this information?*
If the state in which the nurse lives has a child abuse law that covers nurses, it would be CORRECT to say that he/she will be

7.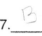

    A. legally liable if a suit for slander is brought by the child's parents
    B. immune from legal action as a consequence of making the report
    C. exempt from appearing in court in defense of the child if a suit develops
    D. none of the above

Questions 8-11.

DIRECTIONS: Questions 8 through 11 are to be answered on the basis of the following information.

Gary Pott, 6 months old, is brought to the clinic by his mother. Gary has phenylketonuria and is on a phenylalanine-controlled diet.

8. The nurse encourages Ms. Pott to keep Gary on the prescribed diet.
The nurse should include in her teaching plan the understanding that phenylketonuria is thought to be the result of

8. ____

    A. insufficient fat intake during early infancy
    B. deficiency of an enzyme needed to utilize galactose during early infancy
    C. inability of the infant to metabolize one of the essential amino acids
    D. abnormal accumulation of lipids in the cells of infants

9. Ms. Pott should be instructed that the food that is HIGHEST in phenylalanine is

9. ____

    A. fruits   B. fats   C. breads   D. jams

10. Ms. Pott tells the nurse that although her husband is working, his salary is small and they are having difficulty covering the cost of Gary's special feedings, along with other expenses.
Which of these actions would BEST exemplify the CORRECT role of the nurse in this situation?

    A. Help Ms. Pott to reassess her budget.
    B. Refer Ms. Pott to the doctor.
    C. Make an appointment for Ms. Pott with the social worker.
    D. Report Ms. Pott's problem to the local department of welfare.

10.____ C

11. All of the following descriptions of Gary's behavior are typical of a normal 6-month-old infant EXCEPT that he

    A. raises himself to a sitting position, but he cannot lie down without help
    B. babbles, but the babbling is not in response to a specific situation
    C. can hold a small object simultaneously in each hand, but he drops one or both of them after a short period
    D. bends his fingers to grasp an object, but he does not use a pincer motion to pick up an object

11.____ A

Questions 12-16.

DIRECTIONS: Questions 12 through 16 are to be answered on the basis of the following information.

One-month-old Susan Black is brought to the well child unit by her mother for her first clinic visit.

12. To assess the adequacy of an infant's weight, the MOST important index is the

    A. age at which the infant doubles his birth weight
    B. relationship between the infant's increase in height and weight
    C. infant's total weight gain since birth
    D. pattern of the infant's weight gain

12.____ D

13. Ms. Black tells the nurse that she gives Susan twice the prescribed amount of a multivitamin preparation because the prescribed amount seems so small.
The nurse's response should MOST certainly include the fact that

    A. it is uneconomical to give vitamins in excess of body requirements
    B. an infant's growth rate can be accelerated by vitamins in excess of the recommended daily requirements
    C. metabolic processes are stimulated by large amounts of vitamins
    D. excessive amounts of fat-soluble vitamins can be toxic

13.____ D

14. Examination reveals a possible congenital dislocation of Susan's left hip.
Which of these observations of an infant would be an early symptom of unilateral congenital dislocation of the hip?

    A. Flexion of the leg on the affected side and extension of the other leg when in the supine position
    B. Absence of a gluteal fold on the affected side

14.____ C

C. Limited abduction of the hip on the affected side
D. Prominence of the hip on the unaffected side

15. Susan is referred to an orthopedic clinic, and a diagnosis of congenital dislocation of the left hip is established. A splint that holds Susan's legs in frog position is used in her initial care.
When Susan is 10 months old, she is admitted to the hospital; and, with closed manipulation, the head of her left femur is placed in the acetabulum. A hip spica cast is then applied. The cast extends from her waistline to below the knee on the left side and to a point above the knee on the right side.
Which of these measures would probably be MOST helpful in preventing Susan from becoming unresponsive and withdrawn while she is hospitalized?

    15.___

A. Placing her in a room with several other infants the same age as she is
B. Providing her with a variety of toys that she can handle
C. Arranging for her mother to help with her care each day
D. Keeping her regimen of care the same each day

16. If treatment for unilateral congenital dislocation of the hip had been delayed for Susan until after she walked, she would have been LIKELY to develop

    16.___

A. scoliosis and scissors gait
B. pigeon toes and knock-knees
C. a limp and lordosis
D. waddling gait and knock-knees

Questions 17-25.

DIRECTIONS: Questions 17 through 25 are to be answered on the basis of the following information.

Mr. Ted Wynn, 17 years old, awakens one night because he is having difficulty breathing and noticeable wheezing on expiration. He is admitted to the hospital. He has a history of asthmatic attacks. His orders include isoproterenol (Isuprel) hydrochloride. Pulmonary function studies and other diagnostic tests will be done after his acute episode subsides.

17. The nurse should observe Mr. Wynn for

    17.___

A. pallor and dyspnea
B. bradycardia and diplopia
C. diarrhea and elevated blood pressure
D. tachycardia and headache

18. All of the following information is provided by Mr. Wynn. The provoking factor of his asthmatic attack is probably that he

    18.___

A. wore a new suit made of a synthetic material two days ago
B. smoked more cigarettes than usual during the past week
C. has been up date at night playing cards with his friends
D. slept on a new feather pillow

19. During the night, Mr. Wynn perspires profusely. The nurse should   19.__D__

    A.   inform the physician
    B.   watch him for signs of hypovolemic shock
    C.   cover him with another blanket
    D.   change his gown and sheets as needed

20. The MAJOR purpose of pulmonary function tests for Mr. Wynn is to   20.__C__

    A.   determine his exercise tolerance
    B.   determine which areas of his lungs are affected
    C.   evaluate the extent of his ventilatory deficiency
    D.   evaluate the adequacy of his cardio-pulmonary circulation

21. The next morning, Mr. Wynn has an acute asthmatic attack. Epinenphrine hydrochloride   21.__B__
(Adrenalin) is administered to him.
The nurse should observe Mr. Wynn for vasoconstricting effects of Adrenalin, which
include

    A.   drowsiness and hypotension
    B.   throbbing headache and tremor
    C.   flushed face and increase in body temperature
    D.   polyuria and urticaria

22. During the asthmatic attack, Mr. Wynn spontaneously assumes an upright sitting posi-   22.__D__
tion, which

    A.   relieves the intrapleural pressure on the diaphragm
    B.   stimulates the pleural reflex
    C.   increases the muscle tone of the bronchioles
    D.   permits a more efficient use of the muscles of respiration

23. All of the following measures should be carried out during Mr. Wynn's asthmatic episode   23.__C__
EXCEPT

    A.   keeping his environment quiet
    B.   offering him sips of water
    C.   teaching him how to deep-breathe and cough
    D.   noting the amount and characteristics of his sputum

24. Mr. Wynn had all of the following diseases during his childhood.   24.__D__
Which one may have had a relationship to his present illness?

    A.   Rheumatic fever   B.   Otitis media
    C.   Chickenpox   D.   Eczema

25. A desensitization program is prescribed for Mr. Wynn. He should be informed that the   25.__C__
outcome of the program is usually MOST dependent upon the

    A.   patient's age
    B.   patient's response to antihistamines
    C.   patient's ability to develop blocking antibodies
    D.   type of serum used for the patient

KEY (CORRECT ANSWERS)

1.	B	11.	A
2.	D	12.	D
3.	D	13.	D
4.	A	14.	C
5.	C	15.	C
6.	B	16.	C
7.	B	17.	D
8.	C	18.	D
9.	C	19.	D
10.	C	20.	C

21.	B
22.	D
23.	C
24.	D
25.	C

TEST 2

DIRECTIONS: Each question or incomplete statement is followed by several suggested answers or completions. Select the one that BEST answers the question or completes the statement. *PRINT THE LETTER OF THE CORRECT ANSWER IN THE SPACE AT THE RIGHT.*

1. The following four children completed their primary tetanus immunization 2 years ago. Which child would be MOST likely to receive a booster dose of toxoid now?   1.___D___

   A. Bill, who sustained several long scratches on his bare legs while climbing on a backyard fence
   B. Sue, who is hospitalized and having emergency treatment for a perforated appendix
   C. John, who is having dental treatment for an abscessed impacted molar
   D. Amy, who walked barefoot around a vacation ranch and cut her foot on a broken bottle

2. The eating habits of most healthy young adolescents probably BEST reflect their need to   2.___A___

   A. conform to peer behavior
   B. look like a favorite adult
   C. spend short periods at a variety of activities
   D. have new experiences

3. A mother calls a neighbor who is a nurse and says that her toddler ate an unknown plant in the backyard and now appears ill.
   In addition to telling the mother to call a doctor immediately, which of the following advice would it be APPROPRIATE for the nurse to give the woman?   3.___D___

   A. Obtain a urine specimen from the child.
   B. Have the child drink an ounce of mineral oil.
   C. Put the child to bed and elevate his extremities.
   D. Make the child vomit and save the vomitus.

4. The CHIEF difficulty in establishing a therapeutic relationship with most children who are autistic stems from the fact that they   4.___C___

   A. have a functional hearing defect
   B. are mentally retarded as well as mentally ill
   C. behave in a manner difficult to understand
   D. are unable to follow directions

5. Which of these measures is the MOST important one to consider in the home management of a young child who is mentally retarded?   5.___C___

   A. Having the same person teach him all new activities
   B. Limiting the amount of stimulation he receives from his environment
   C. Maintaining a consistent routine for the performance of his activities of daily living
   D. Teaching him amenities that will help him to be accepted by others

6. An infant has erythroblastosis fetalis (hemolytic disease of the newborn).   6. C
   The parents should be informed that the development of jaundice in the infant is
   caused by

    A. an overproduction of erythrocytes
    B. an abnormal production of melanin
    C. excessive destruction of red blood cells
    D. hypobilirubinemia

7. A child with an eye infection is to have physiologic saline eye irrigations.   7. B
   When carrying out an eye irrigation, it is CORRECT to

    A. use a solution in which there is a tablespoon of salt in each quart of water
    B. use only enough pressure to maintain a steady flow of solution along the lower
        conjunctival sac
    C. direct the flow of solution toward the inner surface of the upper lid
    D. keep the head flat

Questions 8-14.

DIRECTIONS: Questions 8 through 14 are to be answered on the basis of the following infor-
               mation.

   Lisa Smith, 2 years old, is admitted to the hospital with acute otitis media of the right ear.
Her body temperature is elevated.

8. Lisa's susceptibility to otitis media is due to the fact that the   8. A

    A. eustachian tube is short and wide in children
    B. causitive organism is part of the normal flora in throats of children
    C. external ear in children is less effective in resisting the entrance of foreign objects
    D. inner ear in children is markedly immature

9. Lisa is to have a tepid sponge bath.   9. C
   To achieve the desired outcome of this procedure, the nurse should

    A. stroke Lisa's skin to cause friction
    B. give Lisa warm fluids to drink
    C. allow moisture on Lisa's skin to evaporate
    D. lower the temperature of Lisa's room

10. Lisa has severe pain in her right ear.   10. C
    The pain of acute otitis media is due CHIEFLY to

    A. reduced tension on structures in the vestibular portion of the inner ear
    B. constriction of the endolymphatic spaces in the labyrinth of the inner ear
    C. increased pressure of fluid in the middle ear
    D. irritation of the stapes in the middle ear

11. Lisa is to receive 100,000 U. of an oral suspension of penicillin four times a day. A bottle   11. _B_
containing 300,000 U. of penicillin in 5 cc. of solution is to be used to prepare Lisa's dosage.
How much solution will contain the amount of penicillin prescribed for Lisa?
_____ cc.

    A. 0.7   B. 1.7   C. 2.7   D. 3.7

12. Lisa's condition improves.   12. _C_
Ms. Smith says to the nurse, *I need to go home to see how my mother is making out
with my other children; but each time I try to leave, Lisa gets so upset that I just can't,*
Which of these responses by the nurse would probably be BEST?

    A. Lisa is now well enough to be without you. Why don't you try slipping away when
she falls asleep?
    B. Stress is not good for Lisa even though her condition is improved. Is it possible for
you to find out about the children without leaving Lisa?
    C. Your feeling torn about whether to stay or go is understandable when Lisa needs
you too. Whenever you're ready to go, let me know and I'll stay with her.
    D. Lisa needs to be more independent of you now. Your being away from her for a
while will help her.

13. Lisa has a temper tantrum one morning while her mother is bathing her. Ms. Smith asks   13. _D_
the nurse how the behavior should be handled.
In replying, the nurse should include that this behavior in 2-year-olds

    A. indicates regression
    B. suggests a poorly developed sense of trust
    C. should be controlled by parental discipline
    D. is a normal outlet for tension

14. A member of the nursing team remarks to the team leader,   14. _D_
*Lisa whines and fusses all the time her mother is with her. She quiets down as soon as
she leaves but cries when she comes back. I wonder if it's good for her to visit so
often.*
Which of these responses would probably help the team member MOST to think
through the problem?

    A. This is a characteristic trait of children this age. Haven't you noticed it in others?
    B. This behavior may be indicative of a disturbed mother-child relationship. You
should continue to watch them closely.
    C. Even if the mother upsets the child, she should be encouraged to continue to visit
as often as she can.
    D. Is it possible that her mother's being with her enables her to express her unhappiness?

Questions 15-21.

DIRECTIONS: Questions 15 through 21 are to be answered on the basis of the following information.

When 16-month-old Ann Wolfe is admitted to the hospital, she has a temperature of
104° F. (40° C.), petechiae, and purpuric areas on her skin. A diagnosis of meningococcal meningitis is established.

15. Ann has opisthotonos.
Which of these positions will be BEST for her while she has this symptom?   15. B

   A. Semi-Flowler's   B. Side-lying
   C. Dorsal recumbent   D. Prone

16. While Ann is acutely ill, which of these measures will be ESSENTIAL in her care?   16. A

   A. Reducing environmental stimuli
   B. Maintaining optimum nutrition
   C. Preventing the development of herpetic lesions of the lips
   D. Exercising her extremities passively several times a day

17. Ann is being watched for signs of adrenal insufficiency. Which of these symptoms are   17. C
characteristic of this condition?
_____ blood pressure and _____.

   A. Normal; increasing pulse rate
   B. Rising; weak, thready pulse
   C. Falling; weak, thready pulse
   D. Fluctuating; decreasing pulse rate

18. Ann is receiving both an antibiotic and a sulfonamide. Because she is receiving a sul-   18. B
fonamide, which of these daily measures will be ESPECIALLY important for her?

   A. Weighing her and observing her for edema
   B. Giving her extra fluids and measuring her fluid intake and output
   C. Taking her blood pressure and her apical pulse at regular, specified intervals
   D. Observing her frequently for signs of photophobia and hyperreflexia

19. A spinal tap is done to assess Ann's response to therapy. Which change in Ann's spinal   19. D
fluid would be indicative of improvement in her condition?

   A. *Increase* in cell count
   B. *Increase* in specific gravity
   C. *Decrease* in sugar
   D. *Decrease* in protein

20. Ann responds favorably to treatment and is convalescing. In order to meet Ann's nutri-   20. A
tional needs, her food plan should be based on which of these needs of normal 16-
month-old children?

   A. Their diets should include a variety of foods that they can eat by themselves.
   B. Liquids and semiliquids are best for them.
   C. Preference should be given to their favorite foods.
   D. Milk is of greater importance to them than solids.

21. After Ann recovers, which type of immunity to the meningococcus will she have?   21. D

   A. Passive acquired   B. Cellular
   C. Natural   D. Active acquired

Questions 22-24.

DIRECTIONS: Questions 22 through 24 are to be answered on the basis of the following information.

Suzanne Edwards, 6 years old, is admitted to the hospital for probable repair of a ventricular septal defect. This is Suzanne's third hospital admission.

22. Suzanne has a cardiac catheterization.   22. D
For the first few hours after the cardiac catheterization, which of these nursing measures will be ESSENTIAL for her?

    A. Keeping the head of her bed elevated 30 degrees
    B. Encouraging her to cough forcefully at regular intervals
    C. Checking her temperature every hour
    D. Taking her pulse frequently in the extremity used for the cutdown

23. In preparing Suzanne for the proposed surgery, which characteristic of 6-year-old chil-   23. A
dren should be given GREATEST consideration by the nurse?

    A. Concrete experiences are most meaningful.
    B. The ability to think abstractly is well-developed.
    C. Cause and effect relationships are readily understood.
    D. The ability to distinguish between fantasy and reality is well-developed.

24. Suzanne has open-heart surgery for repair of a ventricular septal defect. She is then   24. B
transferred to the intensive care unit.
During Suzanne's surgery, her femoral arteries were cannulated.
As a result of this procedure, it is ESSENTIAL postoperatively for the nurse to make
frequent checks of Suzanne's

    A. urinary output
    B. pedal pulses
    C. rectal temperature
    D. ability to move her lower extremities

25. A woman phones a nurse at home and says that her son fell and broke his eyeglasses   25. C
and that she thinks some glass may have penetrated one eye.
The nurse advises immediate medical attention and that in the meanwhile it would be
MOST important for the mother to

    A. apply a pressure dressing to the affected eye and keep the child in an erect sitting
       position
    B. examine the affected eye to determine whether any glass can be easily removed
       and apply petrolatum (Vaseline) on the outer surface of the eyelid
    C. loosely cover both eyes and have the child remain quiet
    D. gently irrigate the affected eye with a copious aount of boiled table salt solution that
       has cooled and leave the eye uncovered

KEY (CORRECT ANSWERS)

1.	D		11.	B
2.	A		12.	C
3.	D		13.	D
4.	C		14.	D
5.	C		15.	B
6.	C		16.	A
7.	B		17.	C
8.	A		18.	B
9.	C		19.	D
10.	C		20.	A

21. D
22. D
23. A
24. B
25. C

———

TEST 3

DIRECTIONS: Each question or incomplete statement is followed by several suggested answers or completions. Select the one that BEST answers the question or completes the statement. *PRINT THE LETTER OF THE CORRECT ANSWER IN THE SPACE AT THE RIGHT.*

1. When a primipara's normal first-born infant is brought to her for the first feeding, she says, *He's so little! I'm afraid I'll hurt him.*
   Which of these responses would be MOST helpful from the standpoint of learning?

    A. You can practice taking care of the baby while you're here.
    B. Is there someone at home who can help you with the baby the first few weeks?
    C. You can watch me take care of the baby.
    D. The public health nurse can come to your home to show you how to take care of the baby.

1. _A_

Questions 2-4.

DIRECTIONS: Questions 2 through 4 are to be answered on the basis of the following information.

Ms. Marie DuPont, who was discharged two days ago from the post-partum unit, is visiting her newborn girl on the pediatric unit. Baby girl DuPont has a cleft lip and cleft palate.

2. The nurse should expect that because Ms. DuPont has an infant with an obvious physical defect, Ms. DuPont may

    A. have difficulty loving such an infant and responding warmly to it
    B. overtly express love for the infant because mother love is instinctive
    C. express mixed feelings for the infant that will require psychiatric treatment to overcome
    D. express guilt that will require her visits with the infant to be curtailed

2. _A_

3. Ms. DuPont is concerned about the likelihood of having other children with the same anomaly as her baby girl's. Ms. DuPont should be given which of the following information about her probability of having another child with a cleft palate?

    A. If this mother has close medical supervision during subsequent pregnancies, the anomaly is not likely to occur again.
    B. Since the anomaly is so rare, it is highly unlikely that a mother would have more than one child with such an anomaly.
    C. There is little probability that future children of this mother will have the same anomaly since there is no genetic basis for its development.
    D. A mother's having one child with this anomaly means that there is a greater-than-average possibility of her having other children with the same anomaly.

3. _D_

4. Children with cleft palates are MOST likely to have

    A. abnormal dentition, speech impairments, and recurrent otitis media
    B. inadequate nutrition, poor muscle coordination, and mental retardation
    C. persistent infantile emotional pattern, regression in speech development, and hearing deficit
    D. accelerated caries formation, peer group maladjustment, and maternal overprotection

4. _A_

Questions 5-10.

DIRECTIONS: Questions 5 through 10 are to be answered on the basis of the following information.

John Stone, a 3 1/2-year-old, was admitted to the hospital because of a persistent bleeding from a minor laceration. His condition is diagnosed as classic hemophilia (factor VIII deficiency).

5.   Because of John's age, which of these aspects of hospitalization is likely to be MOST   5.___
traumatic for him?

    A.   Being inhibited from running about freely
    B.   Being separated from his family
    C.   Being placed in an unfamiliar environment
    D.   Having his routines and rituals disrupted

6.   John is an only child. His parents are concerned about the possibility of their future off-   6.___
spring having hemophilia.
His parents should be told that

    A.   male offspring will have the hemophilic trait and will either be carriers or will have
the bleeding tendency; female offspring will not be subject to the condition
    B.   hemophilia is unlikely to occur in female offspring, but they can be carriers; male
offspring have a 50 percent chance of having the condition
    C.   the probability that hemophilia will occur in other offspring is no greater than it is in
the general population
    D.   each of their offspring will have a 25 percent chance of having hemophilia, a 50
percent chance of being a carrier, and a 25 percent chance of being free of the
gene for hemophilia

7.   Before his illness, John had achieved all of the following abilities.   7.___
Which ability did he probably develop MOST recently?

    A.   Throwing a large ball four to five feet
    B.   Putting a spoon in his mouth without spilling the contents
    C.   Speaking in sentences of three or four words
    D.   Alternating his feet while walking upstairs

8.   All of these measures should be considered in feeding John.   8.___
Which one is MOST important in terms of the development needs of a 3 1/2-year-old?

    A.   Using colorful child-size cups and dishes for his food
    B.   Having him sit at a table that is of a height appropriate for his size
    C.   Serving him small portions of food
    D.   Letting him feed himself

9. In discussing dental prophylaxis for John with Mr. and Mrs. Stone, the nurse should tell them that dental visits should be

    9. _C_

    A. scheduled only when definite symptoms occur
    B. preceded by the administration of antihemophilic globulin (AHG) factor VIII
    C. scheduled at regular intervals
    D. started when the deciduous teeth become loose

10. Which of these understandings about John should his parents be helped to gain?

    10. _C_

    A. John's participation in active range-of-motion activities will help to prevent contractures.
    B. John's emotional development will be fostered by a warm, indulgent family, but some curtailment of his physical development may result.
    C. Overprotection may impede John's emotional and physical development.
    D. Children with John's condition tend to limit their own physical activity.

Questions 11-18.

DIRECTIONS: Questions 11 through 18 are to be answered on the basis of the following information.

Ms. Wendy Stevens, 18 years old, is admitted to the hospital with a diagnosis of infectious hepatitis (Type A). Her orders include bed rest and diagnostic studies.

11. On admission, Ms. Stevens should be expected to have which of these early symptoms of infectious hepatitis (Type A)?

    11. _A_

    A. Loss of appetite
    B. Ecchymoses
    C. Shortness of breath on exertion
    D. Abdominal distension

12. Which of these factors in Ms. Stevens' history is MOST likely to be related to her diagnosis?

    12. _C_

    A. Recent recovery from an upper respiratory infection
    B. Being bitten by an insect
    C. Contact with a person who was jaundiced
    D. Eating home-canned foods

13. The nurse should monitor the results of which of these tests that is used to assess Ms. Stevens' liver function?

    13. _A_

    A. Serum transaminase   B. Protein-bound iodine
    C. Creatinine clearance   D. Glucose tolerance

14. All of the following precautionary measures are essential in Ms. Stevens' case EXCEPT

    14. _B_

    A. serving food on disposable dishes
    B. wearing a face mask
    C. carrying out procedures for decontamination of urine and feces
    D. modifying procedures for discarding used syringes and needles

15. The CHIEF purpose of bed rest for Ms. Stevens is to   15. A

    A. minimize liver damage
    B. reduce the breakdown of fats for metabolic needs
    C. decrease the circulatory load to reduce cardiac effort
    D. control the spread of the disease

16. Members of Ms. Stevens' family who have been exposed to infectious hepatitis should be   16. C
given

    A. penicillin
    B. sulfadiazine
    C. immune human serum globulin
    D. irradiated plasma

17. Ms. Stevens' condition improves.   17. C
The nurse is planning Ms. Stevens' care during her convalescent period.
The nurse should expect that Ms. Stevens will have the MOST difficulty with

    A. relieving pain
    B. regulating bowel elimination
    C. maintaining morale
    D. preventing respiratory complications

18. As a result of her having hepatitis, Ms. Stevens should be instructed NEVER to   18. C

    A. smoke   B. eat fried foods
    C. donate blood   D. exercise strenuously

Questions 19-25.

DIRECTIONS: Questions 19 through 25 are to be answered on the basis of the following information.

Alison Wright, 19 months old, is diagnosed by the family doctor as having acute laryngotracheobronchitis. Alison's temperature is 103° F. (39.4° C.) when Ms. Wright brings her to
the hospital. This is Alison's first hospital admission.

19. Two early symptoms that are MOST likely to occur in laryngotracheobronchitis are   19. A

    A. cough and inspiratory stridor
    B. elevated temperature and prostration
    C. Kussmaul respirations and bradycardia
    D. flushed face and labored expirations

20. Ms. Wright tells the nurse, who is filling out a habit record for Alison, that Alison has   20. B
achieved bowel control. Which additional information would it be MOST important for the
nurse to obtain from Ms. Wright at this time?

    A. The extent of Ms. Wright's understanding of the regressive effect of illness and
        hospitalization on bowel-training in children of Alison's age
    B. Alison's toileting routines at home
    C. The age at which Alison's bowel-training was started
    D. Whether Alison has indicated readiness for bladder-training

21. Alison is placed in a Croupette.   21. _D_
    Restraints are to be used on Alison because she continually tries to get out of the
    Croupette. Because Alison requires the restraints, the nurse should

    A. tell Alison's mother that bilateral arm and leg restraints are necessary for toddlers
    B. inform Alison's mother that Alison will probably adjust better to restraints if she is
       left alone for a while after they are applied
    C. explain to Alison the need for the restraints in order to help her adjust to them
    D. watch Alison carefully after the restraints are applied to see whether she struggles
       to the point of negating the value of the therapy

22. Which of these symptoms in Alison could give the EARLIEST indication of increased res-   22. _B_
    piratory difficulty?

    A. Generalized cyanosis
    B. Increased pulse rate
    C. Decreased respiratory rate
    D. Abdominal breathing

23. Alison is to receive a dose of aspirin in liquid form. In view of her condition and her age, it   23. _A_
    would be BEST to

    A. support Alison in a sitting position, hold the medicine glass with the medication to
       her lips, and tell her calmly and firmly to drink it
    B. turn Alison on her side, give her a straw, and tell her to suck the medication from
       the medicine glass
    C. hand Alison the medicine glass containing the drug and tell her to drink it, saying
       that it will taste like candy
    D. mix the medication in a 4-ounce glass of sweetened fruit juice, prop Alison up in a
       sitting position, give her the glass, and tell her in a positive tone to drink the juice

24. Alison's condition improves, and the Croupette is discontinued. Diet as tolerated is   24. _B_
    ordered for her.
    A nurse's aide reports to the nurse that although Alison seems hungry, she pushes the
    aide's hand away and will not eat when the aide tries to feed her. The nurse should
    communicate to the aide that most children of Alison's age

    A. eat better when seated at a table with adults
    B. prefer to feed themselves
    C. have finicky appetites
    D. have strong food preferences

25. A normal 19-month-old child can be expected to   25. _C_

    A. stand briefly on one foot without support and to put together simple jigsaw puzzles
    B. drink through a straw and to know his own sex
    C. manage finger foods and to understand *No, no*
    D. build a tower of 7 blocks and to open doors by turning knobs

KEY (CORRECT ANSWERS)

1. A	11. A
2. A	12. C
3. D	13. A
4. A	14. B
5. B	15. A
6. B	16. C
7. D	17. C
8. D	18. C
9. C	19. A
10. C	20. B

21. D
22. B
23. A
24. B
25. C

EXAMINATION SECTION
TEST 1

DIRECTIONS: Each question or incomplete statement is followed by several suggested answers or completions. Select the one that BEST answers the question or completes the statement. *PRINT THE LETTER OF THE CORRECT ANSWER IN THE SPACE AT THE RIGHT.*

1. A relationship in which a patient becomes dependent on the nurse   1.____

    A. is always unprofessional
    B. is inevitably "bad" for the patient
    C. may be necessary temporarily
    D. impedes learning

2. Anxiety is the CHIEF characteristic of the   2.____

    A. immature personality
    B. psychoneurotic disorder
    C. involutional psychotic reaction
    D. mentally retarded adolescent

3. The mode of psychological adjustment known as regression can BEST be described as   3.____

    A. refusing to think of unpleasant situations
    B. changing to a type of behavior which is characteristic of an earlier period in life
    C. reverting to actions characteristic of an historically early or primitive code of behavior
    D. hostility towards persons or objects that prove frustrating

4. The CHIEF danger in the employment of escape mechanisms as a form of adjustment is that they   4.____

    A. do more harm than good
    B. are socially undesirable
    C. make the experience expensive
    D. leave the basic problem unsolved

5. Of the following, the LEADING cause of *all* adult deaths is   5.____

    A. malignant neoplasms
    B. influenza and pneumonia
    C. heart disease
    D. vascular lesions of the central nervous system

6. Of the following, an overdose of insulin is MOST likely to produce   6.____

    A. nervousness, excessive hunger, weakness and sweating
    B. vomiting, labored respiration and anorexia
    C. polyuria, restlessness and anhydremia
    D. nausea, labored respiration and dyspnea

7. In essential hypertension, there is a(n)   7.____

    A. *increase* in systolic pressure and a *decrease* in diastolic pressure
    B. *decrease* in systolic pressure and an *increase* in diastolic pressure
    C. *increase* in *both* systolic and diastolic pressure
    D. *decrease* in *both* systolic and diastolic pressure

8. The use of mineral oil in low caloric diets should be discouraged CHIEFLY because it   8.____

    A. interferes with the absorption of all fat soluble vitamins
    B. spoils the flavor of food
    C. contains 9 calories per gram
    D. interferes with the absorption of sugar

9. Water is important in the daily intake of the body CHIEFLY because it   9.____

    A. causes the oxidation of food in the body
    B. is a transporting medium for all body substances
    C. cools the air in the lungs
    D. promotes protein metabolism

10. Of the following, the MOST important reason why a nurse should have a basic knowledge of the foods of the foreign-born is that   10.____

    A. many foreign dishes are more nutritious than American foods
    B. such knowledge would prove beyond doubt that poor diet is the cause of poor health among the foreign-born
    C. such knowledge would help the nurse to advise the patient on how to follow the prescribed diet using familiar foods
    D. it is interesting and exciting to eat the exotic dishes of foreign lands

11. Liver should be included in the diet chiefly because it is a GOOD source of   11.____

    A. Vitamin C   B. phosphorus   C. iodine   D. iron

12. Lack of iodine in the diet may result in   12.____

    A. gout   B. simple goiter
    C. arthritis   D. diabetes

13. The one of the following diseases which is the MOST COMMON cause of disability is   13.____

    A. arthritis   B. diabetes
    C. poliomyelitis   D. Parkinson's Disease

14. The glucose tolerance test is a test used to diagnose   14.____

    A. ulcers   B. hypertension
    C. leukemia   D. diabetes

15. When using a sphygmomanometer, the moment that the pulsation can be felt or heard marks the point of   15.____

    A. systolic blood pressure   B. diastolic blood pressure
    C. brachial stenosis   D. vasomotor restriction

16. The *initial* paralysis in cerebral vascular accident, regardless of cause, is the type known as   16.____

    A. spastic   B. paraplegic   C. flaccid   D. rigid

17. Cerebral hemorrhage *most frequently* occurs in males in the age range from   17.____

    A. 20 to 30 years   B. 30 to 40 years
    C. 40 to 50 years   D. 50 years and over

18. The one of the following conditions which is due to dysfunction of the thyroid gland is   18.____

    A. cholecystitis   B. cretinism
    C. dwarfism   D. epilepsy

19. The morbidity rate of tuberculosis is HIGHEST in the age range from   19.____

    A. birth to 20 years   B. 20 to 45 years
    C. 45 to 65 years   D. 65 years and over

20. An IMPORTANT early sign of carcinoma of the larynx is   20.____

    A. chronic hoarseness   B. regurgitation of fluids
    C. difficulty in swallowing   D. respiratory distress

21. Of the following, the MOST common and earliest recognizable sign of cancer of the breast is   21.____

    A. pain in the breast   B. nipple discharge
    C. lump in the breast   D. enlargement of the breast

22. In cancer of the breast, the lesion is MOST frequently found in the   22.____

    A. lower outer quadrant   B. lower inner quadrant
    C. upper inner quadrant   D. upper outer quadrant

23. Of the following, the MOST usual cause of hemoptysis in a 40-year-old male is   23.____

    A. tuberculosis   B. cancer of the lung
    C. congenital ringworm   D. spontaneous pneumothorax

24. Assume that a cardiac patient regularly assigned for nursing care has been receiving digitalis orally. On one of the nurse's regular home visits she finds the patient's radial pulse rate is 58. Nursing orders do not give specific directions regarding pulse. In this situation, it would be MOST advisable for the nurse to   24.____

    A. give no direction to the patient regarding medication but watch his pulse rate more closely on future visits for changes
    B. advise the patient to stop taking medication and tell him that she will report the pulse rate immediately to his physician
    C. report immediately to the physician on her observations as to pulse rate as well as regularity of pulse, patient's appetite, presence or absence of nausea
    D. teach the patient how to take his pulse and instruct hiiri to take digitalis if his pulse rate goes above 60

25. Hereditary progressive muscular dystrophy is a disease characterized by progressive   25._____
weakness and final atrophy of groups of muscles.
Of the following statements about muscular dystrophy, the one which is LEAST accurate is that

    A. there is no known cure for muscular dystrophy at present
    B. muscular dystrophy is a disease of the central nervous system
    C. early signs of muscular dystrophy are frequent falls, difficulty climbing stairs, devel-
opment of lordosis and a waddling gait
    D. therapeutic exercises may have some temporary value in the treatment of muscu-
lar dystrophy

26. The home care program is an extension of the hospital's service into the home on an   26._____
extra-mural basis.
Of the following statements, the one that BEST explains the success of this program is
that it

    A. recognizes the value to the patient and his family of the preservation of normal
family life despite the limitations imposed by the patient's illness
    B. makes more hospital beds available for acute illnesses and emergency care
    C. reduces the cost of hospital care by reducing the number of in-patients
    D. simplifies hospital administration by reducing the number of chronically ill in hospi-
tals

27. The PRIMARY objective of a day care program is to   27._____

    A. provide group care for a child in order to promote his physical or emotional adjust-
ment
    B. insure adequate care, supervision and guidance for a child while his parents are at
work
    C. safeguard a child's home and strengthen and support the family relationships for
the child
    D. give financial assistance to voluntary agencies sponsoring the day care program

28. The MOST important of the following reasons for the rehabilitation of the seriously hand-   28._____
icapped individual is that

    A. hospitalization of the handicapped is usually prolonged and costly to the commu-
nity
    B. beds occupied by such patients reduce the number of hospital beds available for
acutely ill patients
    C. care of chronically ill or handicapped patients is taxing and difficult for the family,
the nurse and the doctor
    D. it is important to the patient that he be as independent and useful as possible

29. There has been a notable increase in the discharge rate from mental institutions in the   29._____
state during recent years.
This change in statistics may be attributed CHIEFLY to

    A. increasing use of psychoanalysis and better trained personnel
    B. new drugs, changes in admission procedures and the "open door" policy
    C. the increase in nursing homes for the elderly
    D. the use of psychotherapeutics and early diagnosis of mental illness

30. The PRINCIPAL and BASIC objective of mental hygiene is to   30.____

    A. modify attitudes as well as unhealthy behavior secondary to unhealthy attitudes
    B. care for the post-hospitalized psychiatric patient at home
    C. increase mental hygiene clinic services
    D. stimulate interest in improved education for doctors, nurses and teachers

---

KEY (CORRECT ANSWERS)

1.	C		16.	C
2.	B		17.	D
3.	B		18.	B
4.	D		19.	D
5.	C		20.	A
6.	A		21.	C
7.	C		22.	D
8.	A		23.	A
9.	B		24.	C
10.	C		25.	B
11.	D		26.	A
12.	B		27.	C
13.	A		28.	D
14.	D		29.	B
15.	A		30.	A

TEST 2

DIRECTIONS: Each question or incomplete statement is followed by several suggested answers or completions. Select the one that BEST answers the question or completes the statement. *PRINT THE LETTER OF THE CORRECT ANSWER IN THE SPACE AT THE RIGHT.*

1. The incidence of syphilis is reported to be rising among teenagers in this country and the disease is still considered to be a major public health problem. Of the following statements about syphilis, the one which is NOT true is that

    A. the treatment most frequently used is penicillin
    B. at one stage of the disease, it causes a skin rash and enlarged lymph nodes
    C. the causative organism is the spirochete, treponema pallidum
    D. syphilis can be transmitted only by sexual intercourse

1. D

2. The one of the following which is the MOST dependable sign of pregnancy is

    A. fetal heart
    B. fetal movements felt by the mother
    C. a positive result on the Aschheim-Zondek test
    D. amenorrhea

2. A

3. An expectant mother states, "I did not plan this pregnancy and I am not making any preparations."
Of the following, the BEST *initial* response for the nurse to make is:

    A. "Don't be upset. You will love your baby just the same."
    B. "Most mothers look forward to a lovely new baby."
    C. "Later when you feel differently you can make the necessary preparations."
    D. "It is not always easy to accept a pregnancy."

3. D

4. A nurse asks you to explain the significance of the Rh negative factor because she is concerned about one of her cases, an expectant mother who is Rh negative.
Of the following, the BEST explanation you could give to this nurse is that

    A. Rh negative is a serious condition in the mother, frequently causing toxic symptoms
    B. if the father is Rh positive, there is no danger to either the mother or the baby
    C. if the baby should be positive, it may be adversely affected by the antibodies from the mother
    D. there is little danger with the Rh factor today because the mother can be treated to prevent the formation of antibodies

4. C

5. A mother who is 7-months pregnant tells the nurse that for the past few days she has been feeling dizzy and has had spots before her eyes. She has an appointment to see her doctor in a week.
Of the following, the BEST advice for the nurse to give this mother is to

    A. not be alarmed but report this to the doctor at her next appointment
    B. rest at least two hours each day and avoid exertion
    C. limit the amount of fluid intake to 3-4 glasses daily
    D. either call the doctor or go to the hospital immediately

5. D

6. Assume that a newly appointed nurse asks you what she should do if she were to find,   6.___
on one of her regular visits, that a mother was in advanced labor.
Of the following, the BEST advice for you to give the nurse is that, in this situation, she
should

    A. go out to the nearest telephone booth and call for an ambulance
    B. apply gentle pressure to the uterus
    C. encourage the mother to bear down
    D. support the baby's head and body as they are delivered

7. To meet the calcium requirement during the second half of pregnancy, it is recommended   7.___
that the diet of a pregnant woman contain

    A. at least two eggs daily
    B. one quart of milk daily
    C. a serving of liver twice weekly
    D. at least two oranges daily

8. A mother seven months pregnant with her first baby asks the nurse how she will know   8.___
when to go to the hospital.
Of the following, the BEST response is that she should go to the hospital when

    A. the membranes rupture, whether or not she has contractions
    B. she has a mucus vaginal discharge
    C. the baby shows marked increase in activity
    D. the baby sinks down into the pelvis and she feels pressure on the bladder and rec-
tum

9. During an in-service education session, a nurse asks for additional information about   9.___
pre-eclamptic toxemia.
Of the following, the MOST accurate information you could give this nurse is that

    A. toxemia usually occurs during the first trimester of pregnancy
    B. overexertion on the part of the mother is known to cause toxemia
    C. pre-eclamptic toxemia is a preventable condition whose cause is well known and
well understood
    D. this condition is usually marked by headache, nausea and vomiting

10. A young nurse asks you how she can help a mother who is breast feeding her baby but   10.___
does not have a sufficient amount of milk.
Of the following, the *most helpful* suggestion the nurse could make to this mother is:

    A. "Nurse the baby every other feeding. This will allow the breasts to fill up between
feedings."
    B. "Plenty of rest and good food will insure a good supply of milk."
    C. "Have the baby empty the breasts completely and regularly before supplementing
with the bottle."
    D. "Many women are too nervous to successfully breast feed."

11. A mother who is 3 months *post partum* has been nursing her baby. She tells the nurse   11.___
that she has not menstruated and asks if it is possible that she is now pregnant.
Of the following, the BEST answer the nurse could give to this mother is:

A. "You cannot become pregnant while you nurse your baby."
B. "You cannot be pregnant until you have your first menstrual period."
C. "You may become pregnant at any time if you have intercourse."
D. "You cannot become pregnant until your uterus has completely involuted."

12. The OUTSTANDING cause of death during the first twenty-four hours of life is   12. B

    A. congenital anomalies   B. prematurity
    C. atelectasis   D. erythroblastosis

13. Of the following, the one which is LEAST characteristic of the eyes of a normal newborn   13. C
child is that

    A. the pupils contract in bright light
    B. sight is confined to the ability to distinguish light from darkness
    C. the lachrymal glands secrete fluid
    D. bright light causes closure of the eyelids

14. Of the following reflexes, the one which is NOT normal in a month-old infant is   14. D

    A. drawing up the legs when startled
    B. grasping an article placed in its hand
    C. sucking
    D. ability to focus the eyes

15. Of the following signs, the one which is MOST helpful in the early diagnosis of congenital   15. C
hip dislocation in the newborn is

    A. marked hip prominence
    B. an even number of gluteal folds
    C. an uneven number of gluteal folds
    D. a grating sound on movement of the hips

16. Egg yolk from a hard cooked egg is added to an infant's diet at the age of three months   16. A
CHIEFLY to

    A. compensate for the low iron content of milk
    B. give bulk to the diet
    C. add protein to the diet
    D. compensate for the low fat content of milk

17. Kicking in a six-month-old baby is *usually* a(n)   17. C

    A. expression of bad temper
    B. sign of excessive restlessness
    C. normal muscular activity which may be a preparation for walking
    D. attempt to attract the attention of the nearest adult

18. Of the following statements with respect to the nutritional needs of children, the one   18. B
which is MOST accurate is that

    A. a four-year-old child requires a minimum of 2000 calories a day
    B. proportionately, children require more protein per pound of body weight than do
       adults

C.   it is better for a child to be slightly underweight than to be overweight
D.   a child whose diet is deficient in Vitamin D may develop scurvy as a result

19.   Cod liver oil is given to children CHIEFLY in order to aid in   19._A_

     A.   absorption of calcium
     B.   carbohydrate metabolism
     C.   prevention of beriberi
     D.   regulation of osmotic pressure

20.   The LEADING cause of death in this country for children from one to four years of age is   20._D_

     A.   influenza and pneumonia
     B.   congenital malformations
     C.   malignant neoplasms of blood and lymph
     D.   accidents

21.   Reconstructive surgery for cleft palate SHOULD be done   21._B_

     A.   at about one month of age
     B.   before the child begins to talk
     C.   when the child is six months old
     D.   when explanation of the procedure can be understood by the child

22.   Separation of a child from his own home and placement in a foster home often arouses   22._B_
adverse reactions in the child.
Of the following, the one which is MOST serious for the child is

     A.   homesickness   B.   withdrawn behavior
     C.   rebellion against authority   D.   dislike of new people

23.   Behavior problems of the adolescent school child can BEST be explained by the fact that   23._D_

     A.   the adolescent suddenly becomes aware of the opposite sex at this time
     B.   the demands made on adolescents by intolerant parents create rebellion against
         authority
     C.   during childhood there is a general disregard of the child's need for independence
         by parents and other adults
     D.   adolescence is a transition period between childhood and adulthood which usually
         creates feelings of insecurity in the adolescent

24.   Of the following, the behavior which is LEAST indicative of serious emotional maladjust-   24._D_
ment in an adolescent boy is

     A.   lying and cheating
     B.   shyness and daydreaming
     C.   gross overweight
     D.   association with a teenage gang

25. The precipitating cause of dental caries is   25. _C_

    A. inadequate cleaning of teeth by toothbrushing
    B. failure to maintain a daily diet containing all of the essential food elements in the right amounts
    C. decalcification of the tooth enamel by acids produced in the fermentation of carbo-hydrates
    D. inherited differences in the ability to resist caries

26. For GREATEST effectiveness, topical application of a fluorine solution should be started   26. _A_

    A. as soon as possible after the deciduous teeth erupt
    B. when the child enters the first grade in school
    C. on the child's first visit to the dentist
    D. when the permanent teeth have erupted

27. The MOST important one of the following contributions that the school nurse can make to the effort to conserve sight and to prevent eye strain in the classroom is to   27. _C_

    A. advise the principal to have the walls painted a light color so as to diffuse the light throughout the classroom
    B. determine whether the school office has in its files the accepted standards for classroom lighting
    C. instruct the teacher and students regarding proper seating and utilization of light in the classroom
    D. provide the teacher with a list of all students in her class who test 20/40 or more on the visual acuity test

28. Of the following statements concerning eyeglasses, the one which is LEAST accurate is that glasses are prescribed in order to   28. _A_

    A. cure infectious diseases of the eye
    B. improve vision and relieve eyestrain
    C. neutralize defects of focus of the eyes
    D. strengthen weak eye muscles

29. Of the following, the BEST description of early symptoms of glaucoma is dimness in visual acuity,   29. _C_

    A. and marked itching of the eyelids
    B. with or without pain in the eye
    C. and haloed lights, with or without pain in the eye
    D. marked itching and redness of the sclera and eyelids

30. Unequal arm or leg lengths, or differences in shoulder height with scapular protrusion, are *early* manifestations of   30. _B_

    A. kyphosis   B. scoliosis   C. torticollis   D. lordosis

KEY (CORRECT ANSWERS)

1.	D	16.	A
2.	A	17.	C
3.	D	18.	B
4.	C	19.	A
5.	D	20.	D
6.	D	21.	B
7.	B	22.	B
8.	A	23.	D
9.	D	24.	D
10.	C	25.	C
11.	C	26.	A
12.	B	27.	C
13.	C	28.	A
14.	D	29.	C
15.	C	30.	B

EXAMINATION SECTION
TEST 1

DIRECTIONS: Each question or incomplete statement is followed by several suggested answers or completions. Select the one that BEST answers the question or completes the statement. *PRINT THE LETTER OF THE CORRECT ANSWER IN THE SPACE AT THE RIGHT.*

1. *What* conceptual model of psychiatric care is PRIMARILY concerned with etiology, pathogenesis, signs and symptoms, differential diagnosis, treatment, and prognosis?

    A. Biological
    B. Psychological
    C. Behavioral
    D. Social
    E. Eclectic

    1. _A_

2. During *what* phase of the life cycle is the problem of immaturity the greatest?

    A. Toddlerhood
    B. Oedipal phase
    C. Latency
    D. Adolescense
    E. Adulthood

    2. _C_

3. *When* is couples group therapy indicated? *When*

    A. their relationship does not appear to be the problem of greatest priority
    B. the couple is not emotionally committed to working out their differences
    C. the problems are experienced both within and outside the marriage
    D. the problems are acute and ego-alien
    E. problems are long-standing and ego-syntonic

    3. _E_

4. *What* is the *most usual* method of medical treatment of schizophrenia?

    A. Reserpine
    B. Thioxanthenes
    C. Phenothiazine
    D. Butyrophenones
    E. Meprobamate

    4. _C_

5. *Which* of the following BEST describes how the nurse should deal with manic patients? *With*

    A. enthusiasm
    B. encouraging support
    C. a reassuring manner that reduces anxiety
    D. understanding
    E. quiet calmness

    5. _E_

6. *Which* of the following is NOT a good technique for the nurse dealing with a patient with hysteria? The nurse should

    A. always refer to the condition by its proper name
    B. not accuse the patient of pretending to be sick
    C. not treat the patient as if the condition was an organic disorder
    D. have an optimistic attitude toward the patient's recovery
    E. encourage participation in ward activities

    6. _A_

7. *Which* of the following defense mechanisms of the ego are *especially characteristic* of obsessional patients?   7. B

      I.   Reaction formation
      II.   Isolation
      III.   Undoing
      IV.   Projection
      V.   Repression
The CORRECT answer is:

   A. I, IV   B. I, II, III   C. II, III, V
   D. II, V   E. I, III, V

8. *Which* of the following is NOT a good interviewing technique?   8. C

   A. A direct approach should be used
   B. Double-edged questions should be avoided
   C. Asking irrelevant questions makes for a good opening
   D. The patient should be allowed to take the initiative
   E. The patient should be allowed to progress at his own pace

9. Nursing management of manipulative behavior involves   9. C

   A. not trying to control the behavior
   B. looking for the situation that has triggered the symptom
   C. understanding the meaning of the behavior and assessing how the patient under-stands it
   D. teaching the patient some of the social skills of how people develop relationships
   E. allotting as much time as possible to the patient in order to help him express his feelings

10. *Which* of the following techniques are *most effective* in interrupting children's hostile behavior in a treatment center?   10. B

      I.   Verbal or physical limits
      II.   Intervening technique
      III.   Removing the cause of the hostility
      IV.   Threatening the loss of privileges
      V.   Ignoring the behavior
The CORRECT answer is:

   A. I, III, V   B. I, II, III   C. I, IV, V
   D. II, III, V   E. I, III, IV

11. All of the following are behavior disorders in adults, termed oral behavior, EXCEPT   11. C

   A. impulsive greed
   B. clinging and demanding behavior
   C. cleanliness or dirtiness
   D. deep feelings of internal division
   E. distrust and reactive rage

12. All of the following are important guidelines for the nurse's notes EXCEPT: 12. E

   A. Avoid lengthy notes
   B. Use the patient's own words

C. Avoid interpretations
D. Answer the four "w's"
E. Avoid the use of technical terminology

13. *Which* of the following are factors indicating high risk or vulnerability to schizophrenia?   13. B
   I. Hyperactivity in the preschool age
   II. Unsocialized aggression among boys and overinhibited hyperconformity among girls during high school
   III. Presence of intimate peer relationships during early adolescense
   IV. Evidence of neuropathology under age 11
   V. Disorganized, disruptive families

The CORRECT answer is:

A. I, II, IV   B. II, IV, V   C. I, II, III
D. I, III, V   E. All of the above

14. *Which* of the following techniques should the nurse use in working with individual   14. B
depressed patients? She *should*

A. be aggressively cheerful
B. indicate the patient's good prognosis
C. push the patient toward making decisions
D. always give elaborate encouragement
E. try to convince the patient that his depression is unjustified by the reality of his life situation

15. *How* does the nurse help the patient re-establish a level of good functioning that has   15. C
been lost to the illness? Through

A. exploratory work   B. direct advice
C. support   D. comradeship bonds
E. education

16. *What* conceptual model of psychiatric care consists of clarifying the psychological mean-   16. B
ing of events, feelings, and behaviors?

A. Biological   B. Psychological
C. Behavioral   D. Social
E. Eclectic

17. During *what* phase of the life cycle is the individual MOST vulnerable to despair?   17. E

A. Oedipal phase   B. Latency
C. Adolescence   D. Adulthood
E. Older adulthood

18. *Which* of the following is used to treat serious depression when drug therapy has failed?   18. A

A. Electroconvulsive therapy
B. Insulin treatment
C. Psychosurgery
D. Hydrotherapy
E. Hypnotic-sedative drugs

19. The psychiatric nurse's responsibility in dispensing medication is   19. _A_

    A. to know the reactions and side effects of the drug
    B. to regulate the dosage
    C. to determine a proper dosage schedule
    D. to keep the patient ignorant of the drugs he is receiving
    E. All of the above

20. *What* should the nurse's reaction be to a manic patient's loud jokes and crude pranks?   20. _E_
She *should*

    A. react with studied prudishness
    B. acknowledge the hilarity
    C. chastise the patient
    D. put restraints on the patient
    E. react with silence, ignoring it

21. *Which* of the following defense mechanisms of the ego is *most pronounced* in paranoid   21. _E_
conditions in which there is an actual break with reality?

    A. Displacement   B. Sublimation
    C. Isolation   D. Regression
    E. Projection

22. *Which* of the following verbal responses is the *most useful* to the therapeutic process?   22. _D_
The _____ response.

    A. evaluative   B. reassuring
    C. probing   D. understanding
    E. hostile

23. *Which* of the following are qualities that distinguish the schizophrenic from the non-   23. _D_
schizophrenic?
    I. A diminished capacity to experience pleasure
    II. A strong tendency to be dependent on others
    III. Awareness that there is a disturbance in mental functioning
    IV. A noteworthy impairment in social competence
    V. Partial loss of adaptation
The CORRECT answer is:

    A. I, II, III   B. I, III, IV   C. I, IV, V
    D. I, II, V   E. II, III, IV

24. An overwhelming number of emotional problems in children are related to   24. _A_
    I. faulty training and faulty life experiences
    II. surface conflicts between children and parents
    III. deeper conflicts within the child
    IV. a difficulty associated with physical handicaps and disorders
    V. difficulties associated with severe mental disorders
The CORRECT answer is:

    A. I, II   B. I, III   C. III, V
    D. II, IV   E. I, IV

25. Strong unconscious feelings of guilt and hostility are *particularly common* in patients with   25. _A_

    A. obsessions
    B. compulsion
    C. phobias
    D. hysteria
    E. hypochondria

26. Adults who withdraw into schizoid and depressive states frequently fail to   26. _D_

    A. resolve the conflict of autonomy vs. shame and doubt
    B. resolve the oedipus complex
    C. master the task of industry
    D. develop basic trust during infancy
    E. establish an identity during adolescence

27. All of the following are defined as antipsychotic or major tranquilizers EXCEPT   27. _C_

    A. Reserpine
    B. Phenothiazines
    C. Tricyclics
    D. Thioxanthenes
    E. Butyrophenones

28. The population felt to be of high risk or vulnerable to schizophrenia are *usually* the children of   28. _E_

    A. disorganized, disruptive families
    B. homosexuals
    C. alcoholics
    D. manic depressives
    E. schizophrenics

29. *Which* of the following is *least likely* to make a suicide attempt?   29. _C_

    A. The patient with a history of suicide attempts
    B. Members of the patient's family having a history of suicide attempts
    C. Patients who obsessively fear that they will commit suicide
    D. Patients who write suicide notes
    E. Patients who have access to suicidal agents

30. The nurse can communicate *move effectively* with small children by   30. _E_

    A. using simple sentences
    B. being specific
    C. being enthusiastic
    D. reflecting feeling tones
    E. all of the above

31. *What* conceptual mode of psychiatric care is more concerned with treating the overt systems (the learned behavior) and not the secondary manifestations of disease or unconscious conflict?   31. _C_

    A. Biological
    B. Psychological
    C. Behavioral
    D. Social
    E. Eclectic

32. The *most helpful* attitude a nurse should have during the therapeutic process is to be _____ the patient.   32. B

    A. reassuring to   B. supportive of
    C. sympathetic to   D. understanding of
    E. a friend to

33. *Which* is the BEST way to treat depression?   33. E

    A. The nurse helps the patient to bear the feelings he doesn't want to bear alone
    B. The nurse helps the patient resolve the feelings that brought on the depression
    C. The nurse encourages the patient to express negative feelings
    D. The nurse teaches the patient how to get the ego supplies he wants
    E. There is no single way to treat depression

34. *Which* of the following psychological disturbances are accompanied by the HIGHEST suicide rate?   34. C

    A. Pick's disease   B. Alzheimer's disease
    C. Huntington's chorea   D. Korsakoff's syndrome
    E. Senile dementia

35. *Which* of the following *should not be displayed* in explaining an anxiety state to the patient?   35. C

    A. Anxiousness
    B. Emotional tension
    C. Nervousness
    D. Wave of emotional tension
    E. Period of anxiousness

36. *What* occurs during the period of development called latency? The   36. D

    A. adolescent gains independence from the family and integrates new-found sexual maturity
    B. individual enters in an involved, reciprocal way with others sexually, occupationally, and socially
    C. child has a growing cognitive ability with the capacity to conceptualize and internalize relationships
    D. child enters into the first major social system outside the family
    E. child experiments with autonomy

37. *How should* the psychiatric nurse handle direct questions from the patient? The nurse should answer   37. D

    A. all questions to substantiate her professional credentials
    B. questions dealing with her personal life
    C. questions about the patient's illness
    D. questions about her behavior that the patient has observed
    E. all questions honestly

38. *What* is the main symptom of hebephrenic schizophrenia?   38. A

    A. The inappropriate affect of the person
    B. The total back of any substantial relationships

C. Abnormal and postural movements
D. Delusions and extreme suspiciousness
E. Undifferentiated symptoms

39. *What* causes neuroses?   39. _B_

A. Depression   B. Emotional turmoil
C. Self-preoccupation   D. Withdrawal
E. Guilt

40. All of the following are good techniques for the nurse dealing with adolescents on psychi- 40. _D_
atric service EXCEPT:

A. She should listen to complaints and criticisms with interest
B. She should use some of the adolescent's jargon
C. The relationship should develop at a rate the adolescent feels comfortable with
D. A social relationship should be developed between nurse and patient
E. Infractions of rules generally should be ignored

41. During what period is narcissim at its height? Between _____ years.   41. _B_

A. 1-2   B. 3-6   C. 7-12
D. 13-19   E. 21-35

42. *Which* of the following is the *most effective* anti-depressant medication?   42. _B_

A. Reserpine   B. Tricyclics
C. Thioxanthenes   D. Miltown
E. Paraldehyde

43. The role of the psychiatric nurse in the care and milieu management of a person who has 43. _D_
a thought disorder *must be*

A. supportive   B. understanding
C. sympathetic   D. flexible
E. rigid

44. *How should* a psychiatric nurse respond when a delusional patient fearfully tells her that 44. _E_
people are waiting outside the hospital to kill him?

A. "You don't have to worry because you are safe here."
B. "You know as well as I do that no one is trying to kill you."
C. "You should go to occupational therapy to take your mind off your fears."
D. "You should rest now and, when you wake up, I'm certain you'll feel less afraid."
E. "I understand how frightened you feel but when you are better you will see things in
a different way."

45. *Which* of the following is a *proper* attitude toward a neurotic patient? The nurse *should* 45. _D_

A. respond emotionally to the patient's behavior
B. pass judgment on the patient
C. express her own feelings and opinions
D. place realistic limits on the patient's behavior
E. not reassure the patient

46. *What* should the psychiatric nurse do when she notices herself becoming tense, rigid, and stilted and wishing that she felt more professional? She *should*   46. A

   A. worry less about trying too hard to follow the book and the prescribed rules, and concentrate on being natural
   B. assay the scope of her judgmental feelings and keep them in check so they do not interfere with the therapeutic process
   C. talk over her feelings with a staff member or supervisor
   D. take time to listen to the patient's requests and his perception of the situation
   E. realize that she is not expected to have all the answers to patients' situations and should consult with her colleagues

47. *What* is the *focus* of behavior therapy? The patient's   47. B

   A. thoughts
   B. overt behavior that is presenting the problem
   C. feelings
   D. behavior
   E. socialization problems

48. *What* is the *most prominent* symptom of senile dementia?   48. D

   A. An impaired time sense ·
   B. Disorientation
   C. Difficulty with abstract reasoning
   D. Impairment in the ability to retain and recall information
   E. Difficulty in identifying people

49. Psychiatric hospitalization is HIGHEST *among*   49. D

   A. single people
   B. married people
   C. widowed people
   D. divorced people
   E. Marital status has not proved to be a factor

50. *Which* of the following is TRUE of the organization of group psychotherapy?   50. B

   A. Divergent age, social and economic backgrounds should be represented
   B. Members should have similar problems
   C. Sexes should be separated into different groups
   D. Active and inactive members should be separated into different groups
   E. Members should be chosen at random

KEY (CORRECT ANSWERS)

1.	A	11.	C	21.	E	31.	C	41.	B
2.	C	12.	E	22.	D	32.	B	42.	B
3.	E	13.	B	23.	D	33.	E	43.	D
4.	C	14.	B	24.	A	34.	C	44.	E
5.	E	15.	C	25.	A	35.	C	45.	D
6.	A	16.	B	26.	D	36.	D	46.	A
7.	B	17.	E	27.	C	37.	D	47.	B
8.	C	18.	A	28.	E	38.	A	48.	D
9.	C	19.	A	29.	C	39.	B	49.	D
10.	B	20.	E	30.	E	40.	D	50.	B

EXAMINATION SECTION
TEST 1

DIRECTIONS: Each question or incomplete statement is followed by several suggested answers or completions. Select the one that BEST answers the question or completes the statement. *PRINT THE LETTER OF THE CORRECT ANSWER IN THE SPACE AT THE RIGHT.*

Questions 1-9.

DIRECTIONS: Questions 1 through 9 are to be answered on the basis of the following information.

Ms. Evelyn Hart, a 75-year-old widow, is admitted to a psychiatric hospital. Her son, who brings her, says that she has been confused and wandered away from home. Also, she has become increasingly careless about her appearance.

1. With a chronic brain syndrome such as Ms. Hart's, the personality changes are MOST often manifested as.

    A. an exaggeration of previous traits
    B. overt pleas for assistance
    C. suspicion and reticence
    D. marked resistance and negativism

2. During the early period following Ms. Hart's admission, the nursing procedure that would be BEST for her is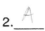

    A. carrying out activities in the same order each day
    B. insisting that she focus her conversation on present events
    C. providing a variety of novel experiences
    D. rotating staff assignments so that she will become acquainted with each member of the nursing staff

3. When Ms. Hart's son comes to visit her the day after admission, Ms. Hart refuses to talk to him. The son goes to the nurse and says, *My mother won't talk to me. Why is she acting like this? I had to do something with her. I couldn't keep her with us. Oh, what a mess!* Which of these responses by the nurse would be MOST appropriate initially?

    A. You feel guilty about having your mother here.
    B. Your mother is having a little difficulty adjusting to the hospital.
    C. This is a difficult situation for you and your mother.
    D. I'm sure you did the best you could under the circumstances.

4. Ms. Hart's son asks the nurse whether he should come to see his mother again on the following day in view of her reaction to his first visit.
Which of these responses would be BEST?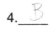

    A. Advising the son to wait until his mother gives some indication that she is ready to see him
    B. Suggesting that the son come back the next day since his continuing interest is important to his mother

C. Telling the son that his mother will not miss him if he doesn't visit because she will become attached to staff members

D. Informing the son that it is important for his mother to have visitors and suggesting that he ask one of her friends to visit her

5. The nurse finds Ms. Hart standing near the lavatory door. She has wet herself - as she does occasionally - because she does not allow herself sufficient time to reach the bathroom. Ms. Hart looks ashamed and turns her head away from the nurse.
Which of these responses by the nurse would be BEST?

    5. _B_

A. Asking, *Can you tell me why you wait so long, Ms. Hart?*
B. Saying, *I know that this is upsetting to you, Ms. Hart. Come with me and I'll get a change of clothes for you*
C. Asking, *Can you think of any way in which we can help you to manage your bathroom trips, Ms. Hart?*
D. Sending Ms. Hart to her room to change her clothing

6. At about 3 P.M. one day, Ms. Hart comes to the nurse and says, *I haven't had a thing to eat all day.* The nurse knows that Ms. Hart did have lunch.
Which of these understandings by the nurse should be BASIC to a response?

    6. _D_

A. Confabulation is used by elderly patients as a means of relieving anxiety.
B. Hunger is symbolic of a feeling of deprivation.
C. Retrospective falsification is a mechanism commonly used by elderly persons who are unhappy.
D. Loss of memory for recent events is characteristic of patients with senile dementia.

7. Ms. Hart is to be encouraged to increase her intake of protein.
The addition of which of these foods to 100 cc. of milk will provide the GREATEST amount of protein?

    7. _B_

A. 50 cc. light cream and 2 tablespoons corn syrup
B. 30 grams powdered skim milk and 1 egg
C. 1 small scoop (90 grams) vanilla ice cream and 1 tablespoon chocolate syrup
D. 2 egg yolks and 1 tablespoon sugar

8. One day when another patient, Mr. Simon, is about to go to the canteen, Ms. Hart says to him, *Bring me a candy bar.* Mr. Simon replies, *Okay, give me the twenty-five cents for it.* Ms. Hart struggles with the idea, taking out a quarter and holding it but not giving it to Mr. Simon. Mr. Simon goes off impatiently, and Ms. Hart looks forlorn.
Which of these responses by the nurse would probably be MOST useful to Ms. Hart?

    8. _B_

A. Ms. Hart, when we get things from the canteen, we have to pay for them. Do you want to buy candy?
B. It was hard for you to decide whether or not to give Mr. Simon the money for the candy. Let's go to the canteen together.
C. I know you are upset about Mr. Simon's going off, but he did have a right to ask you for the money for the candy.
D. You feel you annoyed Mr. Simon. Would you like to talk about it?

9. Ms. Hart tells stories over and over about her childhood. One day she keeps talking   9. _A_
about holidays and how she used to make cookies for visiting children.
Which of the responses by the nurse would be BEST?

    A. That must have been a lot of fun, Ms. Hart. Will you help us make popcorn balls for
the unit party?
    B. I can understand that those things were important to you, Ms. Hart. Now we can
talk about something that is going on in the unit.
    C. Things are different now, Ms. Hart. What does your family serve as party refresh-
ments nowadays?
    D. Those were the good old days. Did you ever go on a hayride?

Questions 10-17.

DIRECTIONS: Questions 10 through 17 are to be answered on the basis of the following information.

    Mr. David Tripp, 28 years old, is brought from his place of work to the emergency depart-
ment of a local general hospital by the police. He had been threatening his supervisor, who
had criticized his work. During the admission procedure, he says, *They're all in on the plot to
lock me up so I can't protect the world from them.*

10. During the early period of Mr. Tripp's hospitalization, which of these plans of care would   10. _D_
probably be BEST for him?

    A. Encourage him to enter into simple group activities.
    B. Establish a daily routine that will help him become oriented to this new environ-
ment.
    C. Plan to cope with his slowness in carrying out his daily schedule.
    D. Assign the same members of the nursing team to care for him each day.

11. Mr. Tripp is on chlorpromazine hydrochloride (Thorazine) 100 mg. t.i.d. and 200 mg. at   11. _C_
h.s.
The CHIEF purpose of chlorpromazine for Mr. Tripp is to

    A. relieve his anxiety
    B. control his aggression
    C. decrease his psychotic symptoms
    D. alleviate his depression

12. Mr. Tripp is walking into the dayroom when a male patient runs toward him screaming,   12. _B_
Let me out! Let me out! A nurse's aide is following the screaming patient and is talking
soothingly to him. Mr. Tripp seems panic-stricken and turns to flee.
Which of these initial responses to Mr. Tripp by the nurse would be BEST?

    A. Don't go, Mr. Tripp. That patient won't hurt you. He is frightened.
    B. It is upsetting to hear someone scream. The aide will help that patient. I will stay
with you for a while, Mr. Tripp.
    C. Don't be upset, Mr. Tripp. That patient is sicker than you are. It's all right for you to
go to your room if you like.
    D. This is nothing to be disturbed about, Mr. Tripp. It is part of that patient's illness.

13. One afternoon, Mr. Tripp is sitting in a small lounge watching a TV news program. During   13. _A_
a biographical sketch of a criminal, Mr. Tripp begins to shout frantically, No, I am not one!
You've no right to say that! Mr. Tripp's response to the program is MOST clearly an example of

    A. an idea of reference   B. an obsession
    C. confabulation   D. negativism

14. Mr. Tripp seems to value his regular sessions with the nurse, but on one occasion he   14. _A_
becomes agitated and suddenly gets up and starts to mumble and pace back and forth.
Which of these actions by the nurse would be BEST when Mr. Tripp does this?

    A. Sit quietly, while remaining attentive to him.
    B. Join him and pace with him.
    C. Leave the room until he calms down.
    D. Get a male nurse's aide to come and stand by and observe Mr. Tripp.

15. Mr. Tripp, who has read widely in the field of psychology, quotes fluently from various   15. _C_
authorities with whose works the nurse is only vaguely acquainted.
Which of these actions by the nurse in this situation would probably be BEST?

    A. Make an attempt to learn more about psychology in order to be able to converse
with Mr. Tripp.
    B. Point out to Mr. Tripp that such theoretical knowledge is of little value unless it is
applied in daily life.
    C. Listen attentively, in a relaxed manner, without attempting to compete with Mr.
Tripp.
    D. Ask Mr. Tripp if he understands why he feels the need to give evidence of his
knowledge of psychology.

16. Mr. Tripp is much improved and is to go home for a weekend. Since he is taking chlorpro-   16. _D_
mazine hydrochloride (Thorazine), he should be given information regarding side-effects
such as

    A. loss of pubic hair and weight gain
    B. agranulocytosis and nausea
    C. gastrointestinal bleeding and gynecomastia
    D. susceptibility to sunburn and potentation of alcohol

17. One day Mr. Tripp remarks to the nurse, *Now that I can concentrate move, I can probably*   17. _C_
hold down a job when I'm discharged from the hospital.
Which of these responses by the nurse would probably be MOST appropriate?

    A. Don't you expect to go back to your old job, Mr. Tripp?
    B. You have improved, Mr. Tripp, but you must be careful not to take on too much.
    C. Have you thought of something you might like to do, Mr. Tripp?
    D. There are agencies that will find work for you when you are ready, Mr. Tripp.

Questions 18-25.

DIRECTIONS: Questions 18 through 25 are to be answered on the basis of the following information.

Ms. Nancy Balm, a 20-year-old former music student, is admitted to a psychiatric hospital. Six months after entering school, she was dismissed for engaging in drug parties and
sexual orgies in the dormitory. She has also been involved in the theft of a car and in several
minor traffic violations. Ms. Balm has grown up in a permissive atmosphere with few controls.

18.   After a few days, it is noted that Ms. Balm frequently seeks the attention of one of the   18. __C__
female nurses; Ms. Balm calls her by her first name, offers to help her with her work, and
frequently tells her that she is the nicest person on the unit.
Based on Ms. Balm's history, it is probably MOST justifiable to say that she

A.   has developed the capacity to be concerned about other people
B.   is asking for help from this nurse
C.   is attempting to use this nurse for her own purposes
D.   genuinely likes this nurse

19.   Ms. Balm is on a locked unit. A new nurse on the unit is about to leave and is holding the   19. __B__
key. Ms. Balm approaches, saying eagerly, *Let me turn the key and unlock the door. The
other nurses let me.*
Which response by the nurse would be MOST appropriate?

A.   Going to the nurse in charge to ask if Ms. Balm's request should be granted
B.   Telling Ms. Balm in a friendly way that this is not permissible
C.   Letting Ms. Balm turn the key in the lock but keeping close to her while she does it
D.   Asking Ms. Balm why she feels that it is important for her to turn the key

20.   One day Ms. Balm talks with the nurse about the events that led up to her hospitalization.   20. __A__
She volunteers the information that she had stolen a car.
Considering the kind of illness she has, which additional comment that she might
make would probably BEST indicate her basic attitude?

A.   I wanted a new sportscar, and that one was just what I had been looking for, so I
took it.
B.   For a long time, I had wanted to steal a car but had been able to control my desire,
but finally it overpowered me.
C.   I knew it was wrong to steal a car, but my friend dared me to.
D.   Once I had driven away in the car, I was sorry I had taken it.

21.   At unit parties, Ms. Balm frequently dances with an elderly man who has chronic brain   21. __D__
syndrome. She is courteous to him, though somewhat condescending. The elderly
patient receives the attention happily.
It would be CORRECT for staff members to make which of these evaluations about
this situation?

A.   Ms. Balm should not be permitted to dance with the elderly patient.
B.   Personnel should let Ms. Balm know that they are aware she is using this means to
get approval.
C.   The elderly patient will terminate their relationship if he ceases to obtain pleasure
from it.
D.   The activity need not be interrupted as long as both Ms. Balm and the elderly
patient receive satisfaction from it.

177

22. A young male nurse who works with Ms. Balm has been going to the unit in the evening   22. A
to see her. When questioned about this, the nurse states that he is fond of Ms. Balm.
It would be ESSENTIAL for the nurse to recognize that

    A. his emotional involvement with Ms. Balm may interfere with his therapeutic effec-
tiveness
    B. Ms. Balm's emotional involvement with him may interfere with her progress
    C. hospital policy prohibits romantic relationships between patients and nurses
    D. Ms. Balm may prove so demanding that he will drop the relationship, thus trauma-
tizing her

23. When Ms. Balm's parents come to see her, they berate her for disgracing them, but they   23. D
demand special privileges for her from the staff.
It is probably MOST justified to say that they

    A. are unable to express their love directly to their daughter
    B. feel protective toward their daughter
    C. feel that a permissive environment would be better for their daughter
    D. have conflicting feelings about their daughter

24. Several patients are in the dayroom singing with a piano accompaniment. Ms. Balm   24. B
enters and interrupts the group by turning on the television set. In addition to turning off
the television set, which of these responses by the nurse would be MOST appropriate?

    A. Ask Ms. Balm if she would like to lead the group singing.
    B. Tell Ms. Balm that she cannot use the television while the group is singing and offer
her a choice of some other activities.
    C. Tell Ms. Balm that she can watch television later.
    D. Tell Ms. Balm that she cannot stay in the dayroom if she continues to disturb the
group.

25. Several weeks after Ms. Balm's admission, a group of patients who have written a play   25. D
for a hospital party ask her to read the script because they know she had a story printed
in the hospital newspaper. Ms. Balm agrees to do so and makes several good suggestions to the group, but does not try to assume control of the project.
It is MOST justifiable to say that she is

    A. expressing a need to be liked
    B. indifferent to this project
    C. using a new method of manipulating the group
    D. showing improvement

KEY (CORRECT ANSWERS)

1.	A	11.	C
2.	A	12.	B
3.	C	13.	A
4.	B	14.	A
5.	B	15.	C
6.	D	16.	D
7.	B	17.	C
8.	B	18.	C
9.	A	19.	B
10.	D	20.	A

21. D
22. A
23. D
24. B
25. D

TEST 2

DIRECTIONS: Each question or incomplete statement is followed by several suggested answers or completions. Select the one that BEST answers the question or completes the statement. *PRINT THE LETTER OF THE CORRECT ANSWER IN THE SPACE AT THE RIGHT.*

Questions 1-9.

DIRECTIONS: Questions 1 through 9 are to be answered on the basis of the following information.

Andrew Miles, 18 years old and living away from home for the first time, is a freshman in college. He is admitted to the hospital because he has been having episodes in which he runs about, screams, and then drops to the floor and lies motionless for a few minutes, after which he gets up, mumbles *I'm sorry,* and behaves normally. His school record has been satisfactory, but his contacts with his peer group have decreased greatly because of these episodes. On the basis of diagnostic studies, it has been determined that Mr. Miles' illness is schizophrenia, catatonic type.

1. Stereotyped behavior such as that shown by Mr. Miles can be BEST explained as a(n)   1. D

    A. way of assuring predictability
    B. device to gain help and treatment
    C. means of increasing interpersonal distance
    D. attempt to control inner and outer forces

2. The behavior demonstrated by patients such as Mr. Miles is USUALLY thought to be indicative of   2. B

    A. damage to the cortex of the brain
    B. an expression of intrapersonal conflict
    C. a deficiency of vitamin B complex in the diet
    D. a disturbance in intellectual functioning

3. Upon Mr. Miles' admission, his needs would BEST be met by a plan that provides   3. B

    A. an introduction to each member of the staff
    B. a climate that makes few demands on him
    C. minimal sensory stimulation
    D. time for him to reflect on his problems without interference

4. The day after Mr. Miles' admission, a nurse, Ms. Caan, is assigned to stay with him for a   4. A
period every day in order to establish a therapeutic nurse-patient relationship.
In carrying out this assignment, it is ESSENTIAL for this nurse to understand that Mr. Miles will probably

    A. be extremely sensitive to the feeling tones of others
    B. be unaware of the nurse's presence
    C. be hostile and verbally abusive
    D. talk if the nurse introduces topics that are of interest to him

5. Which of these insights that Mr. Miles might gain would be MOST basic to his improvement?

    A. Introjection of parental standards in childhood contributed to my personality.
    B. I am a person of worth and value.
    C. My behavior interferes with the development of good relationships.
    D. I require more reassurance than most people do.

5. B

6. One day a nurse finds Mr. Miles and another young male patient.having an argument in the lounge. The other patient says, *Don't criticize me, you phony. You and your fits!* The other patient is pressing the argument, and Mr. Miles has run behind a chair.
Which of these measures by the nurse would probably be BEST?

    A. Attempting to find out who started the argument
    B. Firmly directing each patient to go to his room
    C. Engaging the attention of the dominant patient
    D. Explaining to the other patient that Mr. Miles cannot control his spells

6. C

7. Mr. Miles now carries on brief conversations with Ms. Caan. During one such conversation, he seems relaxed and affable initially but soon begins to shift his position frequently, grasping the arms of his chair so tightly that his fingers blanch. Ms. Caan remarks to Mr. Miles that he seems tense, to which he replies *Yes*.
Which of these responses by the nurse at this time would demonstrate the BEST understanding?

    A. I'm beginning to feel tense too, Mr. Miles.
    B. I wonder if I have said something wrong, Mr. Miles.
    C. Do women usually make you feel nervous, Mr. Miles.
    D. At what point in our talk did you begin to feel uneasy, Mr. Miles?

7. D

8. When Ms. Caan tells Mr. Miles that she will be off duty for two days, he says flatly, *So what. It doesn't matter.* It is MOST accurate to say that Mr. Miles is

    A. incapable of manifesting emotion
    B. confident of his ability to manage without the nurse
    C. controlling expression of his feelings
    D. apathetic toward the nurse

8. C

9. Family therapy is recommended for Mr. Miles. When explaining the purpose of this type of therapy to Mr. Miles' family, which of the following information would it be important to convey to them?

    A. Family members can reinforce the therapist's recommendations between sessions.
    B. Family members need advice in dealing with the identified patient's behavior.
    C. Joint treatment permits equal participation, eliminating anxieties that might otherwise lead to termination of treatment.
    D. Joint treatment alters family interaction, facilitating change in the behavior of the identified patient.

9. D

Questions 10-16.

DIRECTIONS: Questions 10 through 16 are to be answered on the basis of the following information.

Fifty-year-old Mr. Jack Dunn, accompanied by his wife, is brought to the emergency room by the police. He has been despondent because he was not promoted in his job. After calling his son to say goodbye, insisting that he was going to end it all, he locked himself in the bathroom, and the police were called to get him out. Mr. Dunn is admitted to the psychiatric unit.

10. Which of these interpretations of Mr. Dunn's behavior should serve as the basis for formulating his nursing care plan?
He

    A. wants to punish those around him
    B. is trying to manipulate his environment
    C. is attempting to get attention and sympathy
    D. is looking for relief from helplessness and hopelessness

10. ___D___

11. Which of these statements ACCURATELY assesses Mr. Dunn's potential for suicide?
His

    A. sex and present stress suggest a high risk, but the likelihood of suicide is low in his age group
    B. threat suggests that the risk of suicide is minor
    C. age, sex, and present stress suggest a high risk of suicide
    D. sex suggests a low risk since suicide occurs 30 times more often in females than in males

11. ___C___

12. Which of these occurrences would be MOST likely to result in an INCREASE in Mr. Dunn's suicidal thoughts?
His

    A. expressing hostility overtly before he is able to tolerate doing so
    B. entrance into a deeply retarded phase of depression
    C. being required to perform work in the kitchen
    D. being allowed to talk about his morbid ideas

12. ___A___

13. During a staff conference concerning Mr. Dunn's care, a young nursing student says, *Even though I know that* Mr. Dunn's condition requires time to respond to therapy, I feel discouraged when I'm with him. No matter what I do, he talks about his failures and makes no attempt to help himself.
The interpretation of the student's reaction to Mr. Dunn's behavior that is probably MOST justifiable is that the

    A. student's difficulty arises from an attitude of hopelessness toward older persons
    B. student feels that Mr. Dunn's condition is not remediable unless he is willing to help himself
    C. student has set up a failure situation that is detrimental to therapeutic usefulness to Mr. Dunn
    D. student's self-concept as a helping person is being threatened

13. ___D___

14. A nurse finds Mr. Dunn cutting his wrist with a razor blade.   14. _C_
    Which of these actions should the nurse take?

    A. Shout *Stop!* and then say, *Tell me what caused your despair.*
    B. Say, *Think of what it would do to your family!*
    C. Grab Mr. Dunn's arm to stop him and say, *I'm going to stay with you.*
    D. Say, *Why, Mr. Dunn! You've just begun to feel better and now look what you've done.*

15. Mr. Dunn seems improved and is sent home on a trial visit. He is then admitted to the   15. _B_
    intensive care unit for treatment for a self-inflicted gunshot wound in the chest. When he
    is somewhat improved, Mr. Dunn remarks, *Everyone here must think I'm some kind of freak.*
    Which of these responses would be MOST appropriate?

    A. None of us thinks that you are a freak.
    B. You feel that others are judging you.
    C. I understand that you were upset when this happened.
    D. What made you so desperate that you did a thing like this?

16. Mr. Dunn has improved and is discharged. A few days after Mr. Dunn returns to work,   16. _A_
    while he is talking with a co-worker, a number of things go wrong in the office. Mr. Dunn
    slams a book on the table and says, *Dammit!* The co-worker who is present is aware that
    Mr. Dunn has been mentally ill.
    Which of these actions on the part of the co-worker would be BEST?

    A. Wait for Mr. Dunn to cool off and then resume the discussion.
    B. Suggest that Mr. Dunn go home and remain there until he calms down.
    C. Urge Mr. Dunn to take his tranquilizers.
    D. Talk with Mr. Dunn about his particular need for controlling outbursts.

Questions 17-25.

DIRECTIONS: Questions 17 through 25 are to be answered on the basis of the following information.

Ms. Julia Warren, 53 years old and with no previous history of mental illness, is admitted to a private psychiatric hospital because of symptoms, including pacing, wringing her hands, moaning, beating her forehead, and saying, *I'm a terrible woman.* She has been unable to do her job as a bookkeeper and has had to have members of her family stay with her day and night.

17. The extent of the nurse's orientation of Ms. Warren to the hospital environment should be   17. _B_
    based CHIEFLY upon Ms. Warren's

    A. willingness to stay with the nurse
    B. ability to concentrate
    C. persistence in making demands on other patients
    D. acceptance of the need for hospitalization

18. During the acute phase of Ms. Warren's illness, it is ESSENTIAL that the nurse have the   18. __C__
ability to

    A. minimize stimuli in Ms. Warren's environment
    B. interest Ms. Warren in a variety of activities
    C. accept Ms. Warren's self-accusations
    D. strengthen Ms. Warren's intellectual defenses

19. Ms. Warren shows typical distress upon being informed of her impending electric convul-   19. __A__
sive therapy. Which understanding by the nurse would BEST serve as the basis for preparing Ms. Warren psychologically for it?

    A. Misinformation may be contributing to her anxiety.
    B. Emphasizing the safety of the procedure will reduce her fear.
    C. Knowing that most people have the same response is usually comforting.
    D. A high level of anxiety renders an individual more receptive to information given by
       helping persons.

20. Depressions of the type Ms. Warren has usually respond well to electric convulsive ther-   20. __D__
apy, but the consequent memory loss is quite disturbing.
The nurse can be MOST helpful to the patient who has such a loss of memory by

    A. engaging the patient in diversional activities
    B. reporting the problem to the physician
    C. explaining to the patient that other patients receiving this therapy also have this
       problem
    D. reassuring the patient repeatedly that this is an expected and temporary reaction

21. Which of the following defense mechanisms is MOST likely to be used by a person who   21. __A__
is as depressed as Ms. Warren?

    A. Turning against the self
    B. Projection
    C. Rationalization
    D. Displacement of instinctual aims

22. When Ms. Warren learns that occupational therapy has been ordered for her, she scoffs   22. __B__
at the idea, saying it is silly.
If Ms. Warren were to think all of the following thoughts regarding occupational therapy,
which one would be MOST acceptable to her?

    A. This is enjoyable.
    B. I'm helping to pay for my care.
    C. This keeps me from thinking about my failures.
    D. I didn't know that I was so creative,

23. Ms. Warren is assigned to group therapy. Which of these ideas would it be MOST desir-   23. __A__
able for each participant to gain?

    A. Each person's opinion is respected.
    B. Verbalization will help each individual to gain insight.
    C. Each member has a responsibility to other members of the group.
    D. The group work consists of analyzing each other's motivations.

24. Ms. Warren improves and goes out with her husband for the afternoon. That evening, a nurse finds Ms. Warren sitting by herself in the dayroom.
Which of these comments by the nurse would probably be BEST?

    A. Why are you so preoccupied, Ms. Warren?
    B. You look tired, Ms. Warren. Was your afternoon too much for you?
    C. You seem very quiet, Ms. Warren.
    D. You looked happier yesterday, Ms. Warren.

24.___C___

25. Ms. Warren is discharged. The day Ms. Warren goes back to work, Bob, a customer she has known for many years, comes in and says, *Hello there, Julia. Good to see you back! your boss told me that you were sick. What was wrong with you?* Which of these replies by Ms. Warren would indicate that she accepted her illness and has recovered?

    A. I was kind of mixed up for a while, Bob, but I'm all right now.
    B. I just didn't feel good, Bob. Old age coming on, I guess.
    C. I was just down in the dumps, Bob, but my doctor insisted that I go to the hospital. You know how they are.
    D. I'm glad to be back. What can I do for you, Bob?

25.___A___

KEY (CORRECT ANSWERS)

1.	D	11.	C
2.	B	12.	A
3.	B	13.	D
4.	A	14.	C
5.	B	15.	B
6.	C	16.	A
7.	D	17.	B
8.	C	18.	C
9.	D	19.	A
10.	D	20.	D

21. A
22. B
23. A
24. C
25. A

TEST 3

DIRECTIONS: Each question or incomplete statement is followed by several suggested answers or completions. Select the one that BEST answers the question or completes the statement. *PRINT THE LETTER OF THE CORRECT ANSWER IN THE SPACE AT THE RIGHT.*

Questions 1-7.

DIRECTIONS: Questions 1 through 7 are to be answered on the basis of the following information.

When Mark Levine, 5 1/2 years old, goes to school for the first time, he screams and seems terrified when he sees the drinking fountain near his classroom door. Mark's mother tells the school nurse that he has an intense fear of drinking fountains.

1. The understanding of Mark's fear of fountains that is MOST justifiable is that it   1. _B_

    A.   is a symptom common in dyslexic children
    B.   is not subject to his conscious control
    C.   stems from his lack of understanding of plumbing
    D.   results from having learned that his symptoms have a manipulative potential

2. Behavior therapy will be used in treating Mark's symptoms. His plan of care will include   2. _D_

    A.   authoritative instruction
    B.   increased cultural orientation
    C.   direct interpretations
    D.   systematic desensitization

3. Mark's behavior reflects his need to control anxiety by   3. _C_

    A.   refusing to recognize the source of his anxiety
    B.   making a conscious effort to avoid situations that cause anxiety
    C.   substituting a neutral object as the target of his negative feelings
    D.   acting in a manner opposite to his underlying need

4. Parents should be instructed that a child's mental health will BEST be promoted if the love he receives from his parents   4. _B_

    A.   is related to the child's behavior
    B.   is unconditional
    C.   makes externally imposed discipline unnecessary
    D.   is reinforced by unchanging physical demonstrations

5. Ms. Levine calls the community mental health clinic and tells the nurse that Mark has suddenly become terrified of getting into the family car, refuses to do so, and is in the yard screaming uncontrollably.
What would it be BEST for the nurse to tell Ms. Levine to do FIRST?   5. _A_

    A.   Hold Mark snugly and talk softly to him.
    B.   Give Mark a warm bath and put him to bed.
    C.   Bring Mark to the clinic as soon as possible.
    D.   Remind Mark that he has never before been afraid of automobiles.

6. Mark is having play therapy.
The choice of play therapy for children of Mark's age should PROBABLY be based upon their inability to

6. _D_

    A. overcome inhibitors about revealing family conflicts and behaviors
    B. differentiate between reality and fantasy
    C. recognize the difference between right and wrong
    D. adequately describe feelings and experience

7. On a rainy day, after Mark's play-therapy session, Ms. Levine hands Mark his overshoes and says, *Put them on. It's pouring outside.* Mark answers defiantly, *No, they're too hard to put on. I can't.* Then he sits down on a bench and pouts. Ms. Levine looks at the nurse in a perplexed way, saying nothing.
Which of these responses by the nurse would probably be BEST?

7. _B_

    A. Say to Ms. Levine, *Maybe the overshoes are too small to Mark.*
    B. Sit on the bench with Mark and say calmly, *It's raining. You start pulling your overshoes on, and I'll help you with the hard part.*
    C. Hand Mark his overshoes and say to him in a matter-of-fact way, *If you will put the first one one, I'll put on the second one for you.*
    D. Say to Mark, firmly but kindly, *You are trying to test your mother's authority. This behavior will not be tolerated. Put your overshoes on right now.*

Questions 8-14.

DIRECTIONS: Questions 8 through 14 are to be answered on the basis of the following information.

    Ms. Eileen Gray, 33 years old, is admitted to the psychiatric hospital with a diagnosis of obsessive-compulsive reaction. Her chief fear is that her excreta may harm others on the unit. As a result, she spends hours in the bathroom washing not only her hands, arms, vulva, and anal area, but also the walls, toilet, and toilet stall. In the process, she discards wet paper towels in every direction and leaves puddles of water everywhere.

8. Ms. Gray's symptoms are MOST clearly an example of

8. _C_

    A. sublimation of anxiety-producing fantasies and daydreams
    B. compensation for an imaginary object loss
    C. a symbolic expression of conflict and guilt feelings
    D. an infantile maneuver to avoid intimacy

9. On the unit, Ms. Gray carries out her elaborate washing routine several times a day. She says to the nurse, *I guess all this seems awfully silly to you.*
It is MOST justifiable to say that she

9. _C_

    A. is asking the nurse to keep her from performing these unreasonable acts
    B. really believes her acts are completely rational, and she is testing the nurse
    C. is indicating an appreciation of the unreasonable-ness of her behavior
    D. is deliberately putting the nurse in a difficult position

10. The nurse should understand that the probable effect of permitting Ms. Gray to perform   10. D
her washing routines will be to

    A.   confirm a basic delusion
    B.   help Ms. Gray to perceive how illogical her behavior is
    C.   create distrust of the nurse, who ought to symbolize reality
    D.   temporarily reduce Ms. Gray's anxiety

11. Ms. Gray is unable to get to the dining room in time for breakfast because of her washing   11. A
rituals.
During the early period of her hospitalization, it would be MOST appropriate to

    A.   wake Ms. Gray early enough so that she can perform her rituals in time to get to
breakfast
    B.   firmly insist that Ms. Gray interrupt her rituals at breakfast time
    C.   explain to Ms. Gray that her rituals are not helping her to get well
    D.   give Ms. Gray a choice between completing her rituals or going to breakfast

12. During a nursing team conference, staff members voice frustration concerning Ms.   12. B
Gray's constant questions such as *Shall I go to lunch or finish cleaning my room?* and
Should I go to O.T. or mend my coat?
In order to deal effectively with this behavior, team members should know that Ms.
Gray's

    A.   dependence upon staff is a symptom that needs to be interrupted by firm limit-set-
ting
    B.   inability to make decisions reflects her basic anxiety about failure
    C.   indecisiveness is meant to test the staff's acceptance of her
    D.   relentless need to seek attention represents a developmental arrest at the autistic
(prototaxic) level

13. Ms. Gray is being treated by psychotherapy. The physician tells the nurse to expect her to   13. C
be upset at times when she returns from her session with him and to let her be upset.
By this directive, the physician MOST probably wants to

    A.   put Ms. Gray under stress so that she will become more responsive to suggestions
    B.   teach Ms. Gray to be satisfied with advice from only one person
    C.   help Ms. Gray become aware of her feelings
    D.   make Ms. Gray independent, which would not be possible if she were to develop
alliances with members of the nursing staff

14. Ms. Gray is given her first pass to spend the night at home. As the time approaches for   14. B
her to leave the hospital, she seems increasingly tense and says, *Maybe I shouldn't stay
home all night. Maybe I should just stay for dinner and then come back here.* When the
nurse responds nondirectively, Ms. Gray answers, *I'm just sort of anxious about things in
general. It's nothing specific.*
Which of these responses by the nurse would probably be BEST?

    A.   Everyone is scared *of* his first overnight pass. You'll find that it will be easier than
you expect.
    B.   It's understandable that you are concerned about your first night at home. Would it
help if you make the decision after you've been home for a while and see how
things are going?

C. I know how you feel, but the staff think that you are well enough to stay home overnight. Won't you try to do so?
D. It's important for you to try to remain at home overnight. If you are able to do it, it will be a measure of your improvement.

Questions 15-25.

DIRECTIONS: Questions 15 through 25 are to be answered on the basis of the following information.

Ms. Kathy Collins, 47 years old, has been hospitalized several times over a period of years because of episodes of elation and depression. She lives with her mother and sister. She is well known to the nursing staff. While she is again being admitted, she is chainsmoking cigarettes, walking back and forth, and talking loudly and gaily about her romantic successes.

15. Which of these greetings by the nurse who is admitting Ms. Collins would probably be MOST appropriate?   15. B

    A. We're sorry you had to come back, Ms. Collins, but we are glad to see you.
    B. Good morning, Ms. Collins. Your doctor called to say you were coming. I will show you to your room.
    C. Hello, Ms. Collins. You're cheerful this morning.
    D. It's good to see you again, Ms. Collins. You don't seem to mind coming back to the hospital.

16. The nurse who will care for Ms. Collins each day should expect to make use of which of these interventions?   16. A

    A. Distracting and redirecting
    B. Orienting and reminding
    C. Explaining and praising
    D. Evoking anger and encouraging insight

17. Ms. Collins is an overactive patient with a mood disturbance rather than a thought disorder.   17. B
    Because of this type of illness, the nursing care plan should include measures that respond to the fact that she is

    A. disoriented
    B. easily stimulated by what is going on around her
    C. preoccupied with a single idea
    D. likely to be panicked by physical contact

18. Which of these nursing goals is likely to require the MOST attention while Ms. Collins is acutely ill?   18. C

    A. Orientation to time, place, and person
    B. Establishment of a sense of self-esteem
    C. Promotion of adequate rest
    D. Prevention of circulatory stasis

19. Ms. Collins and her roommate are in their room. While passing by, a registered nurse hears them arguing. Ms. Collins says, *You're a slob. How can anybody live in this mess!* The roommate answers, *What right do you have to say that?* and starts to cry. Which of these interventions by the nurse would be appropriate?

    A. Enter the room and say to Ms. Collins, *You have upset your roommate. She's crying.*
    B. Enter and say, *It sounds as if you are both upset.*
    C. Stand in the doorway and say, *It's part of your therapy to learn how to get along together.*
    D. Take the roommate aside and explain to her that Ms. Collins can be expected to be difficult for a few days.

19. B

20. Ms. Collins is not eating sufficient food. Which approach by the nurse would probably be BEST as a first step in trying to get her to eat more?

    A. Giving her foods that she can eat with her fingers while she is moving about
    B. Conveying to her tactfully the idea that she has to eat
    C. Serving her food to her on a tray and telling her firmly but kindly to eat
    D. Assuring her that she can have anything she wants to eat whenever she wants it

20. A

21. The physician orders lithium carbonate for Ms. Collins. To accompany the order for lithium carbonate, the physician is likely to specify that

    A. the patient should lie down for a half hour after each dose
    B. the medication should be evenly distributed throughout each 24-hour period
    C. a salt-free diet should be provided for the patient
    D. the drug level of the patient's blood should be monitored regularly

21. D

22. When their desires are frustrated, patients such as Ms. Collins are likely to

    A. maintain a superficial affability
    B. sulk and retire temporarily from the situation
    C. suddenly show hostility and aggression
    D. seek support from personnel

22. C

23. Group psychotherapy is ordered for Ms. Collins. The CHIEF purpose of this therapy is to help her to

    A. socialize easily with a group
    B. gain self-knowledge through the sharing of problems
    C. identify various types of emotional problems and ways in which people handle them
    D. become acquainted with types of problems that will be encountered after discharge

23. B

24. After several days, Ms. Collins' behavior changes, and she becomes depressed. One night the nurse finds Ms. Collins unconscious in bed with a strip of her sheet tied around her neck. She is cyanotic and her respirations are labored and stertorous. After loosening the constriction around Ms. Collins' neck and signaling for help, which of these actions by the nurse would demonstrate the BEST judgment?

    A. Remain with her.
    B. Place her in the proper position and start artificial respiration.

24. A

C. Give her a vigorous thump on the sternum.
D. Raise the foot of her bed.

25. Ms. Collins is gradually improving, and the team talks of plans for her discharge. 25. _D_
On a visit to the unit, Ms. Collins' mother and sister tell the nurse that Ms. Collins
doesn't seem much better, and they are very hesitant about having her return home
because of the previous problems they've had with her. Which of these actions should
INITIALLY be taken by the nurse?

A. Suggest that the family find a place where Ms. Collins can live by herself after discharge.
B. Elaborate on Ms. Collins' hospital regimen and the normality of her present behavior.
C. Assure the relatives that Ms. Collins is better and refer them to the physician if they have further questions.
D. Listen to Ms. Collins' relatives and suggest that they make an appointment with the family counselor.

KEY (CORRECT ANSWERS)

1.	B	11.	A
2.	D	12.	B
3.	C	13.	C
4.	B	14.	B
5.	A	15.	B
6.	D	16.	A
7.	B	17.	B
8.	C	18.	C
9.	C	19.	B
10.	D	20.	A

21.	D
22.	C
23.	B
24.	A
25.	D

LISTENING COMPREHENSION
EXAMINATION SECTION
TEST 1

DIRECTIONS: In this part a passage will be read orally to you. It is NOT written out in the test booklet so you will have to listen carefully. After the reading of the passage, you will answer the questions that follow. Each question or incomplete statement is followed by several suggested answers or completions. Select the one that BEST answers the question or completes the statement. *PRINT THE LETTER OF THE CORRECT ANSWER IN THE SPACE AT THE RIGHT.*

Listening Passage

(The following speech was delivered by Ronald Roskens at commencement exercises at the University of Nebraska, 1981.)

Thoreau tells us that dreams are the touchstones of our characters. As educated individuals we should understand that the impediments to realizing our aspirations often lie within ourselves. If we are content merely to accept what comes to us and to fashion a life which permits no challenges—mediocrity, or even failure, will be our lot. We will have killed our own dreams, and no matter how much we might have succeeded in the eyes of others, our accomplishments will not have approached the potential which lies within us.

Each of us is human, and the essence of that humanity is that we have, and will persistently exercise, the capacity to make mistakes, to be less than perfect. Human weaknesses are inevitably magnified when subjected to the harsh glare of public scrutiny. The shortcomings of one public official trigger a disregard for all elements of government. One practitioner fails, and an entire profession falls into disrepute.

The Hebrew prayerbook *Ethics of the Fathers* tells us:
> "There are seven marks of an uncultured man, and
> seven of a wise man. The wise man does not speak
> before him who is greater than he in wisdom; and
> does not break in upon the speech of his fellow;
> he is not hasty to answer; he questions according
> to the subject matter, and answers to the point;
> he speaks upon the first thing first, and upon the
> last last; regarding that which he has not under-
> stood he says, I do not understand it, and he
> acknowledges the truth. The reverse of all this
> is to be found in an uncultured man." (End of quote.)

Do you sense the seeds of such wisdom in yourselves? If you do, the University has passed this final examination. If you do not, I hope that you will have found at this University the foundation of such wisdom, and may take comfort in the fact that "learning never ends."

Whatever your answer, you will find that your time at the University has profoundly influenced you. You will, for the rest of your lives, play out your experiences here, even as we continue to reach out to you through your memories and in your skills.

Who is wise? All of us—if we continue to care about learning and learn about caring. For that is the essence of wisdom.

1. According to the speaker, we are frequently kept from reaching our goals by   1.____

   A. our own attitudes
   B. the lack of opportunity
   C. the frustrations of daily life
   D. the lack of education

2. According to this speech, a person's dreams can be destroyed only by   2.____

   A. society   B. passiveness
   C. wealth   D. pressure

3. The speaker says that it is in the nature of humans to   3.____

   A. be too ambitious   B. make errors
   C. distrust public officials   D. despair too easily

4. The speaker states that human weaknesses are inevitably magnified when they are   4.____

   A. questioned   B. acknowledged
   C. publicized   D. despised

5. According to the speaker, the effect of one practitioner's wrongdoings is to   5.____

   A. discredit the entire profession
   B. weaken the government
   C. lead to reform of social institutions
   D. encourage others to commit wrongs

6. The Hebrew prayerbook states that if a man is wise, he will never   6.____

   A. dispute an older person's opinion
   B. speak until spoken to
   C. leave the least important thing until last
   D. speak before someone wiser than he

7. When the Hebrew prayerbook says that a wise man "speaks upon the first things first,   7.____
   and upon the last last," it means that a wise man

   A. states simple things first
   B. saves the best for last
   C. knows the proper value of things
   D. waits for his turn to speak

8. According to the Hebrew prayerbook, the opposite of a wise man is   8.____

   A. an uneducated man   B. an uncultured man
   C. a simple man   D. an insensitive man

9. The speaker says that the University can continue to be valuable in life if one   9.____

   A. does well on final examinations
   B. returns to renew the experience
   C. accepts the truth
   D. remembers and uses what he has learned

10. The speaker says that the essence of wisdom is a combination of 10.____

    A. learning and caring
    B. education and experience
    C. character and ambition
    D. culture and truth

———

KEY (CORRECT ANSWERS)

1.	A	6.	D
2.	B	7.	C
3.	B	8.	B
4.	C	9.	D
5.	A	10.	A

———

TEST 2

DIRECTIONS: In this part a passage will be read orally to you. It is NOT written out in the test booklet so you will have to listen carefully. After the reading of the passage, you will answer the questions that follow. Each question or incomplete statement is followed by several suggested answers or completions. Select the one that BEST answers the question or completes the statement. *PRINT THE LETTER OF THE CORRECT ANSWER IN THE SPACE AT THE RIGHT.*

Listening Passage

(The following speech to a graduating class has been adapted from "Finding America" by George Hartzog.)

History mocks those who suggest that the past is wholly dreadful and ignoble.

It is from beachheads secured at great personal sacrifice by individuals and generations gone before that society has been able to find the higher ground. Each of our lives has been enriched by the works of a Gandhi, a Rembrandt, and a Woody Guthrie.

We must preserve the independence of the youthful spirit and the continuing values of the past. For every future is shaped by the past. Only in knowing the past may we judge wisely what is obsolete and what is not, what to discard and what to preserve.

Aristotle observed that youth has a long time before it and a short past behind: on the first day of one's life one has nothing at all to remember and can only look forward. By contrast, he added, the elderly live by memory rather than hope; for what is left to them of life is little compared with the long past.

The capacity to love and to cherish ideals with intransigent commitment is a marvelous trait of youth. On the other hand, the wisdom and earthbound experience that come with age are necessary balance wheels on the soaring fantasy, the untested ideas and the despair of youth.

As you set out to revise and rebuild the Establishment into which you are about to enter, I suggest that you do not deny your birthright; nor reject the proud heritage which is rightfully yours.

Today is your opportunity for greatness!
Go then. Build your houses of tomorrow.
In them may you experience a new quality of life.

1. Which phrase *most nearly* expresses the MAIN idea of this speech?   1.____

    A. A perspective of the past   B. The generation gap
    C. The ignoble past   D. Aristotle's legacy

2. An underlying principle of the speech seems to be that   2.____

    A. youth is more valuable than age
    B. knowledge is cumulative
    C. the present is identical to the past
    D. Greek philosophers had the answers

3. One specific benefit of the past which is referred to in the speech is   3.____

    A. land acquisition   B. the invention of printing
    C. artistic creation   D. judicial precedent

4. According to this speech, the value of the past is MOST beneficial in   4.____

    A. justifying old people's existence
    B. giving a sense of roots
    C. making reasonable judgments
    D. retaining everything that has been created

5. By quoting Aristotle, the author demonstrates his own belief that   5.____

    A. philosophy is the goal of age
    B. old people are wise
    C. young people are romantic
    D. the past enriches the present

6. According to Aristotle, the CHIEF asset of youth is   6.____

    A. hope   B. strength
    C. experience   D. the past

7. According to the speaker, the experiences of youth could be BEST described as   7.____

    A. new and tranquil   B. extreme and varied
    C. bright and wise   D. restrained and optimistic

8. The speaker indicates that the BEST approach to life for his audience is a   8.____

    A. concentration on the past
    B. reversal of the past
    C. blending of the past and present
    D. concentration on the future

9. The ideas in the speech are developed basically through the technique of   9.____

    A. comparing qualities   B. quoting authorities
    C. understanding suggestions   D. logical deductions

10. The overall tone of this speech can be BEST described as   10.____

    A. despondent   B. cynical
    C. cautious   D. optimistic

KEY (CORRECT ANSWERS)

1.	A	6.	A
2.	B	7.	B
3.	C	8.	C
4.	C	9.	A
5.	D	10.	D

TEST 3

DIRECTIONS: In this part a passage will be read orally to you. It is NOT written out in the test booklet so you will have to listen carefully. After the reading of the passage, you will answer the questions that follow. Each question or incomplete statement is followed by several suggested answers or completions. Select the one that BEST answer the question or completes the statement. *PRINT THE LETTER OF THE CORRECT ANSWER IN THE SPACE AT THE RIGHT.*

Listening Passage

(The following speech by Ray Billington has been adapted from "Cowboys, Indians, and the Land of Promise," *Representative American Speeches,* 1975-1976.)

The persuasive influence of the frontier image is nowhere better exhibited than by the cultists of other nations who try to recapture life in that never-never land of the past. In Paris, western addicts buy "outfits" at a store near the Arch of Triumph called the Western House and spend weekends at Camp Indian clad in Comanche headdresses.

All are responding to the image of the American West projected by twentieth-century films, novels, and television programs: a sun-drenched land of distant horizons, peopled largely by scowling bad men in black shirts, villainous Indians, and those Galahads of the Plains, the cowboys, glamorous in hip-hugging Levis and embroidered shirts, a pair of Colt revolvers worn low about the waist. A land, too, of the shoot-out, individual justice, and sudden death at the hand of lynch mobs. A few months ago an Israeli army psychologist, pleased that his country's soldiers did not use their guns when on leave, expressed delight that "There is no shooting like in the Wild West."

That such an image should be popular today is easy to understand. To empathize with a make-believe land of masculinity and self-realization is to forget momentarily the monotony of a standardized machine civilization, to escape the uncertainties of a turbulent world, and to recapture an unregimented past. The vogue of a "Western" cult demonstrates a universal urge to lessen the controls necessary in today's societies.

1. By his word choice, the speaker suggests that the French buy cowboy outfits in order to   1._____

   A. enjoy a fantasy world
   B. express strong anti-Indian feelings
   C. have a better concept of the American West
   D. relive their own past glory

2. Which are the major sources of the popular frontier image?   2._____

   A. American myths   B. Mass media
   C. Travel brochures   D. Historical accounts

3. In this speech, the depiction of sinister characters is best described as   3._____

   A. accurate   B. conflicting
   C. stereotyped   D. vague

4. According to this speech, most Indians in Western stories are portrayed as   4._____

   A. bad   B. passive
   C. glamorous   D. oppressed

5. The speaker compares the position of the cowboy to that of   5.____

   A. a TV programmer   B. an Israeli soldier
   C. a famous actor   D. a chivalrous knight

6. According to the projected image of the Old West, justice was handled by   6.____

   A. the sheriff   B. each person
   C. the good guys   D. no one

7. According to the speaker, the main reason for the allure of this Western imagery is that   7.____
   the

   A. past provides relief from the present
   B. present is very similar to the past
   C. past serves as a model for the present
   D. achievement of the present outweighs that of the past

8. Throughout this description of the West, a recurring difference from modern day life that   8.____
   is expressed is the

   A. cowboy's knowledge of self-defense
   B. chance to fight evil
   C. individual's control of his life
   D. opportunity to become famous

9. This speech suggests that the projected image of the West is best described as   9.____

   A. realistic   B. understated
   C. changing   D. romantic

10. According to this speech, the largest group that accepts the projected image of the West   10.____
    is

   A. modern ranchers   B. movie viewers
   C. the American public   D. people around the world

KEY (CORRECT ANSWERS)

1.	A		6.	B
2.	B		7.	A
3.	C		8.	C
4.	A		9.	D
5.	D		10.	D

TEST 4

DIRECTIONS: In this part a passage will be read orally to you. It is NOT written out in the test
booklet so you will have to listen carefully. After the reading of the passage,
you will answer the questions that follow. Each question or incomplete statement is followed by several suggested answers or completions. Select the one
that BEST answers the question or completes the statement. *PRINT THE
LETTER OF THE CORRECT ANSWER IN THE SPACE AT THE RIGHT.*

<u>Listening Passage</u>

(The following speech has been adapted from *At Wit's End* by Erma Bombeck.)

The end of summer is to me like New Year's Eve. I sense an end to something carefree
and uninhibited, sandy and warm, cold and melting, barefoot and tanned. And yet I look forward with great expectation to a beginning of schedules and appointments, bookbinders with
little tabs, freshly sharpened pencils, crisp winds, efficiency, and routine.

I am sadly aware of a great rushing of time as I lengthen skirts and discard sweaters that
hit above the wristbones. Time is moving and I want to stop it for just a while so that I may
snatch a quiet moment and tell my children what it is I want for them.

The moment never comes, of course. I must compete with Captain Kangaroo, a baseball
game, a record, a playmate, a cartoon or a new bike in the next block. So I must keep these
thoughts inside.

Too fast....you're moving too fast. Don't be in such a hurry. You're going to own your own
sports car before you've tried to build one out of orange crates and four baby buggy wheels.
You're going to explore the world before you've explored the wonders of your own back yard.

Don't shed your childhood like a good coat that's gotten a little small for you. A full-term
childhood is necessary as are all phases of your growth. Childhood is a time for absorbing
ideas, knowledge, and people like a giant sponge. Childhood is a time when "competition" is
a baseball game and "responsibility" is a paper route.

I want to teach you so much that you must know to find happiness within yourself. Yet, I
don't know where to begin or how.

If I could only be sure all the lessons are sinking in and are being understood. How can I
tell you about disappointments? You'll have them you know. And they'll be painful, they'll hurt,
they'll shatter your ego, lay your confidence in yourself bare, and sometimes cripple your initiative. But people don't die from them. They just emerge stronger. I want you to hear the
thunder, so you can appreciate the calm. I want you to fall on your face in the dirt once in a
while, so you will know the pride of being able to stand tall.

1. To the speaker, the end of summer represents   1._____

    A.   the end of a routine
    B.   a new beginning
    C.   a continuation of her schedule
    D.   an end to childhood

2. To the speaker, summer appears to represent   2._____

    A.   growth   B.   responsibility
    C.   efficiency   D.   freedom

3. To the speaker, fall appears to represent   3._____

     A.   peace   B.   competition
     C.   routine   D.   maturity

4. The speaker's thoughts are not said aloud to her children because she   4._____

     A.   finds no time in their busy schedule
     B.   realizes it would make no difference
     C.   fears rejection
     D.   has too much to say

5. Which statement best expresses the speaker's advice to her audience?   5._____

     A.   Do not think of the future.
     B.   Try to avoid disappointments.
     C.   Listen to experienced people.
     D.   Enjoy the present.

6. The speaker compares childhood to a coat because they both can be   6._____

     A.   altered to fit   B.   put aside
     C.   stored   D.   worn

7. According to the speaker, the positive aspect of disappointments is that they   7._____

     A.   are short-lived   B.   build character
     C.   reveal true friends   D.   make people humble

8. The speaker's feelings about her own ability to help her children can best be described   8._____
as

     A.   uncertain   B.   unrealistic
     C.   sophisticated   D.   matter-of-fact

9. What is the main idea of the speech?   9._____

     A.   Children need some pain in order to become strong.
     B.   Only adults appreciate life.
     C.   People should learn to appreciate all stages of life.
     D.   Competition and responsibility are only for adults.

10. A characteristic of the speaker's style in this speech is that she   10._____

     A.   depends on humor to make her point
     B.   makes the same point in different ways
     C.   uses sentimental appeal to please her audience
     D.   uses irony to emphasize her theme

KEY (CORRECT ANSWERS)

1.	B	6.	B
2.	D	7.	B
3.	C	8.	A
4.	A	9.	C
5.	D	10.	B

———

TEST 5

DIRECTIONS: In this part a passage will be read orally to you. It is NOT written out in the test booklet so you will have to listen carefully. After the reading of the passage, you will answer the questions that follow. Each question or incomplete statement is followed by several suggested answers or completions. Select the one that BEST answers the question or completes the statement. *PRINT THE LETTER OF THE CORRECT ANSWER IN THE SPACE AT THE RIGHT.*

Listening Passage

(The following passage is adapted from "America and the Americans" by John Steinbeck.)

The American dream does not die. The dreams of a people either create folk literature or find their way into it; and folk literature, again, is always based on something that happened. Our most persistent folk tales concern cowboys, gunslinging sheriffs and Indian-fighters. These folk figures did exist and this dream persists. Businessmen in Texas wear the high-heeled boots though they ride in air-conditioned cars and have forgotten the reason for the high heel. Our children play cowboy and Indian. And in these moral tales, virtue does not arise out of reason or orderly process of law - it is imposed by violence and maintained by the threat of violence. Are these stories permanent because we know within ourselves that only the threat of violence makes it possible for us to live together in peace?

Something happened in America to create the Americans. Now we face the danger which in the past has been most destructive to the human: success, plenty, comfort, and ever-increasing leisure. No dynamic people has ever survived these dangers. I wonder about the tomorrow of my people, which is a young people. My questioning is compounded of some fear, more hope, and great confidence.

I have named the destroyers of nations: comfort, plenty and security — out of which grows boredom, in which rebellion against the world as it is, and myself as I am, is submerged in listless self-satisfaction. A dying people tolerates the present, rejects the future and finds its satisfactions in past greatness and half-remembered glory. A dying people arms itself with defense weapons against change. It is in the American negation of these symptoms of extinction that my hope and confidence lie. We are not satisfied. Our restlessness, perhaps inherited from the hungry immigrants of our ancestry, is still with us.

How will the Americans act and react to a new set of circumstances for which new rules must be made? We know from our past some of the things we will do. We will make mistakes; we always have. But from our beginning, our social direction is clear. We have fired to become one people out of many. We have failed sometimes, taken wrong paths, paused for renewals; but we have never slipped back — never.

1. Although not completely attained, the American dream seems to be   1._____

   A. outlived   B. persistent
   C. realistic   D. democratic

2. According to his passage, which statement about folk heroes is most likely true?   2._____

   A. They are based on fact.
   B. They are created in someone's imagination
   C. They are only an American dream.
   D. They are created as a way for Americans to escape reality.

3. The speaker cites the wearing of high heeled boots by Texas businessmen as evidence of their   3.____

    A. ability to buy whatever they want
    B. interest in the work of the cowboy
    C. belief in the dream of folk heroes
    D. desire to return to the past

4. According to the speaker, folk tales indicate that Americans generally do the right thing because of their   4.____

    A. belief in law and order
    B. moral convictions
    C. fear of violence
    D. confidence in the future

5. The speaker implies that success, plenty, and comfort should be regarded with   5.____

    A. amazement   B. confidence
    C. toleration   D. suspicion

6. The speaker believes that a self-satisified nation will   6.____

    A. eventually perish   B. be more comfortable
    C. become revolutionary   D. invent myths

7. According to the speaker, one valuable quality America inherited from its immigrants is   7.____

    A. belief in myths   B. belief in hard work
    C. restlessness   D. stability

8. Past experience suggests that one of the reactions Americans will have to new situations will be to   8.____

    A. give up the American dream   B. make some mistakes
    C. resist any change   D. relive past glories

KEY (CORRECT ANSWERS)

1.	B	5.	D
2.	A	6.	A
3.	C	7.	C
4.	C	8.	B

READING COMPREHENSION
UNDERSTANDING AND INTERPRETING WRITTEN MATERIAL

EXAMINATION SECTION

DIRECTIONS: Each question or incomplete statement is followed by several suggested answers or completions. Select the one that BEST answers the question or completes the statement. *PRINT THE LETTER OF THE CORRECT ANSWER IN THE SPACE AT THE RIGHT.*

TEST 1

Skiing has recently become one of the more popular sports in the United States. Because of its popularity, thousands of winter vacationers are flying north rather than south. In many areas, reservations are required months ahead of time.

I discovered the accommodation shortage through an unfortunate experience. On a sunny Saturday morning, I set out from Denver for the beckoning slopes of Aspen, Colorado. After passing signs for other ski areas, I finally reached my destination. Naturally, I lost no time in heading for the nearest tow. After a stimulating afternoon of miscalculated stem turns, I was famished. Well, one thing led to another, and it must have been eight o'clock before I concerned myself with a bed for my bruised and aching bones.

It took precisely one phone call to ascertain the lack of lodgings in the Aspen area. I had but one recourse. My auto and I started the treacherous jaunt over the pass and back towards Denver. Along the way, I went begging for a bed. Finally, a jolly tavernkeeper took pity, and for only thirty dollars a night allowed me the privilege of staying in a musty, dirty, bathless room above his tavern.

1.   The author's problem would have been avoided if he had   1._____

    A.   not tired himself out skiing
    B.   taken a bus instead of driving
    C.   looked for food as soon as he arrived
    D.   arranged for accommodations well ahead of his trip
    E.   answer cannot be determined from the information given

---

TEST 2

Helen Keller was born in 1880 in Tuscumbia, Alabama. When she was two years old, she lost her sight and hearing as the result of an illness. In 1886, she became the pupil of Anne Sullivan, who taught Helen to *see* with her fingertips, to *hear* with her feet and hands, and to communicate with other people. Miss Sullivan succeeded in arousing Helen's curiosity and interest by spelling the names of objects into her hand. At the end of three years, Helen had mastered the manual and the braille alphabet and could read and write.

2.   When did Helen Keller lose her sight and hearing?   2._____

TEST 3

Sammy got to school ten minutes after the school bell had rung. He was breathing hard and had a black eye. His face was dirty and scratched. One leg of his pants was torn.

Tommy was late to school, too; however, he was only five minutes late. Like Sammy, he was breathing hard, but he was happy and smiling.

3. Sammy and Tommy had been fighting.
   Who probably won?

   3._____

   A. Sammy   B. Tommy
   C. Cannot tell from story   D. The teacher
   E. The school

TEST 4

This is like a game to see if you can tell what the nonsense word in the paragraph stands for. The nonsense word is just a silly word for something that you know very well. Read the paragraph and see if you can tell what the underlined nonsense word stands for.

You can wash your hands and face in <u>zup</u>. You can even take a bath in it. When people swim, they are in the <u>zup</u>. Everyone drinks <u>zup</u>.

4. <u>Zup</u> is PROBABLY

   4._____

   A. milk   B. pop   C. soap   D. water   E. soup

TEST 5

After two weeks of unusually high-speed travel, we reached Xeno, a small planet whose population, though never before visited by Earthmen, was listed as *friendly* in the INTERSTEL-LAR GAZETTEER.

On stepping lightly (after all, the gravity of Xeno is scarcely more than twice that of our own moon) from our spacecraft, we saw that *friendly* was an understatement. We were immediately surrounded by Frangibles of various colors, mostly pinkish or orange, who held out their *hands* to us. Imagine our surprise when their *hands* actually merged with ours as we tried to shake them!

Then, before we could stop them (how could we have stopped them?), two particularly pink Frangibles simply stepped right into two eminent scientists among our party, who immediately lit up with the same pink glow. While occupied in this way, the scientists reported afterwards they suddenly discovered they *knew* a great deal about Frangibles and life on Xeno.

Apparently, Frangibles could take themselves apart atomically and enter right into any other substance. They communicated by thought waves, occasionally merging *heads* for greater clarity. Two Frangibles who were in love with each other would spend most of their time merged into one; they were a bluish-green color unless they were having a lover's quarrel, when they turned gray.

5. In order to find out about an object which interested him, what would a Frangible MOST likely do?   5.____

    A. Take it apart
    B. Enter into it
    C. Study it scientifically
    D. Ask earth scientists about it
    E. Wait to see if it would change color

TEST 6

This is like a game to see if you can tell what the nonsense word in the paragraph stands for. The nonsense word is just a silly word for something that you know very well. Read the paragraph and see if you can tell what the underlined nonsense word stands for.

Have you ever smelled a <u>mart</u>? They smell very good. Bees like <u>marts</u>. They come in many colors. <u>Marts</u> grow in the earth, and they usually bloom in the spring.

6. <u>Marts</u> are PROBABLY   6.____

    A. bugs   B. flowers   C. perfume
    D. pies   E. cherries

TEST 7

Christmas was only a few days away. The wind was strong and cold. The walks were covered with snow. The downtown streets were crowded with people. Their faces were hidden by many packages as they went in one store after another. They all tried to move faster as they looked at the clock.

7. When did the story PROBABLY happen?   7.____

    A. November 28   B. December 1   C. December 21
    D. December 25   E. December 28

TEST 8

THE WAYFARER

The wayfarer,
Perceiving the pathway to truth,
Was struck with astonishment.
It was thickly grown with weeds.
Ha, he said,
I see that no one has passed here
In a long time.
Later he saw that each weed
Was a singular knife,
Well, he mumbled at last,
Doubtless there are other roads.

8. *I see that no one has passed here In a long time.*
   What do the above lines from the poem mean?

   A. The way of truth is popular.
   B. People are fascinated by the truth.
   C. Truth comes and goes like the wind.
   D. The truth is difficult to recognize.
   E. Few people are searching for the truth.

8.____

TEST 9

Any attempt to label an entire generation is unrewarding, and yet the generation which went through the last war, or at least could get a drink easily once it was over, seems to possess a uniform, general quality which demands an adjective. It was John Kerouac, the author of a fine, neglected novel, THE TOWN AND THE CITY, who finally came up with it. It was several years ago, when the face was harder to recognize, but he had a sharp, sympathetic eye, and one day he said, *You know, this is really a beat generation.* The origins of the word *beat* are obscure, but the meaning is only too clear to most Americans. More than mere weariness, it implies the feeling of having been used, of being raw. It involves a sort of nakedness of mind, and, ultimately, of soul; a feeling of being reduced to the bedrock of consciousness. In short, it means being undramatically pushed up against the wall of oneself. A man is beat whenever he goes for broke and waters the sum of his resources on a single number; and the young generation has done that continually from early youth.

9. What does the writer suggest when he mentions a *fine, neglected novel*?

   A. Kerouac had the right idea about the war
   B. Kerouac had a clear understanding of the new post-war generation
   C. Kerouac had not received the recognition of THE TOWN AND THE CITY that was deserved
   D. Kerouac had the wrong idea about the war.
   E. All of the above

9.____

TEST 10

One spring, Farmer Brown had an unusually good field of wheat. Whenever he saw any birds in this field, he got his gun and shot as many of them as he could. In the middle of the summer, he found that his wheat was being ruined by insects. With no birds to feed on them, the insects had multiplied very fast. What Farmer Brown did not understand was this: A bird is not simply an animal that eats food the farmer may want for himself. Instead, it is one of many links in the complex surroundings, or environment, in which we live.

How much grain a farmer can raise on an acre of ground depends on many factors. All of these factors can be divided into two big groups. Such things as the richness of the soil, the amount of rainfall, the amount of sunlight, and the temperature belong together in one of these groups. This group may be called <u>nonliving factors</u>. The second group may be called <u>living factors</u>. The living factors in any plant's environment are animals and other plants. Wheat, for example, may be damaged by wheat rust, a tiny plant that feeds on wheat, or it may be eaten by plant-eating animals such as birds or grasshoppers...

It is easy to see that the relations of plants and animals to their environment are very complex, and that any change in the environment is likely to bring about a whole series of changes.

10. What does the passage suggest a good farmer should understand about nature?   10._____

   A.   Insects are harmful to plants
   B.   Birds are not harmful to plants
   C.   Wheat may be damaged by both animals and other plants
   D.   The amount of wheat he can raise depends on two factors: birds and insects
   E.   A change in one factor of plants' surroundings may cause other factors to change

11. What important idea about nature does the writer want us to understand?   11._____

   A.   Farmer Brown was worried about the heavy rainfall
   B.   Nobody needs to have such destructive birds around
   C.   Farmer Brown did not want the temperature to change
   D.   All insects need not only wheat rust but grasshoppers
   E.   All living things are dependent on other living things

TEST 11

For a 12-year-old, I've been around a lot because my father's in the Army. I have been to New York and to Paris. When I was nine, my parents took me to Rome. I didn't like Europe very much because the people don't speak the same language I do. When I am older, my mother says I can travel by myself. I think I will like that. Ever since I was 13, I have wanted to go to Canada.

12. Why can't everything this person said be TRUE?   12._____

   A.   12-year-olds can't travel alone
   B.   No one can travel that much in 12 years
   C.   There is a conflict in the ages used in the passage
   D.   9-year-olds can't travel alone
   E.   He is a liar

TEST 12

Between April and October, the Persian Gulf is dotted with the small boats of pearl divers. Some seventy-five thousand of them are busy diving down and bringing up pearl-bearing oysters. These oysters are not the kind we eat. The edible oyster produces pearls of little or no value. You may have heard tales of divers who discovered pearls and sold them for great sums of money. These stories are entertaining but not accurate.

13. The Persian Gulf has many   13._____

     A. large boats of pearl divers
     B. pearl divers who eat oysters
     C. edible oysters that produce pearls
     D. non-edible oysters that produce pearls
     E. edible oysters that do not produce pearls

TEST 13

Art says that the polar ice cap is melting at the rate of 3% per year. Bert says that this isn't true because the polar ice cap is really melting at the rate of 7% per year.

14. We know for certain that   14._____

     A. Art is wrong
     B. Bert is wrong
     C. they are both wrong
     D. they both might be right
     E. they can't both be right

TEST 14

FORTUNE AND MEN'S EYES

Shakespeare

1.   When, in disgrace with fortune and men's eyes,
2.   I all alone beweep my outcast state,
3.   And trouble deaf heaven with my bootless cries,
4.   And look upon myself and curse my fate,
5.   Wishing me like to one more rich in hope,
6.   Featured like him, like him with friends possessed
7.   Desiring this man's art, and that man's scope,
8.   With what I most enjoy contented least;
9.   Yet in these thoughts myself almost despising,
10. Haply I think on thee; and then my state,
11. Like to the lark at break of day arising
12. From sullen earth, sings hymns at heaven's gate;
13. For thy sweet love remembered, such wealth brings
14. That then I scorn to change my state with kings.

15. What saves this man from wishing to be different than he is?   15._____

     A.   Such wealth brings
     B.   Hymns at heaven's gate
     C.   The lark at break of day
     D.   Thy sweet love remembered
     E.   Change my state with kings

TEST 15

My name is Gregory Gotrocks, and I live in Peoria, Illinois. I sell tractors. In June 1952, the Gotrocks Tractor Company (my dad happens to be the president) sent me to Nepal-Tibet to check on our sales office there.

Business was slow, and I had a lot of time to kill. I decided to see Mt. Everest so that I could tell everyone back in Peoria that I had seen it.

It was beautiful; I was spellbound. I simply had to see what the view looked like from the top. So I started up the northwest slope. Everyone know that this is the best route to take. It took me three long hours to reach the top, but the climb was well worth it.

16. Gregory Gotrocks went to see Mt. Everest so that he could   16._____

     A.   see some friends
     B.   sell some tractors
     C.   take a picture of it
     D.   plant a flag at its base
     E.   entertain his friends back home

TEST 16

Suburbanites are not irresponsible. Indeed, what is striking about the young couples' march along the abyss is the earnestness and precision with which they go about it. They are extremely budget-conscious. They can rattle off most of their monthly payments down to the last penny; one might say that even their impulse buying is deliberately planned. They are conscientious in meeting obligations and rarely do they fall delinquent in their accounts.

They are exponents of what could be called budgetism. This does not mean that they actually keep formal budgets – quite the contrary. The beauty of budgetism is that one doesn't have to keep a budget at all. It's done automatically. In the new middle-class rhythms of life, obligations are homogenized, for the overriding aim is to have oneself precommitted to regular, unvarying monthly payments on all the major items.

Americans used to be divided into three sizable groups: those who thought of money obligations in terms of the week, of the month, and of the year. Many people remain at both ends of the scale; but with the widening of the middle class, the mortgage payments are firmly geared to a thirty-day cycle, and any dissonant peaks and valleys are anathema. Just as young couples are now paying winter fuel bills in equal monthly fractions through the year, so they seek to spread out all the other heavy seasonal obligations they can anticipate. If vendors will not oblige by accepting equal monthly installments, the purchasers will smooth out the load themselves by floating loans.

It is, suburbanites cheerfully explain, a matter of psychology. They don't trust themselves. In self-entrapment is security. They try to budget so tightly that there is no unappropriated funds, for they know these would burn a hole in their pocket. Not merely out of greed for goods, then, do they commit themselves; it is protection they want, too. And though it would be extreme to say that they go into debt to be secure, carefully chartered debt does give them a certain peace of mind – and in suburbia this is more coveted than luxury itself.

17. What is the *abyss* along which the young couples are marching?   17._____

    A. Nuclear war   B. Unemployment
    C. Mental breakdown   D. Financial disaster
    E. Catastrophic illness

18. What conclusion does the author reach concerning carefully chartered debt among   18._____
young couples in the United States today?
It

    A. is a symbol of love
    B. brings marital happiness
    C. helps them to feel secure
    D. enables them to acquire wealth
    E. provides them with material goods

TEST 17

Read the verse and fill in the space beside the object described in the verse.

You see me when I'm right or wrong;
My face I never hide.
My hands move slowly round and round
And o'er me minutes glide.

19. A. ___ Book   B. ___ Clock   C. ___ Record   19.____
     D. ___ Table   E. ___ Lock

———

TEST 18

Until about thirty years ago, the village of Nayon seems to have been a self-sufficient agricultural community with a mixture of native and sixteenth century Spanish customs. Lands were abandoned when too badly eroded. The balance between population and resources allowed a minimum subsistence. A few traders exchanged goods between Quito and the villages in the tropical barrancas, all within a radius of ten miles. Houses had dirt floors, thatched roofs, and pole walls that were sometimes plastered with mud. Guinea pigs ran freely about each house and were the main meat source. Most of the population spoke no Spanish. Men wore long hair and concerned themselves chiefly with farming.

The completion of the Guayaquil-Quito railway in 1908 brought the first real contacts with industrial civilization to the high inter-Andean valley. From this event gradually flowed not only technological changes but new ideas and social institutions. Feudal social relationships no longer seemed right and immutable; medicine and public health improved; elementary education became more common; urban Quito began to expand; and finally, and perhaps least important so far, modern industries began to appear, although even now on a most modest scale.

In 1948-49, the date of our visit, only two men wore their hair long; and only two old-style houses remained. If guinea pigs were kept, they were penned; their flesh was now a luxury food, and beef the most common meat. Houses were of adobe or fired brick, usually with tile roofs, and often contained five or six rooms, some of which had plank or brick floors. Most of the population spoke Spanish. There was no resident priest, but an appointed government official and a policeman represented authority. A six-teacher school provided education. Clothing was becoming citified; for men it often included overalls for work and a tailored suit, white shirt, necktie, and felt hat for trips to Quito. Attendance at church was low, and many festivals had been abandoned. Volleyball or soccer was played weekly in the plaza by young men who sometimes wore shorts, blazers, and berets. There were few shops, for most purchases were made in Quito, and from there came most of the food, so that there was a far more varied diet than twenty-five years ago. There were piped water and sporadic health services; in addition, most families patronized Quito doctors in emergencies.

The crops and their uses had undergone change. Maize, or Indian corn, was still the primary crop, but very little was harvested as grain. Almost all was sold in Quito as green corn to eat boiled on the cob, and a considerable amount of the corn eaten as grain in Nayon was imported. Beans, which do poorly here, were grown on a small scale for household consumption. Though some squash was eaten, most was exported. Sweet potatoes, tomatoes, cabbage, onions, peppers, and, at lower elevations, sweet yucca, and arrowroot were grown extensively for export; indeed, so export-minded was the community that it was almost impossible to buy locally grown produce in the village. People couldn't be bothered with retail scales.

20. Why was there primitiveness and self-containment in Nayon before 1910? 20.____

    A. Social mores   B. Cultural tradition
    C. Biological instincts   D. Geographical factors
    E. Religious regulations

21. By 1948, the village of Nayon was 21.____

    A. a self-sufficient village
    B. out of touch with the outside world
    C. a small dependent portion of a larger economic unit
    D. a rapidly growing and sound social and cultural unit
    E. a metropolis

22. Why was Nayon originally separated from its neighbors? 22.____

    A. Rich arable land
    B. Long meandering streams
    C. Artificial political barriers
    D. Broad stretches of arid desert
    E. Deep rugged gorges traversed by rock trails

TEST 19

Read the verse and fill in the space beside the object described in the verse.

    I have two eyes and when I'm worn
    I give the wearer four.
    I'm strong or weak or thick or thin -
    Need I say much more?

23.   A. ___ Clock   B. ___ Eyeglasses   C. ___Piano   23.____
       D. ___ Thermometer   E. ___ I don't know

TEST 20

Scarlet fever begins with fever, chills, headache, and sore throat. A doctor diagnoses the illness as scarlet fever when a characteristic rash erupts on the skin. This rash appears on the neck and chest in three to five days after the onset of the illness and spreads rapidly over the body. Sometimes the skin on the palm of the hands and soles

of the feet shreds in flakes. Scarlet fever is usually treated with penicillin and, in severe cases, a convalescent serum. The disease may be accompanied by infections of the ear and throat, inflammation of the kidneys, pneumonia, and inflammation of the heart.

24. How does the author tell us that scarlet fever may be a serious disease?   24.____

    A. He tells how many people die of it.
    B. He tells that he once had the disease.
    C. He tells that hands and feet may fall off.
    D. He tells how other infections may come with scarlet fever.
    E. None of the above

TEST 21

Read the verse and fill in the space beside the object described in the verse.

    I have no wings but often fly:
    I come in colors many.
    From varied nationalities
    Respect I get a-plenty.

25. A. ___ Deck of cards   B. ___ Eyeglasses   C. ___ Flag   25.____
      D. ___ Needles   E. ___ None of the above

KEY (CORRECT ANSWERS)

1.	D		11.	E
2.	B		12.	C
3.	B		13.	D
4.	D		14.	E
5.	B		15.	D
6.	B		16.	E
7.	C		17.	D
8.	E		18.	C
9.	C		19.	B
10.	E		20.	D

21.	C
22.	E
23.	B
24.	D
25.	C

WORD MEANING
COMMENTARY

DESCRIPTION OF THE TEST

On many examinations, you will have questions about the meaning of words, or vocabulary.

In this type of question you have to state what a word or phrase means. (A phrase is a group of words.) This word or phrase is in CAPITAL letters in a sentence. You are also given for each question five other words or groups of words — lettered A, B, C, D, and E — as possible answers. One of thes words or groups of words means the same as the word or group of words in CAPITAL letters. Only one is right. You are to pick out the one that is right and select the letter of your answer.

HINTS FOR ANSWERING WORD-MEANING QUESTIONS

Read each question carefully.

Choose the best answer of the five choices even though it is not the word you might use yourself.

Answer first those that you know. Then do the others.

If you know that some of the suggested answers are not right, pay no more attention to them.

Be sure that you have selected an answer for every question, even if you have to guess.

SAMPLE QUESTIONS

DIRECTIONS: For the following questions, select the word or group of words lettered A, B, C, D, or E that means MOST NEARLY the same as the word in capital letters. Indicate the letter of the CORRECT answer for each question.

SAMPLE QUESTIONS 1 AND 2

1.   The letter was SHORT. SHORT means *MOST NEARLY*   1.____

     A. tall   B. wide   C. brief   D. heavy   E. dark

EXPLANATION

SHORT is a word you have used to describe something that is small, or not long, or little, etc. Therefore you would not have to spend much time figuring out the right answer. You would choose C. brief.

2.   The young man is VIGOROUS. VIGOROUS means *MOST NEARLY*   2.____

     A. serious   B. reliable   C. courageous
     D. strong   E. talented

EXPLANATION

VIGOROUS is a word that you have probably used yourself or read somewhere. It carries with it the idea of being active, full of pep, etc. Which one of the five choices comes closest to meaning that? Certainly not A. serious, B. reliable, or E. talented; C. courageous — maybe, D. strong — maybe. But between courageous or strong, you would have to agree that strong is the better choice. Therefore, you would choose D.

WORD MEANING
EXAMINATION SECTION
TEST 1

DIRECTIONS: For the following questions, select the word or group of words lettered A, B, C, D, or E that means MOST NEARLY the same as the word in capital letters. *PRINT THE LETTER OF THE CORRECT ANSWER IN THE SPACE AT THE RIGHT.*

1. To SULK means MOST NEARLY to   1.____

    A. cry   B. annoy   C. lament   D. be sullen   E. scorn

2. To FLOUNDER means MOST NEARLY to   2.____

    A. investigate B. label   C. struggle   D. consent   E. escape

3. PARLEY means MOST NEARLY   3.____

    A. discussion   B. thoroughfare
    C. salon   D. surrender
    E. divsion

4. MAESTRO means MOST NEARLY   4.____

    A. official   B. ancestor   C. teacher   D. watchman   E. alien

5. MEANDERING means MOST NEARLY   5.____

    A. cruel   B. adjusting   C. winding   D. smooth   E. combining

6. GNARLED means MOST NEARLY   6.____

    A. angry   B. bitter
    C. twisted   D. ancient
    E. embroidered

7. TEMPERANCE means MOST NEARLY   7.____

    A. moderation   B. climate
    C. carelessness   D. disagreeableness
    E. rigidity

8. A PRECARIOUS position is one that is   8.____

    A. foresighted   B. careful
    C. modest   D. headstrong
    E. uncertain

9. COVETOUS means MOST NEARLY   9.____

    A. undisciplined   B. grasping
    C. timid   D. insincere
    E. secretive

10. PRIVATION means MOST NEARLY   10.____

    A. reward   B. superiority in rank
    C. hardship   D. suitability of behavior
    E. solitude

TEST 2

DIRECTIONS: For the following questions, select the word or group of words lettered A, B, C, D, or E that means MOST NEARLY the same as the word in capital letters. *PRINT THE LETTER OF THE CORRECT ANSWER IN THE SPACE AT THE RIGHT.*

1. To INFILTRATE means MOST NEARLY to   1._____

   A. pass through   B. stop   C. consider
   D. challenge openly   E. meet secretly

2. REVOCATION means MOST NEARLY   2._____

   A. certificate   B. repeal   C. animation   D. license   E. plea

3. LOQUACIOUS means MOST NEARLY   3._____

   A. grim   B. stern
   C. talkative   D. lighthearted
   E. liberty-loving

4. APERTURE means MOST NEARLY   4._____

   A. basement   B. opening   C. phantom
   D. protective coloring E. light refreshment

5. A PUNGENT odor is one that is   5._____

   A. biting   B. smooth
   C. quarrelsome   D. wrong
   E. proud

6. To CORROBORATE means MOST NEARLY to   6._____

   A. deny   B. elaborate   C. confirm   D. gnaw   E. state

7. BENEVOLENCE means MOST NEARLY   7._____

   A. good fortune   B. well-being   C. inheritance
   D. violence   E. charitableness

8. PETULANT means MOST NEARLY   8._____

   A. rotten   B. fretful   C. unrelated   D. weird   E. throbbing

9. DERELICT means MOST NEARLY   9._____

   A. abandoned B. widowed   C. faithful   D. insincere   E. hysterical

10. INCISIVE means MOST NEARLY   10._____

   A. stimulating B. accidental C. brief   D. penetrating E. final

_____

TEST 3

DIRECTIONS: For the following questions, select the word or group of words lettered A, B, C, D, or E that means MOST NEARLY the same as the word in capital letters. *PRINT THE LETTER OF THE CORRECT ANSWER IN THE SPACE AT THE RIGHT.*

1. To LAUD means MOST NEARLY to   1._____

    A. praise   B. cleanse   C. replace   D. squander   E. frown upon

2. To TAUNT means MOST NEARLY to   2._____

    A. jeer at   B. tighten   C. rescue   D. interest   E. ward off

3. DEITY means MOST NEARLY   3._____

    A. renown   B. divinity   C. delicacy   D. destiny   E. futility

4. GRAVITY means MOST NEARLY   4._____

    A. displeasure   B. thankfulness   C. suffering
    D. roughness   E. seriousness

5. A CONTEMPTUOUS author is one that is   5._____

    A. thoughtful   B. soiled   C. dishonorable
    D. scornful   E. self-satisfied

6. To WAIVE means MOST NEARLY to   6._____

    A. exercise   B. swing   C. claim   D. give up   E. wear out

7. To ASPIRE means MOST NEARLY to   7._____

    A. fade away   B. excite   C. desire earnestly
    D. breathe heavily   E. roughen

8. PERTINENT means MOST NEARLY   8._____

    A. related   B. saucy   C. quick   D. impatient   E. excited

9. DEVASTATION means MOST NEARLY   9._____

    A. desolation   B. displeasure   C. dishonor
    D. neglect   E. religious fervor

10. IMMINENT means MOST NEARLY   10._____

    A. sudden   B. important   C. delayed   D. threatening E. forceful

TEST 4

DIRECTIONS: For the following questions, select the word or group of words lettered A, B, C, D, or E that means MOST NEARLY the same as the word in capital letters. *PRINT THE LETTER OF THE CORRECT ANSWER IN THE SPACE AT THE RIGHT.*

1. CONTROVERSIAL means MOST NEARLY   1._____

    A. faultfinding B. pleasant   C. debatable D. ugly   E. talkative

2. GHASTLY means MOST NEARLY   2._____

    A. hasty   B. furious   C. breathless D. deathlike E. spiritual

3. A BELLIGERENT attitude is one that is   3._____

    A. worldly   B. warlike
    C. loudmouthed   D. furious
    E. artistic

4. PROFICIENCY means MOST NEARLY   4._____

    A. wisdom   B. oversupply
    C. expertness   D. advancement
    E. sincerity

5. COMPASSION means MOST NEARLY   5._____

    A. rage   B. strength of character   C. forcefulness
    D. sympathy   E. uniformity

6. DISSENSION means MOST NEARLY   6._____

    A. treatise   B. pretense   C. fear   D. lineage   E. discord

7. To INTIMATE means MOST NEARLY to   7._____

    A. charm   B. hint   C. disguise   D. frighten   E. hum

8. To BERATE means MOST NEARLY to   8._____

    A. classify   B. scold   C. underestimate
    D. take one's time   E. evaluate

9. DEARTH means MOST NEARLY   9._____

    A. scarcity   B. width   C. affection   D. wealth   E. warmth

10. To MEDITATE means MOST NEARLY to   10._____

    A. rest   B. stare
    C. doze   D. make peace
    E. reflect

TEST 5

DIRECTIONS: For the following questions, select the word or group of words lettered A, B, C, D, or E that means MOST NEARLY the same as the word in capital letters. *PRINT THE LETTER OF THE CORRECT ANSWER IN THE SPACE AT THE RIGHT.*

1. BONDAGE means MOST NEARLY   1._____

   A. poverty   B. redemption C. slavery   D. retirement   E. complaint

2. AGILITY means MOST NEARLY   2._____

   A. wisdom   B. nimbleness C. agreeable   D. simplicity   E. excitement

3. To ABDICATE means MOST NEARLY to   3._____

   A. achieve   B. protest   C. renounce   D. demand   E. steal

4. To STIFLE means MOST NEARLY to   4._____

   A. talk nonsense   B. sidestep
   C. depress   D. smother
   E. stick

5. EDICT means MOST NEARLY   5._____

   A. abbreviation   B. lie
   C. carbon copy   D. correction
   E. decree

6. AMITY means MOST NEARLY   6._____

   A. ill will   B. hope   C. pity   D. friendship   E. pleasure

7. COERCION means MOST NEARLY   7._____

   A. force   B. disgust   C. suspicion   D. pleasure   E. criticism

8. To ABASH means MOST NEARLY to   8._____

   A. embarrass   B. encourage   C. punish   D. surrender   E. overthrow

9. TACITURN means MOST NEARLY   9._____

   A. weak   B. evil   C. tender   D. silent   E. sensitive

10. REMISS means MOST NEARLY   10._____

   A. memorable   B. neglectful C. useless   D. prompt   E. exact

TEST 6

DIRECTIONS: For the following questions, select the word or group of words lettered A, B, C, D, or E that means MOST NEARLY the same as the word in capital letters. *PRINT THE LETTER OF THE CORRECT ANSWER IN THE SPACE AT THE RIGHT.*

1. STAGNANT means MOST NEARLY   1._____

   A. inactive   B. alert   C. selfish   D. difficult   E. scornful

2. MANDATORY means MOST NEARLY   2._____

   A. instant   B. obligatory   C. evident   D. strategic   E. unequaled

3. INFERNAL means MOST NEARLY   3._____

   A. immodest   B. incomplete
   C. domestic   D. second-rate
   E. fiendish

4. To EXONERATE means MOST NEARLY to   4._____

   A. free from blame   B. warn
   C. drive out   D. overcharge
   E. plead

5. ARBITER means MOST NEARLY   5._____

   A. friend   B. judge
   C. drug   D. tree surgeon
   E. truant

6. ENMITY means MOST NEARLY   6._____

   A. boredom   B. puzzle   C. offensive language
   D. ill will   E. entanglement

7. To DISCRIMINATE means MOST NEARLY to   7._____

   A. fail   B. delay   C. accuse   D. distinguish   E. reject

8. DERISION means MOST NEARLY   8._____

   A. disgust   B. ridicule   C. fear   D. anger   E. heredity

9. EXULTANT means MOST NEARLY   9._____

   A. essential   B. elated   C. praiseworthy
   D. plentiful   E. high-priced

10. OSTENSIBLE means MOST NEARLY   10._____

   A. vibrating   B. odd   C. apparent   D. standard   E. ornate

TEST 7

DIRECTIONS: For the following questions, select the word or group of words lettered A, B, C, D, or E that means MOST NEARLY the same as the word in capital letters. *PRINT THE LETTER OF THE CORRECT ANSWER IN THE SPACE AT THE RIGHT.*

1. To ABHOR means MOST NEARLY to   1.____

    A. hate   B. admire   C. taste   D. skip   E. resign

2. DUTIFUL means MOST NEARLY   2.____

    A. lasting   B. sluggish   C. required   D. soothing   E. obedient

3. ZEALOT means MOST NEARLY   3.____

    A. breeze   B. enthusiast   C. vault
    D. wild animal   E. musical instrument

4. A MAGNANIMOUS attitude is one that is   4.____

    A. high-minded   B. faithful
    C. concerned   D. individual
    E. small

5. To CITE means MOST NEARLY to   5.____

    A. protest   B. depart   C. quote   D. agitate   E. perform

6. OBLIVION means MOST NEARLY   6.____

    A. hindrance   B. accident
    C. courtesy   D. forgetfulness
    E. old age

7. CARDINAL means MOST NEARLY   7.____

    A. independent   B. well-organized   C. subordinate
    D. dignified   E. chief

8. To DEPLETE means MOST NEARLY to   8.____

    A. restrain   B. corrupt   C. despair
    D. exhaust   E. spread out

9. To SUPERSEDE means MOST NEARLY to   9.____

    A. retire   B. replace   C. overflow   D. bless   E. oversee

10. SPORADIC means MOST NEARLY   10.____

    A. bad-tempered   B. infrequent
    C. radical   D. reckless
    E. humble

TEST 8

DIRECTIONS: For the following questions, select the word or group of words lettered A, B, C, D, or E that means MOST NEARLY the same as the word in capital letters. *PRINT THE LETTER OF THE CORRECT ANSWER IN THE SPACE AT THE RIGHT.*

1. To NEUTRALIZE means MOST NEARLY to   1.____

   A. entangle   B. strengthen   C. counteract   D. combat   E. converse

2. To INSINUATE means MOST NEARLY to   2.____

   A. destroy   B. hint   C. do wrong   D. accuse   E. release

3. DIMINUTIVE means MOST NEARLY   3.____

   A. proud   B. slow   C. small   D. watery   E. puzzling

4. PLIGHT means MOST NEARLY   4.____

   A. departure   B. weight
   C. conspiracy   D. predicament
   E. stamp

5. An ILLICIT relationship is one that is   5.____

   A. unlawful   B. overpowering   C. ill-advised
   D. small-scale   E. unreadable

6. A BENIGN manner is one that is   6.____

   A. contagious   B. fatal   C. ignorant   D. kindly   E. decorative

7. REVERIE means MOST NEARLY   7.____

   A. abusive language   B. love song   C. backward step
   D. daydream   E. holy man

8. APPREHENSIVE means MOST NEARLY   8.____

   A. quiet   B. firm   C. curious   D. sincere   E. fearful

9. To RECOIL means MOST NEARLY to   9.____

   A. shrink   B. attract   C. electrify   D. adjust   E. fear

10. GUISE means MOST NEARLY   10.____

    A. trickery   B. request   C. innocence
    D. misdeed   E. appearance

TEST 9

DIRECTIONS: For the following questions, select the word or group of words lettered A, B, C, D, or E that means MOST NEARLY the same as the word in capital letters. *PRINT THE LETTER OF THE CORRECT ANSWER IN THE SPACE AT THE RIGHT.*

1. To RELINQUISH means MOST NEARLY to   1._____

    A. regret   B. abandon   C. pursue   D. secure   E. penetrate

2. INJUNCTION means MOST NEARLY   2._____

    A. error   B. attack   C. injustice   D. suggestion   E. order

3. ADVENT means MOST NEARLY   3._____

    A. attachment   B. reference   C. arrival   D. excitement   E. vent

4. BICAMERAL means MOST NEARLY   4._____

    A. dealing with life forms   B. meeting on alternate years
    C. over-sweet   D. having two legislative branches
    E. having two meanings

5. A PERVERSE attitude is one that is   5._____

    A. contrary   B. stingy   C. unfortunate   D. hereditary   E. easygoing

6. To THWART means MOST NEARLY to   6._____

    A. assist   B. whimper   C. slice   D. escape   E. block

7. DEVOID means MOST NEARLY   7._____

    A. empty   B. illegal   C. affectionate   D. pious   E. annoying

8. A BLAND manner is one that is   8._____

    A. gentle   B. guilty   C. salty   D. unfinished   E. majestic

9. To OSTRACIZE means MOST NEARLY to   9._____

    A. flatter   B. scold   C. show off   D. banish   E. vibrate

10. CANDOR means MOST NEARLY   10._____

    A. sociability   B. outspokenness
    C. grief   D. light
    E. flattery

TEST 10

DIRECTIONS: For the following questions, select the word or group of words lettered A, B, C, D, or E that means MOST NEARLY the same as the word in capital letters. *PRINT THE LETTER OF THE CORRECT ANSWER IN THE SPACE AT THE RIGHT.*

1. ACQUIT means MOST NEARLY

    A. increase   B. harden   C. clear   D. sharpen   E. sentence

    1.____

2. DEXTERITY means MOST NEARLY

    A. conceit   B. skill
    C. insistence   D. embarrassment
    E. guidance

    2.____

3. ASSIMILATE means MOST NEARLY

    A. absorb   B. imitate   C. maintain   D. outrun   E. curb

    3.____

4. DESPONDENCY means MOST NEARLY

    A. relief   B. gratitude   C. dejection   D. hatred   E. poverty

    4.____

5. A BUOYANT manner is one that is

    A. conceited   B. cautioning   C. youthful   D. musical   E. cheerful

    5.____

6. CULINARY means MOST NEARLY

    A. having to do with cooking   B. pertaining to dressmaking
    C. fond of eating   D. loving money
    E. tending to be secretive

    6.____

7. CAPRICE means MOST NEARLY

    A. wisdom   B. ornament   C. pillar   D. whim   E. energy

    7.____

8. DETERRENT means MOST NEARLY

    A. restraining   B. cleansing   C. deciding
    D. concluding   E. crumbling

    8.____

9. A PUGNACIOUS attitude is one that is

    A. sticky   B. cowardly
    C. precise   D. vigorous
    E. quarrelsome

    9.____

10. ABSCOND means MOST NEARLY

    A. detest   B. reduce   C. swallow up   D. dismiss   E. flee

    10.____

TEST 11

DIRECTIONS: For the following questions, select the word or group of words lettered A, B, C, D, or E that means MOST NEARLY the same as the word in capital letters. *PRINT THE LETTER OF THE CORRECT ANSWER IN THE SPACE AT THE RIGHT.*

1.   DOLDRUMS means MOST NEARLY   1.____

    A.   delirium   B.   rage   C.   saturation
    D.   incarceration   E.   listlessness

2.   DOUR means MOST NEARLY   2.____

    A.   gloomy   B.   cowardly   C.   untidy   D.   stingy   E.   doubtful

3.   DRAGOON means MOST NEARLY   3.____

    A.   defy   B.   enlist   C.   surrender   D.   lead   E.   persecute

4.   EMPIRICAL means MOST NEARLY   4.____

    A.   experiential   B.   undeniable   C.   melancholy
    D.   territorial   E.   traditional

5.   ENCOMIUM means MOST NEARLY   5.____

    A.   antidote   B.   adage   C.   anteroom   D.   eulogy   E.   bombast

6.   ENTOMOLOGIST means MOST NEARLY student of   6.____

    A.   insects   B.   fish   C.   words   D.   fossils   E.   reptiles

7.   EPHEMERAL means MOST NEARLY   7.____

    A.   persistent   B.   useless   C.   effete   D.   visionary   E.   short-lived

8.   ETIOLOGY means MOST NEARLY   8.____

    A.   epitome   B.   inertia   C.   astronomy   D.   disease   E.   cause

9.   FETISH means MOST NEARLY   9.____

    A.   tuft of hair above horse's hoof   B.   embryo of an animal
    C.   object of excessive devotion   D.   spirit of a festival
    E.   feast of the Haitians

10.   GAMUT means MOST NEARLY   10.____

    A.   gamble   B.   alphabet
    C.   keys   D.   chess move
    E.   range

———

TEST 12

DIRECTIONS: For the following questions, select the word or group of words lettered A, B, C, D, or E that means MOST NEARLY the same as the word in capital letters. *PRINT THE LETTER OF THE CORRECT ANSWER IN THE SPACE AT THE RIGHT.*

1. HALLOW means MOST NEARLY   1._____

   A. shout aloud   B. make sacred
   C. haunt   D. reveal
   E. hole out

2. HEGEMONY means MOST NEARLY   2._____

   A. flight   B. restraint   C. nationalism D. autonomy   E. leadership

3. HERMETIC means MOST NEARLY   3._____

   A. air-tight   B. protruding
   C. sequestered   D. briskly
   E. ascetic

4. IBID means MOST NEARLY   4._____

   A. that is   B. as an example   C. the same
   D. see above   E. and so forth

5. IMPUGN means MOST NEARLY   5._____

   A. enhance   B. attribute
   C. assail   D. compromise
   E. defend

6. INCIPIENT means MOST NEARLY   6._____

   A. tasteless   B. annoying
   C. unyielding   D. ultimate
   E. commencing

7. INEXORABLE means MOST NEARLY   7._____

   A. hateful   B. conciliatory   C. unresponsive
   D. relentless   E. pliant

8. INTREPID means MOST NEARLY   8._____

   A. awesome   B. bellicose   C. undisciplined
   D. courageous   E. pacific

9. INVECTIVE means MOST NEARLY   9._____

   A. self study   B. geometrical analysis   C. verbal abuse
   D. hard-won victory   E. indecision

10. INVEIGLED means MOST NEARLY   10._____

   A. ensnared   B. terrified   C. coerced
   D. corrupted   E. incarcerated

TEST 13

DIRECTIONS: For the following questions, select the word or group of words lettered A, B, C, D, or E that means MOST NEARLY the same as the word in capital letters. *PRINT THE LETTER OF THE CORRECT ANSWER IN THE SPACE AT THE RIGHT.*

1. ITERANT means MOST NEARLY   1._____

    A. distant   B. repeating   C. directed   D. wandering   E. errant

2. LAMPOON means MOST NEARLY   2._____

    A. magazine   B. satire   C. clown   D. lament   E. shade

3. LAPIDARY means MOST NEARLY one who   3._____

    A. collects butterflies   B. breaks up large estates
    C. indulges the senses   D. judges the quality of beverages
    E. cuts precious stones

4. MERETRICIOUS means MOST NEARLY   4._____

    A. according to the metric system   B. deserving
    C. scholarly   D. indigent
    E. tawdry

5. MITIGATE means MOST NEARLY   5._____

    A. exonerate   B. handicap   C. aggravate   D. appease   E. defile

6. MORES means MOST NEARLY   6._____

    A. beginnings   B. conglomerations   C. curses
    D. mutations   E. customs

7. NOSTRUM means MOST NEARLY   7._____

    A. ocean sea   B. paternity   C. remedy   D. pungency   E. family

8. OBJURGATE means MOST NEARLY   8._____

    A. chide   B. sacrifice   C. oppose   D. purge   E. repeat

9. OSSIFY means MOST NEARLY   9._____

    A. vacillate   B. harden   C. categorize D. tipple   E. abstain

10. PARLOUS means MOST NEARLY   10._____

    A. wise   B. bargaining C. talkative   D. dangerous   E. partial

TEST 14

DIRECTIONS: For the following questions, select the word or group of words lettered A, B, C, D, or E that means MOST NEARLY the same as the word in capital letters. *PRINT THE LETTER OF THE CORRECT ANSWER IN THE SPACE AT THE RIGHT.*

1. ADVENTITIOUS means MOST NEARLY   1.____

    A. opportunistic   B. daring   C. helpful
    D. deceptive   E. extrinsic

2. AMBIVALENT means MOST NEARLY   2.____

    A. helpful in walking   B. equally skillful with both hands
    C. simultaneously hating and loving   D. ambiguous in origin
    E. equivalent

3. AMORPHOUS means MOST NEARLY   3.____

    A. inelegant   B. clamorous   C. quiescent   D. ardent   E. formless

4. ANATHEMA means MOST NEARLY   4.____

    A. despair   B. benevolence
    C. disputation   D. anomaly
    E. curse

5. APIARY means MOST NEARLY   5.____

    A. bee house   B. pear-shaped figure   C. main-traveled road
    D. monkey cage   E. bird house

6. APOCRYPHAL means MOST NEARLY of   6.____

    A. scholarly pursuits   B. sacred origin
    C. ancient beginnings   D. ecclesiastical power
    E. doubtful authenticity

7. APOSTASY means MOST NEARLY   7.____

    A. confirmation   B. defection   C. supposition
    D. canonization   E. deification

8. ASCETIC means MOST NEARLY   8.____

    A. exclusive   B. sharp   C. fragrant   D. austere   E. authentic

9. BADINAGE means MOST NEARLY   9.____

    A. indifference   B. song   C. banter   D. mucilage   E. autarchy

10. BOGGLE means MOST NEARLY   10.____

    A. dampen   B. hesitate   C. undermine   D. disarrange   E. haggle

TEST 15

DIRECTIONS: For the following questions, select the word or group of words lettered A, B, C, D, or E that means MOST NEARLY the same as the word in capital letters. *PRINT THE LETTER OF THE CORRECT ANSWER IN THE SPACE AT THE RIGHT.*

1. BUCOLIC means MOST NEARLY

    A. rustic
    B. flatulent
    C. angry
    D. loud
    E. bureaucratic

1.____

2. CAESURA means MOST NEARLY

    A. genesis
    B. referring to Caesar
    C. tyranny
    D. domain
    E. break

2.____

3. CAREEN means MOST NEARLY

    A. lurch
    B. wail
    C. pour
    D. contain
    E. corrode

3.____

4. CARET means MOST NEARLY

    A. measure of weight
    B. sign of omission
    C. technique in ballet
    D. growth of root
    E. notice for caution

4.____

5. CARIES means MOST NEARLY

    A. treatment
    B. convalescent
    C. decay
    D. chemicals
    E. roots

5.____

6. CASUIST means MOST NEARLY

    A. sophistical reasoner
    B. careless worker
    C. innocent victim
    D. habitual late-comer
    E. frenzied lawyer

6.____

7. CHIMERICAL means MOST NEARLY

    A. scientific
    B. debasing
    C. well-ordered
    D. maniacal
    E. fanciful

7.____

8. CLABBER means MOST NEARLY

    A. gossip
    B. climb
    C. crop
    D. entwine
    E. curdle

8.____

9. COMME IL FAUT means MOST NEARLY

    A. unnecessary
    B. erroneous
    C. proper
    D. mixed
    E. illegal

9.____

10. CRYPTIC means MOST NEARLY

    A. succinct
    B. astringent
    C. death-like
    D. crotchety
    E. occult

10.____

TEST 16

DIRECTIONS: For the following questions, select the word or group of words lettered A, B, C, D, or E that means MOST NEARLY the same as the word in capital letters. *PRINT THE LETTER OF THE CORRECT ANSWER IN THE SPACE AT THE RIGHT.*

1. CYNOSURE means MOST NEARLY

1._____

    A. act of completion   B. occupation of ease
    C. attitude of doubt   D. center of attraction
    E. cynical statement

2. DEBENTURE means MOST NEARLY

2._____

    A. written acknowledgment of debt
    B. sale of preferred stock
    C. illegal sale of securities
    D. dividend on stocks or bonds
    E. disclaimer in a prospectus

3. DEMURRER means MOST NEARLY

3._____

    A. promotion   B. objection   C. interrogation
    D. retainer   E. demerit

4. DERELICTION means MOST NEARLY

4._____

    A. general decline   B. damaging criticism
    C. probable cause   D. abandoned vessel
    E. failure in duty

5. DESCRIED means MOST NEARLY

5._____

    A. delimned   B. defined   C. rejected   D. erred   E. discerned

6. DESIDERATUM means MOST NEARLY

6._____

    A. final outcome   B. hearty approval   C. last remnant
    D. desired object   E. prescribed treatment

7. DISCRETE means MOST NEARLY

7._____

    A. separate   B. reserved   C. foresighted
    D. unbounded   E. tactful

8. DISINGENUOUS means MOST NEARLY

8._____

    A. unsophisticated   B. skillful   C. apathetic
    D. naive   E. insincere

9. DISSIDENT means MOST NEARLY

9._____

    A. malodorous   B. amoral   C. discordant
    D. unfeeling   E. divisive

10. EGREGIOUS means MOST NEARLY

10._____

    A. debased   B. inconsequential   C. incorrigible
    D. egotistical   E. prominent

TEST 17

DIRECTIONS: For the following questions, select the word or group of words lettered A, B, C, D, or E that means MOST NEARLY the same as the word in capital letters. *PRINT THE LETTER OF THE CORRECT ANSWER IN THE SPACE AT THE RIGHT.*

1.   EMPATHY means MOST NEARLY   1._____

     A.   comatose condition   B.   sympathetic understanding
     C.   depressed feeling   D.   political subdivision
     E.   patriotic devotion

2.   ESOTERIC means MOST NEARLY   2._____

     A.   abstruse   B.   intestinal   C.   lively   D.   joining   E.   essential

3.   ESPERANTO means MOST NEARLY   3._____

     A.   fabled country   B.   artificial language
     C.   European peace manifesto   D.   place of abandoned hope
     E.   pertaining to the Elysian Fields

4.   EUPHEMISM means MOST NEARLY   4._____

     A.   pleasant sight   B.   right direction
     C.   verbal platitude   D.   buoyant feeling
     E.   inoffensive expression

5.   FINICAL means MOST NEARLY   5._____

     A.   blundering   B.   fastidious   C.   conclusive
     D.   maniacal   E.   extravagant

6.   GUERDON means MOST NEARLY   6._____

     A.   debacle   B.   shield
     C.   fruit   D.   obstacle
     E.   recompense

7.   GYVES means MOST NEARLY   7._____

     A.   gallows   B.   chains   C.   barbs   D.   vegetables E.   jives

8.   HEDONIST means MOST NEARLY   8._____

     A.   reviler   B.   recluse
     C.   pleasure-seeker   D.   savage
     E.   hermit

9.   HIATUS means MOST NEARLY   9._____

     A.   flower   B.   gap   C.   mistake   D.   digression E.   hearsay

10.   IMBROGLIO means MOST NEARLY   10._____

     A.   secluded dwelling   B.   impassioned plea
     C.   rampant destruction   D.   petit point
     E.   complicated situation

TEST 18

DIRECTIONS: For the following questions, select the word or group of words lettered A, B, C, D, or E that means MOST NEARLY the same as the word in capital letters. *PRINT THE LETTER OF THE CORRECT ANSWER IN THE SPACE AT THE RIGHT.*

1. IMPALPABLE means MOST NEARLY not   1.____
   A. truthful   B. concrete   C. throbbing
   D. deviating   E. suggestive

2. IMPECUNIOUS means MOST NEARLY   2.____
   A. poor   B. wayward
   C. troublesome   D. inordinate
   E. ingenuous

3. IMPORTUNATE means MOST NEARLY   3.____
   A. critical   B. empty-handed   C. disastrous
   D. pusillanimous   E. pressing

4. IMPRIMIS means MOST NEARLY   4.____
   A. church dignitary B. sanction   C. manuscript
   D. sacred song   E. in the first place

5. INURED means MOST NEARLY   5.____
   A. belligerent   B. hardened   C. apprehensive
   D. irreverent   E. injured

6. INVIDIOUS means MOST NEARLY   6.____
   A. obscure   B. unconquerable   C. offensive
   D. niggardly   E. invariable

7. JOCOSE means MOST NEARLY   7.____
   A. intemperate   B. contemptuous   C. morose
   D. nugatory   E. facetious

8. LACHRYMOSE means MOST NEARLY   8.____
   A. milky   B. disdainful   C. comic   D. tearful   E. comatose

9. LISSOME means MOST NEARLY   9.____
   A. nimble   B. comely   C. laughable
   D. lackadaisical   E. aggressive

10. MERCURIAL means MOST NEARLY   10.____
    A. thermal   B. coy   C. volatile
    D. ponderous   E. unchangeable

235

KEYS (CORRECT ANSWERS)

TEST 1
1.	D	6.	C
2.	C	7.	A
3.	A	8.	E
4.	C	9.	B
5.	C	10.	C

TEST 2
1.	A	6.	C
2.	B	7.	E
3.	C	8.	B
4.	B	9.	A
5.	A	10.	D

TEST 3
1.	A	6.	D
2.	A	7.	C
3.	B	8.	A
4.	E	9.	A
5.	D	10.	D

TEST 4
1.	C	6.	E
2.	D	7.	B
3.	B	8.	B
4.	C	9.	A
5.	D	10.	E

TEST 5
1.	C	6.	D
2.	B	7.	A
3.	C	8.	A
4.	D	9.	D
5.	E	10.	B

TEST 6
1.	A	6.	D
2.	B	7.	D
3.	E	8.	B
4.	A	9.	B
5.	B	10.	C

TEST 7
1.	A	6.	D
2.	E	7.	E
3.	B	8.	D
4.	A	9.	B
5.	C	10.	B

TEST 8
1.	C	6.	D
2.	B	7.	D
3.	C	8.	E
4.	D	9.	A
5.	A	10.	E

TEST 9
1.	B	6.	E
2.	E	7.	A
3.	C	8.	A
4.	D	9.	D
5.	A	10.	B

TEST 10
1.	C	6.	A
2.	B	7.	D
3.	A	8.	A
4.	C	9.	E
5.	E	10.	E

TEST 11
1.	E	6.	A
2.	A	7.	E
3.	E	8.	E
4.	A	9.	C
5.	D	10.	E

TEST 12
1.	B	6.	E
2.	E	7.	D
3.	A	8.	D
4.	C	9.	C
5.	C	10.	A

TEST 13
1.	B	6.	E
2.	B	7.	C
3.	E	8.	A
4.	E	9.	B
5.	D	10.	D

TEST 14
1.	E	6.	E
2.	C	7.	B
3.	E	8.	D
4.	E	9.	C
5.	A	10.	B

TEST 15
1.	A	6.	A
2.	E	7.	E
3.	A	8.	E
4.	B	9.	C
5.	C	10.	E

TEST 16
1.	D	6.	D
2.	A	7.	A
3.	B	8.	E
4.	E	9.	C
5.	E	10.	E

TEST 17
1.	B	6.	E
2.	A	7.	B
3.	B	8.	C
4.	E	9.	B
5.	B	10.	E

TEST 18
1.	B	6.	C
2.	A	7.	E
3.	E	8.	D
4.	E	9.	A
5.	B	10.	C

SENTENCE COMPLETION
EXAMINATION SECTION
TEST 1

DIRECTIONS: Each question in this part consists of a sentence in which one word is missing; a blank line indicates where the word has been removed from the sentence. Beneath each sentence are five words, one of which is the missing word. You are to select the number of the missing word by deciding which one of the five words BEST fits in with the meaning of the sentence. *PRINT THE LETTER OF THE CORRECT ANSWER IN THE SPACE AT THE RIGHT.*

1. Although they had little interest in the game they were playing, rather than be _____, they played it through to the end.   1._____

    A. inactive   B. inimical   C. busy
    D. complacent   E. vapid

2. That he was unworried and at peace with the world could be, perhaps, observed from his _____ brow.   2._____

    A. unwrinkled   B. wrinkled   C. furrowed
    D. twisted   E. askew

3. Among the hundreds of workers in the assembly plant of the factory, one was _____ because of his skill and speed.   3._____

    A. steadfast   B. condemned   C. consistent
    D. outstanding   E. eager

4. The story of the invention of many of our best known machines is a consistent one: they are the result of a long series of experiments by many people; thus, the Wright Brothers in 1903 _____ the airplane rather than invented it.   4._____

    A. popularized   B. regulated   C. perfected
    D. contrived   E. developed

5. As soon as the former political exile returned to his native country, he looked up old supporters, particularly those whom he knew to be _____ and whose help he might need.   5._____

    A. potent   B. pusillanimous   C. attentive
    D. free   E. retired

6. A recent study of the New Deal shows that no other man than the President could have brought together so many _____ interests and combined them into so effective a political organization.   6._____

    A. secret   B. interior   C. predatory
    D. harmonious   E. conflicting

7. A study of tides presents an interesting _____ in that, while the forces that set them in motion are universal in application, presumably affecting all parts of our world without distinction, the action of tides in particular areas is completely local in nature.   7._____

    A. phenomenon   B. maneuver   C. paradox
    D. quality   E. spontaneity

8. Many of the facts that are found in the ancient archives constitute _____ that help shed   8._____
   light upon human activities in the past.

    A.   facts   B.   reminders   C.   particles
    D.   sources   E.   indications

9. It is a regrettable fact that in a caste society which deems manual toil a mark of _____,   9._____
   rarely does the laborer improve his social position or gain political power.

    A.   inferiority   B.   consolation   C.   fortitude
    D.   hardship   E.   brilliance

10. As a generalization, one can correctly say that crises in history are caused by the re-   10._____
    opening of questions which have been safely _____ for long periods of time.

    A.   debated   B.   joined   C.   recondite
    D.   settled   E.   unanswered

KEY (CORRECT ANSWERS)

    1.   A
    2.   A
    3.   D
    4.   C
    5.   A

    6.   E
    7.   C
    8.   D
    9.   A
  10.   A

TEST 2

DIRECTIONS: Each question in this part consists of a sentence in which one word is missing; a blank line indicates where the word has been removed from the sentence. Beneath each sentence are five words, one of which is the missing word. You are to select the number of the missing word by deciding which one of the five words BEST fits in with the meaning of the sentence. *PRINT THE LETTER OF THE CORRECT ANSWER IN THE SPACE AT THE RIGHT.*

1. We can see in retrospect that the high hopes for lasting peace conceived at Versailles in 1919 were _____.

    A. ingenuous   B. transient   C. nostalgic
    D. ingenious   E. species

    1.____

2. One of the constructive effects of Nazism was the passage by the U.N. of a resolution to combat _____.

    A. armaments   B. nationalism   C. colonialism
    D. genocide   E. geriatrics

    2.____

3. In our prisons, the role of _____ often gains for certain inmates a powerful position among their fellow prisoners.

    A. informer   B. clerk   C. warden
    D. trusty   E. turnkey

    3.____

4. It is the _____ liar, experienced in the ways of the world, who finally trips upon some incongruous detail.

    A. consummate   B. incorrigible   C. congenital
    D. flagrant   E. contemptible

    4.____

5. Anyone who is called a misogynist can hardly be expected to look upon women with _____ contemptuous eyes.

    A. more than   B. nothing less than   C. decidedly
    D. other than   E. always

    5.____

6. Demagogues such as Hitler and Mussolini aroused the masses by appealing to their _____ rather than to their intellect.

    A. emotions   B. reason   C. nationalism
    D. conquests   E. duty

    6.____

7. He was in great demand as an entertainer for his _____ abilities: he could sing, dance, tell a joke, or relate a story with equally great skill and facility.

    A. versatile   B. logical   C. culinary
    D. histrionic   E. creative

    7.____

8. The wise politician is aware that, next to knowing when to seize an opportunity, it is also important to know when to _____ an advantage.

    A. develop   B. seek   C. revise   D. proclaim   E. forego

    8.____

9. Books on psychology inform us that the best way to break a bad habit is to _____ a new habit in its place. 9.____

    A. expel
    B. substitute
    C. conceal
    D. curtail
    E. supplant

10. The author who uses one word where another uses a whole paragraph, should be considered a _____ writer. 10.____

    A. successful
    B. grandiloquent
    C. succinct
    D. prolix
    E. experienced

_____

KEYS (CORRECT ANSWERS)

    1. A
    2. D
    3. A
    4. A
    5. D

    6. A
    7. A
    8. E
    9. B
  10. C

_____

TEST 3

DIRECTIONS: Each question in this part consists of a sentence in which one word is missing; a blank line indicates where the word has been removed from the sentence. Beneath each sentence are five words, one of which is the missing word. You are to select the number of the missing word by deciding which one of the five words BEST fits in with the meaning of the sentence. *PRINT THE LETTER OF THE CORRECT ANSWER IN THE SPACE AT THE RIGHT.*

1. The prime minister, fleeing from the rebels who had seized the government, sought _____ in the church.   1.____

   A. revenge   B. mercy   C. relief
   D. salvation   E. sanctuary

2. It does not take us long to conclude that it is foolish to fight the _____, and that it is far wiser to accept it.   2.____

   A. inevitable   B. inconsequential C. impossible
   D. choice   E. invasion

3. _____ is usually defined as an excessively high rate of interest.   3.____

   A. Injustice   B. Perjury   C. Exorbitant
   D. Embezzlement   E. Usury

4. "I ask you, gentlemen of the jury, to find this man guilty since I have _____ the charges brought against him."   4.____

   A. documented   B. questioned   C. revised
   D. selected   E. confused

5. Although the critic was a close friend of the producer, he told him that he could not _____ his play.   5.____

   A. condemn   B. prefer   C. congratulate
   D. endorse   E. revile

6. Knowledge of human nature and motivation is an important _____ in all areas of endeavor.   6.____

   A. object   B. incentive   C. opportunity
   D. asset   E. goal

7. Numbered among the audience were kings, princes, dukes, and even a maharajah, all attempting to _____ one another in the glitter of their habiliments and the number of their escorts.   7.____

   A. supersede   B. outdo   C. guide
   D. vanquish   E. equal

8. There seems to be a widespread feeling that peoples who are located below us in respect to latitude are _____ also in respect to intellect and ability.   8.____

   A. superior   B. melodramatic   C. inferior
   D. ulterior   E. contemptible

9. This should be considered a(n) _____ rather than the usual occurrence.   9.____

    A. coincidence ✓   B. specialty   C. development
    D. outgrowth   E. mirage

10. Those who were considered states' rights aherents in the early part of our history   10.____
espoused the diminution of the powers of the national government because they had
always been _____ of these powers.

    A. solicitous   B. advocates   C. apprehensive ✓
    D. mindful   E. respectful

KEYS (CORRECT ANSWERS)

1. E
2. A
3. E
4. A
5. D

6. D
7. B
8. C
9. A
10. C

TEST 4

DIRECTIONS: Each question in this part consists of a sentence in which one word is missing; a blank line indicates where the word has been removed from the sentence. Beneath each sentence are five words, one of which is the missing word. You are to select the number of the missing word by deciding which one of the five words BEST fits in with the meaning of the sentence. *PRINT THE LETTER OF THE CORRECT ANSWER IN THE SPACE AT THE RIGHT.*

1. The life of the mining camps as portrayed by Bret Harte - boisterous, material, brawling - was in direct _____ to the contemporary Eastern world of conventional morals and staid deportment depicted by other men of letters.

    A. model   B. parallel   C. antithesis
    D. relationship   E. response

    1.____

2. The agreements were to remain in force for three years and were subject to automatic _____ unless terminated by the parties concerned on one month's notice.

    A. renewal   B. abrogation   C. amendment
    D. confiscation   E. option

    2.____

3. In a democracy, people are recognized for what they do rather than for their _____.

    A. alacrity   B. ability   C. reputation
    D. skill   E. pedigree

    3.____

4. Although he had often loudly proclaimed his _____ concerning world affairs, he actually read widely and was usually the best informed person in his circle.

    A. weariness   B. complacency   C. condolence
    D. indifference   E. worry

    4.____

5. This student holds the _____ record of being the sole failure in his class.

    A. flagrant   B. unhappy   C. egregious
    D. dubious   E. unusual

    5.____

6. She became enamored _____ the acrobat when she witnessed his act.

    A. of   B. with   C. for   D. by   E. about

    6.____

7. This will _____ all previous wills.

    A. abrogates   B. denies   C. supersedes
    D. prevents   E. continues

    7.____

8. In the recent terrible Chicago _____, over ninety children were found dead as a result of the fire.

    A. hurricane   B. destruction   C. panic
    D. holocaust   E. accident

    8.____

9. I can ascribe no better reason why he shunned society than that he was a _____.

    A. mentor   B. Centaur   C. aristocrat
    D. misanthrope   E. failure

    9.____

10. One who attempts to learn all the known facts before he comes to a conclusion may most aptly be described as a   10.____

    A. realist
    D. pessimist
    B. philosopher
    E. skeptic
    C. cynic

KEY (CORRECT ANSWERS)

1. C
2. A
3. E
4. D
5. D

6. A
7. C
8. D
9. D
10. E

TEST 5

DIRECTIONS: Each question in this part consists of a sentence in which one word is missing; a blank line indicates where the word has been removed from the sentence. Beneath each sentence are five words, one of which is the missing word. You are to select the number of the missing word by deciding which one of the five words BEST fits in with the meaning of the sentence. *PRINT THE LETTER OF THE CORRECT ANSWER IN THE SPACE AT THE RIGHT.*

1. The judge exercised commendable _____ in dismissing the charge against the prisoner. In spite of the clamor that surrounded the trial, and the heinousness of the offense, the judge could not be swayed to overlook the lack of facts in the case.   1.____

   A. avidity   B. meticulousness   C. clemency
   D. balance   E. querulousness

2. The pianist played the concerto _____, displaying such facility and skill as has rarely been matched in this old auditorium.   2.____

   A. strenuously   B. deftly   C. passionately
   D. casually   E. spiritedly

3. The Tanglewood Symphony Orchestra holds its outdoor concerts far from city turmoil in a _____, bucolic setting.   3.____

   A. spectacular   B. atavistic   C. serene
   D. chaotic   E. catholic

4. Honest satire gives true joy to the thinking man. Thus, the satirist is most _____ when he points out the hypocrisy in human actions.   4.____

   A. elated   B. humiliated   C. ungainly
   D. repressed   E. disdainful

5. She was a(n) _____ who preferred the company of her books to the pleasures of cafe society.   5.____

   A. philanthropist   B. stoic   C. exhibitionist
   D. extrovert   E. introvert

6. So many people are so convinced that people are driven by _____ motives that they cannot believe that anybody is unselfish!   6.____

   A. interior   B. ulterior   C. unworthy
   D. selfish   E. destructive

7. These _____ results were brought about by a chain of fortuitous events.   7.____

   A. unfortunate   B. odd   C. harmful
   D. haphazard   E. propitious

8. The bank teller's _____ of the funds was discovered the following month when the auditors examined the books.   8.____

   A. embezzlement   B. burglary   C. borrowing
   D. assignment   E. theft

245

9. The monks gathered in the _____ for their evening meal.   9.____

    A. lounge   B. auditorium   C. refectory
    D. rectory   E. solarium

10. Local officials usually have the responsibility in each area of determining when the need   10.____
is sufficiently great to _____ withdrawals from the community water supply.

    A. encourage   B. justify   C. discontinue
    D. advocate   E. forbid

KEY (CORRECT ANSWERS)

  1. D
  2. B
  3. C
  4. A
  5. E

  6. B
  7. D
  8. A
  9. C
10. B

BASIC FUNDAMENTALS OF ENGLISH EXPRESSION

TABLE OF CONTENTS

BASIC FUNDAMENTALS OF ENGLISH EXPRESSION

A. FUNCTIONAL INTRODUCTION TO GRAMMAR

For examination purposes, there are two clear-cut and yet related divisions in grammar: classification and syntax.

Classification refers to the required nomenclature for the proper identification and description of the uses of words or groups of words. Syntax refers to the relations of words and groups of words with one another in sentences.

The more usual terms of Classification are the following:

CLASSIFICATION

1. Nominative Absolute
2. Nominative of Direct Address
3. Nominative of Exclamation
4. Predicate Nominative
5. Predicate Adjective
6. Object of a Verb
7. Indirect Object
8. Object of a Preposition
9. Objective Complement
10. Adverbial Objective
11. Retained Object
12. Noun in Apposition
13. Auxiliary Verb
14. Copulative Verb
15. Progressive Forms of the Verb
16. Past Participle
17. Mood
18. Tense
19. Subject - complete subject, including modifiers
20. Predicate - verb and all modifiers and complements
21. Verbals

The more outstanding and the more frequently occurring types of syntactical relationships are defined in the illustrations appearing hereafter.

SYNTAX

I. Uses of the Noun
   A. Nominative Case:
      1. Subject of a verb: MARY bought a hat.
      2. Predicate Nominative: (Double Function)
         a. With a copulative verb: He became PRESIDENT. Is that the SORT of a person you take me for?
         b. With a verb in the passive voice: He was chosen PRESIDENT.
      3. Independent Constructions:
         a. Noun in Apposition with a noun in the nominative case: My sister, CLARA, is going with me.
         b. Nominative Absolute: The TRAIN having stopped, the passengers got out. James stood before me, his HANDS in his pocket
         c. Nominative of Direct Address: MARY, open the door.
         d. Nominative of Exclamation: What a MAN!

B. Possessive Case:
   1. To show ownership: MARY'S hat is brown.
   2. To indicate the relation of the doer to an act expressed in a particular noun: MARY'S having her homework saved the day. (See Predicate Complement of Copulative Verbal, below)
C. Objective Case: (Complements)
   1. Object of a
      a. Verb: The child ate the APPLE.
      b. Verbal:
         1. Infinitive: At times, it's a pleasure to eat an APPLE.
         2. Participle: Having lost the larger PART of his fortune, my friend found that economy was necessary.
         3. Participial Noun: Eating an APPLE is a pleasure.
      c. Preposition: She gave the book to CLARA.
      d. Cognate Object: He spoke his SPEECH well.
      e. Secondary Object of a Verb or Verbal: He told John the ANSWER. He asked John a QUESTION. He paid his workers good WAGES. (Differs from the indirect object because the secondary object can be dropped.)
   2. Indirect Object of a
      a. Verb: We gave JOHN our books.
      b. Verbal:
         1. Infinitive: He asked us to give CATHERINE the money.
         2. Participle: Giving my FRIEND the money I had borrowed, I heaved a sigh of relief.
         3. Participial Noun: Giving PEOPLE money makes most people happier.
   3. Subject of an Infinitive: I expect JOHN to be present. Let ME rest!
   4. Objective Complement: (See Predicate Nominative with Passive Verb) We elected him PRESIDENT. The Romans called Caesar FRIEND.
   5. Retained Object:(See 2a.)John was given our BOOKS.
   6. Adverbial Objective: I wanted to go HOME. The child is three YEARS old.
   7. Predicate Complement of Copulative Verbals:
      a. Referring back to the Subject of the Infinitive: I believed Allen to be the MAN.
      b. Referring back to the noun modified by a participle:
         Or lonely house,
         Long held the witches' HOME.
      c. Referring back to the Possessive with the Participial Noun: There is sense in your hoping to be SECRETARY. I was sure of John's being the AGGRESSOR.
   8. Noun in Apposition with a noun in the objective case: I gave the song, SOPHISTICATED LADY, to my friend to play.

II. Uses of the Pronoun
   A. Personal Pronouns: Similar to nouns in use, but, in addition, they must agree with the antecedent in person, number, and gender.
      1. Nominative Case:
         a. Subject of a verb: SHE bought a hat.
         b. Predicate Nominative with Copulative Verb: It is I
         c. Independent Construction:
            1. Nominative Absolute: SHE being ill, we decided to go.

           2.   Nominative of Direct Address: YOU, will you come!

           3.   Nominative of Exclamation: I! You cannot accuse me!

    2.   Possessive Case:

        a.   To show ownership: HER hat is brown.

        b.   To indicate relation of doer to an act or state expressed in a participial noun: HIS having a car saved the day.

    3.   Objective Case:

        a.   Object of a

           1.   Verb: The child ate IT.

           2.   Verbal:

               a.   Infinitive: At times it is a pleasure to eat IT.

               b.   Participle: Having lost IT, we hunted for another.

               c.   Participial Noun: Taking IT in large doses is bad.

           3.   Preposition: She referred me to HIM for an answer.

        b.   Indirect Object of a

           1.   Verb: We gave HIM our books.

           2.   Verbal:

               a.   Infinitive: He asked us to give HER the money.

               b.   Participle: Giving HIM the money I had borrowed, I heaved a sigh of relief.

               c.   Participial Noun: Giving HIM money made him unhappy.

        c.   Subject of the Infinitive: I expected HIM to be present.

        d.   Retained Object: He was given IT for his own use.

B.   Uses of "it":

    1.   Impersonal Pronoun, subject of a verb when no definite subject is expressed: IT rains.

    2.   Expletive, serving to introduce the verb "is" when the real subject is in the Predicate: IT may be true that he did not commit the crime.

C.   Compound Personal Pronouns:

    1.   Intensively: I, MYSELF, will go.

    2.   Reflexively: I have harmed MYSELF. The neighbors left us severely to OUR-SELVES.

D.   Interrogative Pronouns: Similar to personal pronouns in use, but, in addition, they assist in asking a question. WHO is that? WHOSE is that? WHOM do you expect? WHICH is the better student? WHAT is your aim in life? He asked me WHAT I had meant by that statement.(Indirect) WHO do you consider is the best agent the company has?

E.   Adjective (Demonstrative) Pronouns: Similar to personal pronouns in use. THIS is a new hat. THESE are very interesting books. The mountains of Colorado are higher than THOSE. I bought ONE, too.

F.   Relative Pronouns: Similar to personal pronouns in use, but, in addition, they <u>connect</u> the adjective clauses they introduce with the nouns or pronouns modified.

      That is the girl WHO is going with me.

      The men WHOM you see there are marines.

      The men WHOSE lights are lit are seniors.

      Ask her for the book WHICH I recommended.

      Tell her WHAT you have told me. (That which)

      That's WHAT I did it for.

      The book THAT I gave her is lost.

      This is the pillow THAT I asked for.

Who do you consider is the best agent (THAT) the company has?
(Elliptical use)
Adjective clauses are also introduced by relative adverbs:
There was one time WHEN I almost caught you.
That is the house WHERE I was born.
G. Compound relative pronouns:
I will go with WHOEVER is going my way. (Implies own antecedent: HIM WHO)
III. Uses of the Adjective
A. Modifier of a noun (pronoun): That was an ORIENTAL rug. This dress is plainer than that PRETTY one. I must have the test-tube CLEAN. Of dark BROWN gardens and of PEEPING flowers.
B. Predicate Adjective:
1. With copulative verb: She was LAZY. This apple is RIPE.
2. Passive Voice: This man was pronounced GUILTY.
C. Objective Complement: I called the ship UNSEAWORTHY. I will make assurance doubly SURE. She wiped the plate DRY.
IV. Uses of the Adverb
A. Modifier of a verb: She walked RAPIDLY. This matter must be acted UPON.
B. Modifier of a verbal:
1. Infinitive: She attempted to walk RAPIDLY.
2. Participle: Having arrived SILENTLY, she overheard the conversation.
3. Participial Noun: Passing COMMENDABLY is our aim.
C. Modifier of an adjective: The ice was UNUSUALLY smooth this winter.
D. Modifier of another adverb: The wheels revolved VERY swiftly.
E. Modifier of a phrase or clause: He arrived JUST in time. That is EXACTLY what I expected of him.
F. As a relative or conjunctive adverb, introducing a clause and modifying the verb in this clause: I passed the house WHERE he was born. AS he rose from his chair, the audience burst into wild applause.
G. As an interrogative adverb, asking a direct or indirect question and modifying the verb: WHEN did you arrive? Tell us WHY he is always successful.
V. Uses of Verbals: Verbals take adverbial modifiers and complements.
A. The Infinitive.
1. As a noun
a. Nominative Case:
1. Subject of Verb: TO EXIST is a hard job these days.
2. Predicate Nominative: Copulative Verb: To work is TO EAT.
3. Independent Constructions: Apposition: Our ambition, TO ACT, was never realized.
4. Nominative Absolute: To ENJOY ourselves being impossible, we left the theatre.
5. Exclamation: TO SOAR! TO SOAR above the earth with wings!
b. Objective Case:
1. Object of a verb: The child asked TO SING. They expect TO TAKE one.
2. Object of a verbal:(Infinitive) It is never safe to ask TO GO. (Participle) Having asked TO LEAVE, he refused when the chance came. Bill Brown came asking
TO BE ADMITTED to the house. (Participial Noun) Learning TO FLY is amusing.

3. Object of a Preposition: There was nothing to do but TO GO.
4. Retained Object: He was told TO GO.
5. Apposition with noun in objective case: We never realized our ambition, TO ACT.
6. Special Use: With an object noun or pronoun as its subject: I wrote for him TO COME.(Such phrases introduced by "for" are used as nouns.) He felt the ground TREMBLE.

2. As an adjective
   a. Modifying a noun: Houses TO RENT are scarce this year.
   c. Predicate Adjective: Our plan seemed TO WORK each day.
3. As an adverb
   a. Modifying a verb: Folks would laugh TO SEE a cindermaid at a court ball.
   b. Modifying an adjective: The army was ready TO MARCH.
   c. Modifying a verbal: (Participle) Having gone out TO SHOP, he could not be found. (Participial Noun) Trying TO STUDY is impossible.
4. As part of the complement of a verb or preposition with a noun as subject: Let me GO!
5. As an Independent Expression: TO LIVE! To live in utter forgetfulness.

B. The Participle: The participial form of a verb used as an adjective: The men HAVING WORKED steadily, the company decided to give them a raise. (Predicate Adjective) He appeared PANTING. (Objective Complement) I must have the test-tube CLEANED. Special Case: (1) With a noun in the nominative absolute construction: The day HAVING DAWNED, we started on our trip. (2) In rare cases, as an adverb: He ran CRYING down the street.

C. The Participal Noun: The participial form of a verb used as a noun. (Subject) SEEING is believing. (Predicate Nominative)Seeing is BELIEVING. (Apposition) The sport, SKATING, is an exciting one. (Nominative Absolute) SKATING being over, the children went home. (With Possessive Pronoun) MARY'S swimming did not succeed very well. (Object of verb) I love SKATING. (Object of Verbal) He wanted to go SKATING. (Object of a Preposition) The pleasure lies in EATING. We went SKATING. (Retained Object) The children were given WEAVING to do. (Adverbial Objective) That is worth THINKING about. The water was BOILING hot.

VI. Uses of Phrases
   A. As nouns:
      1. The Infinitive Phrase: His aim is TO BE WELL.
      2. Participial Noun Phrase: His only pleasure is BEING WELL. MENDING BROKEN CHINA was his occupation.
   B. As adjectives:
   1. Prepositional Phrase:(Modifier of a Noun) The trees OF THE FOREST are fading. (Predicate Adjective) The sun is IN ITS SPLENDOR.
   2. Infinitive Phrase: (Modifier of a Noun) The house TO BE SOLD was burned. (Predicate Adjective) The house was TO BE SOLD.
   3. Participial Phrase: (Modifier of Noun) RUNNING AWAY, he was shot.
   C. As adverbs:
      1. Prepositional Phrase: Frank came A-RUNNING. Tom ran crying DOWN THE STREET. The room was full OF PEOPLE.
      2. Infinitive Phrase: Folks would laugh TO SEE a cindermaid at a ball.
   D. As Independent Elements: It is true, TO BE SURE. It is better, IN MY OPINION, to face the situation directly.

VII. Uses of Subordinate Clauses
   A. Noun Clauses: Introduced by subordinating conjunctions such as THAT, WHETHER; interrogative pronouns in indirect questions, such as WHO, WHICH, WHAT; interrogative adverbs in indirect questions, such as WHERE, WHEN, WHY, HOW; all illustrated below.
      1. Subject of a Verb: THAT WE HAVE SURVIVED THE ORDEAL is evident.
      2. Predicate Nominative: The truth is THAT HE FAILED TO PASS.
      3. Noun in Apposition: The fact THAT THE EARTH IS ROUND is never disputed.
      4. Object of a Verb or Verbal: Tell me WHERE IS FANCY BRED. I wish HE WOULD HELP ME, I begged him to tell me WHAT HE WANTED. I asked him just WHAT HE REPORTED.
      5. Object of a Preposition: I am going there no matter WHAT YOU SAY. We came to the conclusion from WHAT WE KNOW.
      6. Retained Object: He was asked just WHAT HE REPORTED. I was asked WHETHER I ENJOY READING.
      7. Special Construction: In apposition with the expletive IT: It is commonly known THAT HE CANNOT BE TRUSTED.
   B. Adjective Clauses: Introduced by relative pronoun, WHO, WHICH, WHAT, THAT; relative adverb, WHERE, WHEN, AFTER.
      1. Modifier of a Noun: Thrice is he armed WHO HATH HIS QUARREL JUST. There is society WHERE NONE INTRUDES. I remember the house WHERE I WAS BORN. Who do you consider is the best agent THE COMPANY HAS?
   C. Adverbial Clauses: Introduced by relative (or conjunctive) adverbs; subordinating conjunctions such as BECAUSE, IF, SINCE, THOUGH.
      1. Modifier of a Verb, Verbal, Adjective, Adverb: Try AS WE MAY, we cannot swim to that rock. I intend to leave WHEN YOU GO. We are glad THAT YOU ARE WITH US. WHERE THE BEE SUCKS, there suck I.
   D. Independent Clause Element: Who DO YOU CONSIDER is the best agent the company has? He is, I THINK, able to do the work well.
VIII. Uses of the Verb
   A. Types of verbs
      1. Transitive verbs
         a. These require direct objects to complete the meaning: John ATE the apple, (direct object)
      2. Intransitive verbs
         a. These do not require an object to complete the meaning: The boy RAN down the mountain. (Common causes of error are the misuse of the intransitive verbs RISE, LIE, and SIT and/or the transitive verbs RAISE, LAY, and SET: She LAID on the bed, for She LAY on the bed.
      3. Copulative verbs
         a. These verbs, especially forms of the verb TO BE, are used to express simply the relationship between the subject and the predicate (or complement): She LOOKS good; The meat SMELLS bad; I FEEL better. (The most common copulative verbs are: BE, SEEM, PROVE, FEEL, SOUND, LOOK, APPEAR, BECOME, TASTE.)
      4. Auxiliary verbs
         a. These verbs assist in forming the voices, modes, and tenses of other verbs: She SHOULD go; They HAVE BEEN gone a month; We WERE given the information. (The most common auxiliary verbs are: BE,

HAVE, DO, SHALL, WILL, MAY, CAN, MUST, OUGHT, with all their inflectional forms.)
- B. Tenses of verbs (Verbs appear in different forms to indicate the time of the action):
  1. Present tense: The boy CARRIES the book; She EATS cookies.
  2. Past tense: The men COMPLETED the job; We VISITED him at home.
  3. Future tense: We WILL DO the job tomorrow; I SHALL GO alone.
     a. In speech and in informal writing, WILL and WOULD are now commonly used for all three persons except for the use of SHOULD to express obligation.
     b. In formal writing and careful usage, the following distinctions are observed between SHALL and WILL:
        1. To express simple futurity, use SHALL (or SHOULD) with the first person, and WILL (or WOULD) with the second or third persons: I SHALL be glad to go; They WOULD like to go.
        2. To express determination, intention, etc., use WILL (or WOULD) with the first person, and SHALL (or SHOULD) with the second and third persons: I WILL do it; You SHALL not go; They SHALL not pass.
        3. In questions, use SHALL with the first person: SHALL we see you tonight? SHALL I do it now? With the second person, use the form that is expected in the answer: WILL you lend us the car? (The answer that is expected here is: I WILL or I WILL not.) With the third person, use WILL to express simple futurity: WILL there be someone to meet him at the train?
        4. In indirect discourse, use the auxiliary that would be used if the discourse were direct: The company asked him whether he WOULD pay the bill. (Direct discourse: WILL you pay the bill?) He stated that he WOULD undertake the mission. (Direct discourse: I WILL undertake the mission.) His wife asked him whether he SHOULD be late for supper. (Direct discourse: SHALL you be late for supper?)
  4. Present perfect tense: I HAVE BEEN LIVING here for three years.
  5. Past perfect tense: He HAD BEEN CONVICTED of a crime many years ago.
  6. Future perfect tense: Before you arrive, I SHALL HAVE BAKED the pie.
- C. Mood (Mode) (The forms of a verb that indiqate the manner of the action):
  1. Indicative Mood (used to state a fact or to ask a question): The man FELL; ARE you well?
  2. Imperative Mood (used to express a command or an urgent request): DO it at once; ANSWER the telephone.
  3. Subjective Mood (used to express a wish, a supposition, a doubt, an exhortation, a concession, a condition contrary to fact): Wish: If only I WERE able to run faster!
     Supposition: They will be married provided their parents CONSENT. Condition contrary to fact: If you HAD more experience, you would know how to handle the problem.

IX. Special Uses
- A. Common Words Used as Different Parts of Speech:
  1. But: as relative pronoun: There is none BUT will answer.
     as adverb: You are BUT half awake, (only)
     as a preposition: Every man BUT him may leave, (except)
     I cannot BUT feel cherful.(except to feel)

as a coordinating conjunction: He leaves BUT I stay.

2. Like: (Never used as a conjunction)
   as a preposition: He talks LIKE his mother,
   as a verb: I LIKE his manner of speech.

3. As: as a relative pronoun: You own the same AS I.
   as an adverb: I am AS young as you are.
   as a subordinating conjunction: I am as young AS you are.
   as a preposition: He has frequently appeared AS Hamlet.

4. Than: as a preposition: He loves money more THAN learning.
   as a subordinating conjunction: He knows more THAN I.

B. BASIC SYNTAX

(NOTE: Rules are numbered for reference.)

A noun is the name of a person, place, object, or Idea.

A pronoun is a word used in place of a noun.

Nouns and pronouns are called .substantives.

1. The subject of a verb is in the nominative case.
   The boy threw the ball.

Transitive verbs express action upon an object or product.

2. The direct object of a transitive verb is in the objective (accusative) case. Whom shall I fear?

Intransitive verbs are often followed by substantives which rename their subject. Such complements are called predicate nominatives, predicate nouns, or attribute complements.

3. A substantive used as attribute complement agrees in case with the subject to which it refers.
   It is I. Whom do you take me to be?

A substantive which helps to complete a verb but renames the object of the verb is called an objective comp1ement.

4. An objective complement is in the objective case.
   The class elected him president.

5. The object of a preposition is in the objective case.
   Give it to me. The cat is under the stove.

The receiver of an action may sometimes be thought of as the principal word in an adverbial phrase from which the preposition to or for is omitted. Such a complement is called an indirect object.

6. An indirect object is in the objective case (dative object). Bring me a chair.

Infinitives and participles do not really assert action or being, but they imply it, and in this sense may have subjects.

Verbs of wishing, desiring, commanding, believing, declaring, perceiving, etc., are likely to be followed by objects which are at the same time subjects of verbals. It is this objective relation which justifies Rule 7.

7. The subject of a verbal is in the objective case.(Except in independent phrases.)
   She has me to protect her. We thought him to be honest.

8. Substantives used with verbals in independent phrases are in the nominative case. ("Absolute.")
   His friends advising it, he resigned.

An appositive is a noun or pronoun used as explanatory of or equivalent to another noun or pronoun.

9. An appositive takes the case of the substantive to which it is attached.
   The book was his, Peter's. (Possessive.)
   'Tis I, Hamlet, the Dane. (Nominative.)

Give it to me your brother.(Objective.)

10. A noun or pronoun <u>independent by address</u> is in the <u>nominative </u>case. ("Vocative".)
<u>"Hens of Athens.</u> Him declare I unto you."
<u>Mr. President,</u> I rise to a point of order.

11. A noun or pronoun used <u>independently with a following adjective, adverb, or</u> <u>phrase</u> may best be regarded as in the objective case, since it is virtually the object in a prepositional phrase from which the preposition is omitted.
<u>Hat in hand,</u> he stood waiting
<u>Beard unkempt, clothes threadbare,</u> he looked down and out.
<u>Fences down, weeds everywhere,</u> the place was desolate.

12. Nouns or pronouns showing ownership are in the <u>possessive </u>case.
<u>John's</u> farm; <u>your</u> shoes.

13. When an inanimate thing is personified, the <u>gender</u> of its noun or pronoun is determied by custom.
<u>She's</u> a good old boat! (Feminine.)
The <u>sun</u> is hiding <u>his</u> head. (Masculine.)

14. <u>Collective nouns are plural</u> when their units act separately as individuals; <u>singular</u> when the units act together as one. <u>Plural</u> <u>titles</u> are in this sense singular nouns.
The class has had its picture taken. (All together.)
The class have had their pictures taken. (Each person by himself.)
"The Newcomes" is by Thackeray.

15. <u>Nouns used adverbially</u> to measure time or distance are in the <u>objective case.</u> <u>(Adverbial objective.)</u>
We walked an <u>hour</u>, travelled four <u>miles.</u>

16. A <u>substantive</u> used as an exclamation is commonly held to be <u>nominative.</u> But if the exclamation repeats an idea already used, it will take the case of the term repeated.
We shall be rich. We! think of that!
"We'll make you do it!" <u>Me!</u> I guess not!

17. A <u>pronoun</u> must agree with its antecedent in <u>number, gender.</u> and <u>person.</u> Collective nouns take singular pronouns when the units act separately
The Ship of State has refused to obey <u>her</u> rudder.
<u>That</u> is <u>he</u> <u>whom</u> you seek. (All three are in 3rd Person, Masculine Gender, Singular Number.)
The <u>case</u> of a pronoun does not depend upon its antecedent, but upon its use in the sentence.
A verb is a word which asserts. (Tells something of its subject.)

18. A verb agrees with its subject in person and number. *I* am: You <u>are;</u> He <u>is;</u> She goes; They <u>go</u> .

19. A compound subject with <u>and</u> takes a singular verb if the idea of the combined subject is of <u>one</u> thing; if the compound subject is made of parts acting separately, the verb is <u>plural.</u>
Roosevelt and Wilson <u>were</u> of opposing parties.
The sum and substance of the matter <u>is</u> this.

20. A <u>distributive</u> subject with each, <u>every, everyone, either, neither.</u> etc., requires a verb in the <u>singular;</u> a disjunctive subject with <u>either-or. neither-nor,</u> takes a verb in the <u>singular</u> if the substantives are singular.
<u>Either</u> the book or the teacher <u>is</u> wrong.
<u>Each</u> of us must use his own judgment.

21. <u>Nouns plural in form</u> but singular in meaning commonly take a verb in the <u>singular.</u>
Hydraulics <u>is</u> a practical study nowadays.

Mumps <u>is</u> contagious.

The news <u>is</u> discouraging.

22. When the subject acts upon an object, the verb is in the ac<u>tive voice;</u> when the subject is a receiver or product of action, the verb is <u>passive.</u>

The hunter <u>shot</u> the door. (Active.)

The deer <u>was shot</u> by the hunter. (Passive.)

23. The <u>indicative mood</u> is used in questions and in simple assertions of factor matter thought of as possible fact.

<u>Were</u> you there?

You <u>were</u> there.

If you <u>were</u> there, I did not see you.(See subjunctive mood, Rule 24.)

24. The <u>subjunctive mood</u> expresses a wish, or a <u>condition contrary to fact.</u>

Would he <u>were</u> here!

If he <u>were</u> here, we would know about it.

(Implying denial. He has.not been here.)

25. The <u>imperative mood</u> states a command or request. Please_go at once.

The subject of an imperative verb is you understood; the <u>you</u> is seldom expressed, unless the mood is emphatic.

26. <u>Infinitives</u> may be used as <u>subject, object of verb, attribute complement, object of preposition, appositive, adjective modifier, adverbial modifier,</u> or in an <u>independent phrase.</u>

For examples, see discussion of <u>Verbals</u> in this section.

27. <u>Gerunds</u> (Verbal nouns in ing) have the uses of <u>nouns</u> together with the power of implying action, being or condition.

Examples have been given under <u>uses</u> of Verbals.

28. <u>Participles</u> may be used as <u>adjectives, adverbs, subjective complements, objective complements, following a preposition,</u> or in <u>absolute phrases.</u>

See examples under Verbals.

29. The comparative degree of adjectives and adverbs, not the superlative degree, is used in comparing two persons or things.

He is the <u>taller</u> of the two; in fact, the <u>tallest</u> of the three.

30. A <u>coordinating conjunction</u> connects words, phrases, or clauses of like rank, grammatically independent of each other.

I will come if I can <u>and</u> if the weather is good.

31. A <u>subordinating conjunction</u> joins a dependent clause to a principal one.

Make hay <u>while</u> the sun shines.

32. <u>Interjections</u> commonly have no grammatical relation in the sentence. In certain constructions, however, the interjection seems to have a phrasal modifier.

"Ah! for the pirate's dream of fight!"

33. Verbs <u>become, feel, look,</u> see, <u>smell, taste, sound, grow</u> may take an <u>attribute complement</u> to describe the subject, or an adverb to modify the assertion of the verb.

He grew <u>tall</u>. Poisonous mushrooms taste <u>good.</u>

"He looks <u>well</u>" may describe his own condition, and so the word <u>well</u> may be a predicate adjective relating to the subject; or the sentence may mean that he <u>searches thoroughly.</u> in which sense <u>well</u> is an adverb modifying <u>looks.</u>

34. <u>Assertions of Simple Futurity</u> take the form

I, we	shall
You	will
He, they	will

<u>Assertions of Strong Purpose, Promise, Threat, Consent</u> take the form I, we will You shall He, they shall

35. Adjectives should not take the place of adverbs, nor adverbs the place of adjectives.

36. The six tenses of English verbs in the Active Voice, Indicative Mood, are built up from the "principal parts" as follows:

Present Tense. Past Tense, as in Principal Parts, Future Tense, shall or will (Rule 34) with Present Infinitive (less "to").

Present Perfect, have or has. with Past Participle Past Perfect, had, with Past Participle.

Future Perfect, shall or will (Rule 34), with Present Perfect, the "have" form.

37. The six tenses of English verbs in the Passive Voice, Indicative Mood, invariably use the past participle of the given verb, preceded by an appropriate form of the verb "be."

38. Gerunds, being verbal nouns, are modified by adjectives and possessive pronouns.

Now do it without my watching you.

C. COMMON ERRORS IN USAGE

(Numbers refer to rules in the preceding section. Correct forms are given first.)

	RULE
This is the better of the two. *NOT* this is the best of the two	(29)
You and I, did it. *NOT* you and me did it, *NOR* me and you.	(1)
We boys will be there. *NOT* us boys will be there.	(1)
It was I, she, he, they. *NOT* me, her, him, them.	(3)
We believed it to be her, him, them. *NOT* she, he, they.	(3)
Between you and me. *NOT* between you and I.	(5)
She is taller than I, (am).*NOT* she is taller than me.	(1)
It was known to be he. *NOT* him. He agrees with "It."	(3)
We were sure of its being him. (Usage divided.)	(3,5)
Let everybody bring his own lunch. *NOT* their own.	(14,17,24)
We should all bring our lunches.(Action concerted.)	(17)
Every boy and girl should do his best. Their would be incorrect.	
His or her is correct, for formal,	(17)
Each of us has his problems.*NOT* have their.	(20)
The actor whom you saw was Otis Skinner. *NOT* who.	(2)
Whom did you call for? *NOT* who.	(5)
Whom did you select?*NOT* who.	(2)
Who do you suppose it is? Who agrees with it.	(3)
Who do you think I am? *NOT* whom. Agrees with I.	(3)
Whom did you.take me to be? Whom agrees with me.	(3)
The tree looks beautiful. *NOT* beautifully.	(33)
The apple tastes good. *NOT* well.	(33)
The tune sounds harsh.	(33)
Roses smell sweet. *NOT* sweetly.	(33)
She looks charming. *NOT* charmingly.	(33)
We shall be drowned if we go there. NOT we will be	(34)
I shall be pleased to help you. *NOT* will be.	(34)
The senate has adjourned. *NOT* have adjourned.	(14)
There are all sorts of graft in town. *NOT* there is all sorts.	(18)
Here are wealth and beauty. *NOT* here is. (Unless taken separately.)	(18)
Neither of the men shows signs of giving in.*NOT* neither show.	(18)
In both cases, there are bad birth and misfortune. *NOT* there is. (Unless taken separately.)	(18)
Our class poet believes in symbolism. *NOT* believe.	(18)

He is one of the best actors <u>that have ever</u> been *here. NOT* <u>has</u>. (17,18)

Let <u>him</u> who will, come. *NOT* let <u>he</u>. (2)

The congregation were free to express their opinions, *OR* was free to express its opinions. (14)

I <u>saw</u>. *NOT* I <u>seen</u>. (36)

I <u>did</u>. *NOT* I *done.* (36)

We <u>have gone</u>. *NOT* have went. (36)

We <u>were</u>. *NOT* we <u>was</u>. (18)

You <u>began</u> it. *NOT* you <u>begun</u> it. (36)

The wind <u>blew</u>. *NOT* the wind <u>blowed</u>. (36)

The glass is <u>broken</u>. *NOT* <u>broke</u>. (37)

I <u>caught, have caught</u>. *NOT* <u>catched, have catched</u>. (36)

Have been <u>chosen</u>. *NOT* have been <u>chose</u>. (37)

We <u>came</u> along. *NOT* we <u>come</u>. (36)

We <u>have</u> come. *NOT* <u>have</u> came. (36)

The-baby <u>crept</u>. *NOT* <u>creeped</u>. (36)

You've <u>done</u> it. *NOT* you've <u>did</u> it. (36)

We <u>drew</u>. *NOT* we <u>drawed</u>. (36)

He <u>has drunk</u> a glassful. *NOT* <u>has drank</u> (36)

<u>Have driven</u>. *NOT* <u>have drove</u>. (36)

<u>Have eaten</u>. *NOT* <u>have ate</u>. (36)

I <u>ate</u> my dinner. *NOT* <u>eat</u> (36)

Eas <u>fallen</u>. *NOT* has fell. (36)

The boys <u>fought</u>. *NOT* fit. (36)

Has <u>flown</u>, *NOT* has <u>flew</u>. (36)

I've <u>forgotten</u>. *NOT* <u>forgot</u>. (36)

It <u>grew</u>. *NOT* it <u>growed</u>. (36)

You <u>lie</u> low. *NOT* lay low. (Lie, to recline; lay, to put down.) (36)

Have <u>ridden</u>. *NOT* have <u>rode</u>. (36)

We <u>rang</u> the bell. *NOT* we <u>rung</u> it. (36)

Had <u>risen</u>. *NOT* had <u>rose</u>. (36)

And then I <u>ran</u> away. *NOT* then I <u>run</u> away. (36)

Ve <u>sang</u> a song. NOT we <u>sung</u> it. (36)

Troubles <u>sprang</u> up. *NOT* troubles <u>sprung</u> up. (36)

Somebody has <u>stolen</u> my hat. *NOT* has <u>stole</u>. (36)

The place <u>stunk</u>. *NOT* <u>stank</u>. (36)

We <u>swam</u> a mile. *NOT* we <u>swum</u>. (36)

Who's <u>taken</u> my hat? *NOT* who's <u>took</u>? (36)

Have <u>torn</u>. .*NOT* have <u>tore</u>. (36)

Have <u>written</u>. *NOT* have <u>wrote</u>. (36)

Say it <u>slowly</u>. *NOT* <u>slow</u>. (35)

We can do that as <u>easily</u> as you please. *NOT* as <u>easy</u>. (35)

The horse threw my brother and <u>me</u> out.*NOT* my brother and <u>I</u>. (2)

We chose the foreman <u>who</u> we thought could handle the *men. NOW* whom. (1)

I never saw a taller man than <u>he</u>. *NOT* <u>him</u>. (1)

There isn't another girl in town so handsome as she. *NOT* <u>her</u>. (1)

MOSSES FROM AN OLD MANSE <u>is</u> a collection of essays and stories.
    NOT <u>are</u> a collection. (14)

Now skate without <u>my</u> helping you. *NOT* <u>me</u> helping. (38)

We ought to keep still about <u>his</u> being here. *NOT* <u>him</u> being. (38)

MODERN SURGICAL DEVELOPMENT AND TERMINOLOGY

CONTENTS

MODERN SURGICAL DEVELOPMENT AND TERMINOLOGY

I. THE DEVELOPMENT OF MODERN SURGICAL PRACTICES

SECTION A—EARLY HISTORY

1-1. Primitive Surgery. Surgery was one of the early practices associated with the ancient art of healing. To a degree its history paralleled that of civilization. In spite of enlightened teachings of a few physicians during earlier periods, for more than a thousand years following the fall of the Roman Empire, surgery was practiced as a lowly form of manual labor. Major obstacles to advancement were lack of knowledge of anatomy and a lack of means of controlling hemorrhage, infection, and pain.

1-2. The Renaissance. Major changes began to take place during the last years of the Dark Ages. The revival of learning and science influenced and brought about changes in all branches of medicine. Leonardo da Vinci (1452-1519), in his attempts to accurately portray the human form, dissected bodies and did detailed sketches of organs and their relationship to each other. Da Vinci's drawings were not published until 1796; in the meantime, Andreas Vesalius (1514-1564) published his *De Humani Corpus Fabrica.*

SECTION B—CONTROL OF HEMORRHAGE

1-3. The Development of Ligatures. As the secrets of anatomy were probed, physiological phenomena were also revealed. Michael Servetus (1511-1553) described the fact that blood moved from the heart to the lungs and returned to the left ventricle. Ambroise Pare (1510-1590) upset the abusive practice of cauterization. He discontinued the use of boiling oil and hot cautery. As an alternative, he reinstated the use of ligatures and the washing of wounds. William Harvey (1578-1657) developed the theory that blood circulates throughout the body, with the heart acting as a pump. Man then possessed the knowledge that the heart forces a limited supply of blood throughout the body and that this supply can be contained by simply tying off several blood vessels. The emergency conditions of military surgery prompted the use of the tourniquet in 1674.

1-4. Other Methods of Hemostasis. In the later part of the 19th century Lister described chromatization of catgut sutures and Kocher and Pean designed their arterial forceps. Halsted contributed to surgical skill through his use of fine silk sutures and fine hemostats. Harvey Cushing introduced silver clips in 1911; and in 1928, Bovie perfected the electro-surgical unit. More recent advances in biochemistry have led to the manufacture of products that produce hemostasis when they are applied locally. And so, as the ligature, tourniquet, hemostat, electro-cautery, silver clip, and finally the biochemical agent became realities, the way was paved for the bloodless surgical procedures we know today.

SECTION C—CONTROL OF INFECTION

1-5. Cleanliness. The high incidence of infection was a major obstacle to the progress of surgery. Although surgeons were developing a great deal of skill and speed, infection caused a high rate of mortality. A few men realized that cleanliness was important and insisted that hands and instruments be washed. In 1874, Ignaz Semmelweis decreased the prevalence of puerperal fever by the simple practice of washing his hands before examining each obstetrical patient.

1-6. Bacteriology. During the latter part of the 17th century, Leeuwenhoek discovered the world of microbes while experimenting with his homemade microscope. Louis Pasteur made perhaps the greatest contribution to medicine in the 19th century by developing the science of bacteriology. He demonstrated the microbial cause of certain disease conditions. This led the way for Lord Lister's contribution: using an antiseptic in surgery. A carbolic spray was used continuously during the operation, and wet carbolic dressings were applied after surgery was completed. As more was learned about bacteria, Lister's methods gradually gave way to less irritating techniques.

1-7. The Beginning of Aseptic Technique. The work of many bacteriologists, surgeons, and nurses has added to the development of aseptic surgery. Dr. William Halsted (1852-1922) introduced the use of rubber gloves in surgery when harsh antiseptics irritated the surgical nurse's hands. In 1866, Von Bergman "pasteurized" instruments by boiling them.

1–8. Additional Barriers. The patient's skin and the operator's hands were washed with soap and water. And by 1894 Halsted's rubber gloves were being used to further protect the surgical wound from the hands of the entire surgical team. The older, intricately carved instruments were replaced by smooth, simple instruments that were less difficult to clean. After the invention of the steam sterilizer it was possible to sterilize dressings, gowns, towels, etc. Caps became a part of surgical attire, and masks were adopted gradually when it was realized that contamination might be caused by bacteria from the nose and mouth of operators.

1–9. Current Methods. These were the innovations and inventions that were forerunners of modern aseptic technique; of chemical disinfection; and of sterilization by prevacuum high temperature steam, by gas, and by radiation. With the advent of antibiotics, man was able to treat many of the infections that precede surgery or that escape our preventive measures. And during recent years it has become possible to create a completely sterile environment around the operative site with the use of transparent, synthetic, tent-like enclosures (germ-free isolators). Improved housekeeping, more efficient architectural designs, and ventilation systems have been important contributions in the continuous struggle for the control of infection.

SECTION D—CONTROL OF PAIN

1–10. Early Anesthesia. The development of surgery was also hampered by a third major obstacle—pain. In spite of the fact that some of the modern anesthetic agents were known and described as early as the 16th century, it wasn't until the mid-19th century that they were accepted and put into general use.

a. *Ether.* This anesthetic was known in the 16th century and named by a German chemist in 1730, but it was not used as an adjunct to surgery until much later. In 1842 its anesthetic quality was successfully demonstrated by Dr. Crawford Long. Dr. Long did not publish his findings, so credit was given to Dr. William Morton, a dentist, who gave a public demonstration of ether inhalation at Massachusetts General Hospital in 1846. A few years later, Oliver Wendell Holmes named the process "anesthesia."

b. *Nitrous Oxide and Oxygen.* These anesthetics were discovered by Joseph Priestly in the 18th century. Dr. Humphrey Davy, an English surgeon, did scientific experiments with nitrous oxide in 1799 and suggested its use for surgery. Soon thereafter equipment was developed that facilitated its administration.

c. *Chloroform.* This anesthetic was introduced in England by Simpson in the late 1840's. But it was not fully accepted by the public until it was administered to Queen Victoria during the birth of Prince Leopold in 1853. Its advantages were soon recognized in the United States where it was used extensively during the Civil War.

1–11. Early Anesthetic Problems. The courtship of anesthesia and surgery was not completely blissful. There were discomforts associated with ether induction, danger of liver damage from chloroform, and problems with the crude equipment used to administer the various agents. But these imperfections only prompted scientists to experiment with other gases and gadgets that would allow safer and easier administration.

1–12. Current Practices. As time went on, anesthetists learned the importance of mixing proper proportions of oxygen along with one or more of the gases or volatile liquids. With further advances in pharmacology, other methods of administration were discovered.

a. *Avertin* was given by rectum, and barbiturates were injected directly into the bloodstream. With *pentothal*, one of the most effective of these intravenous agents, the patient could be put to sleep rapidly and would awaken soon after the drug was discontinued.

b. Safety and comfort were increased with the refined use of *preanesthesia medication to reduce anxiety and salivation* and by the use of drugs that reduce postoperative nausea. It was found that the addition of curare with the intravenous solution brought about muscle relaxation that made the work of the surgeon much easier. Hypothermia and anticoagulants were important in the development of cardiovascular surgery and organ transplants.

c. The discovery of *novocain* opened the door to regional and local anesthesia, thus eliminating certain dangers for patients whose heart or lungs could not tolerate general anesthesia. The derivatives of novocain are now used extensively for spinals, caudals, nerve blocks, and local infiltration. To add further refinement to the administration of inhalation anesthesia, machines have been devised that can be regulated so that they automatically force a prescribed mixture of anesthetic agents at a set rate to the patient. Finally, in an effort to reduce the danger from cardiac arrest, the techniques of open and closed cardiac massage were devised. And cardiac defibrillators and pacemakers help ensure the return of normal heart rhythm following such emergencies.

SECTION E—ADVANCES IN OPERATIVE SURGERY

1-13. Development of New Procedures. Only after hemostasis, sterility, and anesthesia had become realities was it possible for surgeons to advance the state of operative surgery much beyond the stage that had been reached hundreds of years before. As the death rate due to surgery began to drop, surgeons started perfecting old procedures and attempting new ones. It became feasible to do elective surgery inside the peritoneal cavity, the brain, and the chest, as well as reconstructive procedures on bones and joints.

1-14. Interdependence With Other Departments. With each passing year, surgeons have added to the feats of the past. It's a bit hard sometimes to give credit where it's due because each surgical innovation is so dependent on what has gone before. A look at the hospital chart of today's surgical patient also shows how dependent we have become on the biological sciences. Without radiology and laboratory reports, no surgeon would attempt most surgical procedures. Information about the physiological requirements for oxygen, adequate blood volume, electrolyte balance, and nutrition has greatly enhanced the chances that patients will receive the support their body needs during surgical procedures. Last but not least, a great deal of credit must go to the engineers who have designed so many mechanical and electronic devices for use in the operating and recovery rooms. Without the contributions of all types of scientific and technological experts, we wouldn't be doing cryosurgery, cutting with the laser, or oxygenating the blood with a pump oxygenator. There would be no artificial heart valves, cardiac pacemakers, or many of the prosthetic devices that are so necessary for the performance of reconstructive surgery.

SECTION F—THE SURGICAL TEAM

1-15. The Patient. The focal point of all operating room activity is the patient. The sole purpose of a hospital is to provide treatment for patients; the sole purpose of the operating suite is to provide treatment for patients whose problems can be corrected through surgical intervention. Therefore, it is well to remember that even though a great many activities may not directly involve patients, their safety is the primary purpose of an endless number of tasks. Each of these tasks will have some relationship to the primary function of supplying the surgeon with the necessary equipment and supplies to perform the operative procedures, of controlling pain and hemorrhage in the patient, and of creating an environment that is free from infectious agents.

1-16. The Chief of Surgical Services. The Chief of Surgical Services has the overall responsibility for all activities carried out within the operating suite. (Figure 1-1 is a functional chart of operating room personnel.) Obviously, other surgeons perform operative procedures and other personnel carry out tasks according to their training and ability. But the Chief

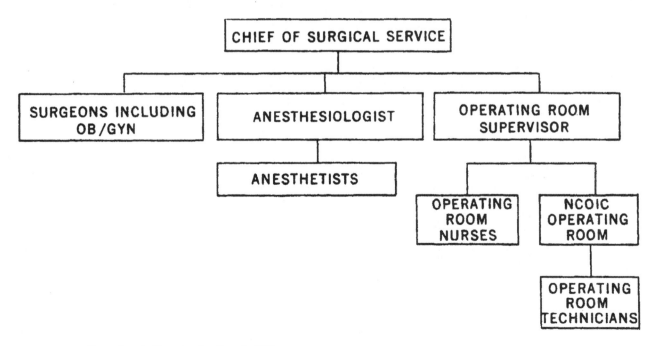

Figure 1-1. Functional Chart—the Surgical Team.

of Surgical Services must exercise administrative control and supervisory authority to assure safe and effective patient treatment.

1–17. The Surgeon. The surgeon is always the leader of the team when an operative procedure is in process. It is the responsibility of all team members to support his or her activities and carry out requests.

1–18. Anesthesiologists. Anesthesiologists are medical doctors who have specialized in the field of anesthesia. They are qualified in the administration of all types of agents which are used to alleviate pain during surgical procedures.

1–19. Anesthetists. Anesthetists are professional nurses who have studied the techniques and practices of administering anesthesia and have passed a national examination. Air Force nurse anesthetists work under the direction of an anesthesiologist or surgeon.

1–20. Operating Room Nurses. Operating room nurses are professional nurses with postgraduate courses or experience in operating room nursing. The *operating room supervisor* is in charge of all nursing activities and directs the administrative and nursing functions of the unit.

1–21. Operating Room Technicians. Operating room technicians are individuals who have received technical training in the performance of nursing functions in the operating room. The *NCOIC of the Operating Room,* under the direction of the operating room supervisor, performs administrative functions and supervises the operating room technicians.

———

II. SURGICAL TERMINOLOGY

SECTION A—PREFIXES, SUFFIXES, AND ROOT WORDS

1. Introduction. A great number of the words used in medicine and surgery are formed by combining units of prefixes, suffixes, and root words. The names of parts of the human body, which are considered root words, are also used as prefixes. This is especially true when the suffix refers to a type of operative procedure; for example, *gastrectomy: gastro* is the prefix and root word meaning *stomach*, and *ectomy* is the suffix meaning *to remove*. So *gastrectomy* is the *removal* of the *stomach*.

2. Common Prefixes. The following is a list of those syllables or groups of syllables which often come at the beginning of medical terms:

a-, an-	absence of
ab-, abs-	away, from
ad-	to, toward, near
aer-	air
ambi-	both
ante-	before
anti-	against
auto-	self
bi-	two
bio-	life
brady-	slow
circum-	around
contra-	against, opposed
de-	from, not
deca-	ten
demi-	half
di-	two
dis-	negative, apart
dys-	difficult, painful
ecto-	on the outside
en-	in
endo-	within
epi-	upon
erythro-	red
eu-	well, normal
ex-, e-, exo-	away from, without
exo-	outside
extra-	outside, beyond
fore-	in front of
glyco-	sugar
hemi-	half
hetero-	other
homo-	same, similar
hydra-, hydro-	water
hyp-, hypo-	below, less
hyper-	above, excessive, over
in-	not, in

infra-	below, beneath
inter-	between
intra-	within
iso-	equal
latero-	side
leuco-, leuko-	white
macro-	large
mal-	bad, disordered
med-	middle
meg-, mego-	great, large
melan-	black
meno-	monthly
meta-	beyond
micro-	small
mono-	single
multi-	many
neo-	new
olig-	little
pan-	all
para-	beside
peri-	around
poly-	many, much
post-	after
pre-	before
pro-	before, in front of
pseud-, pseudo-	false
retro-	backward, behind
semi-	half
sub-	under
super-	above, excess
supra-	over, above
sum-, syn-	with, together
tachy-	fast
topo-	place
tox-	poison
therm-, thermo-	heat
trans-	across, through
tri-	three
ultra-	excess
uni-	one

3. Prefixes Relating to the Human Body. Below is a list of syllables or groups of syllables that often come at the beginning of words which relate to the human body:

adeno-	gland
angi, angio-	blood vessel
arterio-	artery
arthro-	joint
audio-	pertaining to hearing
bili-	relating to bile
broncho-	pertaining to bronchus
cardi-	heart
cephalo-	pertaining to the head
chole-, chol-, cholo-	bile
cholecyst-	gallbladder
chondro-	cartilage
col-	colon (large bowel)

colpo-	vagina
costo-	rib
cranio-	skull
cyst-, cysto-	urinary bladder, sac
dent-	relating to teeth
derma-	skin
duodeno-	duodenum (small intestine)
encephalo-, cephalo-	brain, head
entero-	intestine
gastro-	stomach
hem-, hema-, hemato-	blood
hepato-	liver
hernio-	rupture
hystero-	uterus (womb)
ileo-	ileum (small intestine)
jejuno-	jejunum (small intestine)
kerato-	cornea (of eye)
lapara-	loin, abdomen
laryng-, laryngo-	larynx (voice box)
latero-	side
lith-	stone
lymph-	watery fluid from glands
mast-	breast
metra-, metro-	uterus
myel- myelo-	bone marrow, spinal cord
myo-	muscle
necro-	relating to death
nephra-, nephro-	kidney
neu-, neuro-	nerve
oculo-	eye
oophor-	ovary
ophthalmo-	eye
opto-	relating to vision
orchi-	testicle
os-	bone or opening (mouth)
oste-. osteo-	bone
oto-	ear
path-, patho-	relating to disease
phlebo-	vein
physio-	relating to nature, life
pneumo-	lung or air
pulmo-	lung
procto-	rectum
psych-	soul, mind
pyelo-	pelvis of kidney
pyo-	pus
rhino-	nose, nasal
sacro-	sacrum (vertebra)
salpingo-	tube, fallopian tube
teno-	tendon
thoraco-	chest
thyro-	thyroid gland
trachelo-	cervix
tracheo-	trachea (windpipe)
uretero-	ureters
urino, uro-	relating to urine or urinary organs
vaso-	blood vessel
ventro-	abdomen
vesico-	urinary bladder

4. Suffixes Pertaining to Medicine and Surgery. The following list contains many of the syllables or groups of syllables which make up the endings of medical and surgical terms:

Suffix	Meaning	Example
-algia	pain	neuralgia
-asthenia	weakness	myasthenia
-biotic	living matter	antibiotic

Suffix	Meaning	Example
-cele	tumor. cyst, hernia	hydrocele
-cide	causing death	germicide
-cyte	cell	leukocyte
-desis	surgical fixation	arthrodesis
-ectomy	removal of	appendectomy
-emia	blood	septicemia
-esthesia	feeling. sensation	anesthesia
-gene, -genic	production. origin	pathogenic
-gram	a tracing, a mark	electrocardiogram
-graph(y)	a writing, a record	radiography
-itis	inflammation	tonsillitis
-ize	to treat by special method	cauterize
-litho	stone, calculus	fecalith
-logy	science of	physiology
-lysis	setting free	tenolysis
-meter	measure	thermometer
-oid	form. shape. resemblance	lymphoid
-oma	tumor	carcinoma
-orrhaphy	repair of	herniorrhaphy
-osis	process (usually disease process)	necrosis
-pathy	disease, suffering	osteopathy
-penia	lack	leukopenia
-pexy	fastening, fixation	nephropexy
-plasty	to shape, mold	rhinoplasty
-rhagia	hemorrhage, flow	menorrhagia
-rhaphy	a suturing, a stitching	perineorrhaphy
-rhea	flow, discharge	diarrhea
-scope	instrument for examining	cystoscope
-scopy	see, examine	bronchoscopy
-stasis	a standing still	hemostasis
-stomy	to form an opening	colostomy
-tomy	incision into	thoracotomy
-uria	relating to urine	oliguria

SECTION B—ABBREVIATIONS

5. The Value of Abbreviations. In addition to the features of terminology already presented, there is another aspect of medical language involving the use of abbreviations. The value of a system of abbreviations is that it saves time and space in the writing of doctors' orders and other medical records. Personnel who work with medical records must be familiar with the most commonly used abbreviations.

6. List of Abbreviations. The following list shows the abbreviations, the foreign derivative, and the English translation. NOTE: Unless otherwise specified, all foreign derivatives are Latin.

Abbreviation	Foreign Derivative	English Translation
a or aa	ana (Greek)	of each
a,c.	ante cibos	before meals
ad lib	ad libitum	as desired
aq	aqua	water
b.i.d.	bis in die	twice a day
b.i.n.	bis in noctus	twice a night
c̄	cum	with
C	centigrade	centigrade
cap	capsula	capsule
cm³	cubic centimetre (French)	cubic centimeter
cm	centimetre (French)	centimeter

Abbreviation	Foreign Derivative	English Translation
CO_2	carbo (Latin) disoxys (Greek)	carbon dioxide
comp	compositus	compound
def	defaecatio	defecation
dil	dilue	dilute
dr	drachma	dram or drams
elix	(Arabic)	elixir
et	et	and
F	Fahrenheit (German)	Fahrenheit (proper name)
fl	fluidus	fluid
fl dr	fluidrachma	fluid dram
fl oz	fluidus uncia	fluid ounce
fort	fortis	strong
gm	gramma	gram
gr	granum	grain
gtt	gutta	drop
h	hora	hour
h. s.	hora somni	at bedtime; hour of sleep
hypo	(Greek)	under (hypodermic)
IM	intramusculus	intramuscular
IV	intravenosus	intravenous
lb	libra	pound
M	metre (French)	meter
m	minimum	minim
mg; mgm	milligramma	milligram
mist	mistura	mixture
ml	mille (Latin) litre (French)	milliliter
mm	mille (Latin) metre (French)	millimeter
no	numero	number
non rep	non repetatur	don't repeat
noct	nocte	at night
O_2	oxysgennan (Greek)	oxygen
ocul	oculus	eye
O.D.	oculo dextro	right eye
O.S.	oculo sinistro	left eye
O.L.	oculo laevo	left eye
O.U.	oculi unitas	both eyes
os	os; ora	mouth
oz	uncia	ounce
P	pulsus	pulse
p.c.	post cibum	after food; after meals
per	per	through or by
pil	pilula	pill
p.m.	post meridiem	afternoon

Abbreviation	Foreign Derivative	English Translation
p.o.	per os	by mouth
p.r.n.	pro re nata	as needed; as desired
pulv	pulvis	powder
q.	quaque	every; each
q.d.	quaque die	every day
q.h.	quaque hora	every hour
q 2h	quaque secunda hora	every 2 hours
q.i.d.	quater in die	four times a day
q.s.	quantum sufficiat	sufficient quantity
rub	ruber	red
Rx	recipe	take thou (prescription)
rep	repatatur	let it be repeated
ꙅ	sans	without
s.c.; subc	sub cutis	subcutaneously
sol	solutio	solution
s.o.s.	si opus sit	if necessary
sp frum	spiritus frumenti	whisky
sp gr	species gravitus	specific gravity
ss	semis	half
stat	statim	immediately; at once
T	temperatura	temperature
tab	tabella	tablet
t.i.d.	ter in die	three times a day
tr. tinct	tinctura	tincture
ung	unguentum	ointment
wt		weight

SECTION C—WEIGHTS AND MEASUREMENTS

7. **Systems of Weights and Measurements.** There are several systems of weight and measurement; the field of medicine has almost universally adopted the metric system. The use of the metric system for ordering and dispensing drugs is mandatory in Air Force hospitals. The metric system and the apothecary system are used in the operating room. Therefore, operating room personnel must be familiar with the basic features of the two systems.

a. *Linear Measure (Distance).* The American measures of length consist of:

inches		feet		yards		rods		furlongs		miles
12	=	1								
36	=	3	=	1						
198	=	16½	=	5½	=	1				
7920	=	660	=	220	=	40	=	1		
63360	=	5208	=	1760	=	320	=	8	=	1

b. *Basic Unit of Length.* The basic unit of length of the metric system is the *meter* (m), which is one ten millionth part of the distance along a meridian from the equator to the pole. The meter is 39 inches long. All of the other measurements are then related to the meter as follows:

1 millimeter = 1/1000 meter
1 centimeter = 1/100 meter

1 decimeter = 1/10 meter
1 decameter = 10 meters
1 hectometer = 100 meters
1 kilometer = 1,000 meters
1 myriameter = 10,000 meters

c. *Equivalents Between the Two Systems.* The approximate equivalents of the American measures of distance and the metric system are as follows:

1 kilometer	=	5/8 mile		1 yard	=	92 centimeters
1 meter	=	39 inches		1 foot	=	30.5 centimeters
1 centimeter	=	3/8 inch		1 inch	=	2.5 centimeters
1 millimeter	=	1/25 inch		1 inch	=	25 millimeters
1 mile	=	1 3/5 kilometers				

d. *Cubic Measure (Volume)*. In the US apothecary system, amounts of liquid are referred to as volume:

minims		fluid drachms		fluid ounces		pints		quarts		gallons
60	=	1								
480	=	8	=	1						
7680	=	128	=	16	=	1				
15360	=	256	=	32	=	2	=	1		
61440	=	1024	=	128	=	8	=	4	=	1

e. *Metric System Volume*. The unit of volume in the metric system is a *liter* (cubic decimeter). The subdivisions are:

liter	deciliter	centiliter	milliliter
1	$\frac{1}{10}$	$\frac{1}{100}$	$\frac{1}{1000}$

Here you will note the same decimal system as is used in metric linear measure.

f. *Basic Unit of Weight*. The gram is the basic metric unit of weight. All of the other weights are related to the gram, as follows:

1 milligram = 1/1000 gram
1 kilogram = 1,000 grams

g. *Approximate Equivalents Metric-Apothecary:*

metric		apothecary	example
1 milliliter (ml.)*	=	15 minims	(hypodermic syringe unit)
30 milliliters	=	1 fluid ounce	(medicine glass size)
500 milliliters	=	16 fluid ounces	(1 pint or blood unit)
1000 milliliters	=	32 fluid ounces	(1 quart or IV fluid unit)

---

* milliliter is the same as cubic centimeter (cm³)

h. *Table of Equivalents*. In approximating the equivalents of these two systems, the following table may serve as a ready reference:

apothecary	metric
1/60 grain (gr)	1.0 milligram (mg)
1/20 grain	3.0 milligrams
1/16 grain	4.0 milligrams
1/4 grain	15.0 milligrams
1 grain	60.0 milligrams
3 grains	0.2 gram (gm)
5 grains	0.3 gram
7 1/2 grains	0.5 gram
15 grains	1.0 gram
22 grains	1.5 grams
30 grains	2.0 grams
60 grains	4.0 grams

SECTION D—OTHER MEASURES

8. Centigrade and Fahrenheit Temperature Measurement. Both the Fahrenheit and centigrade thermometer are used in hospitals. Figure 2–1 shows comparative temperature scales and some differences between Fahrenheit and centigrade readings. *To convert a reading from Fahrenheit to centigrade* subtract 32 from the Fahrenheit reading, divide by 9, and multiply by 5; the resulting figure is the centigrade temperature. For example:

$$98.6°F. - 32 = 66.6$$
$$66.6 \div 9 = 7.4$$
$$7.4 \times 5 = 37.0°C.$$

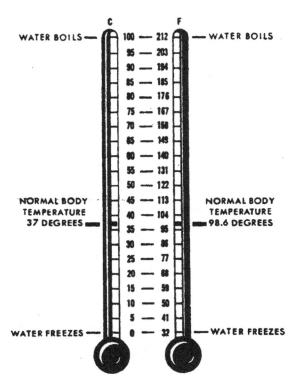

C | F

WATER BOILS — 100 — 212 — WATER BOILS
95 — 203
90 — 194
85 — 185
80 — 176
75 — 167
70 — 158
65 — 149
60 — 140
55 — 131
50 — 122

NORMAL BODY
TEMPERATURE
37 DEGREES — 45 — 113
40 — 104

NORMAL BODY
TEMPERATURE
98.6 DEGREES — 35 — 95
30 — 86
25 — 77
20 — 68
15 — 59
10 — 50
5 — 41

WATER FREEZES — 0 — 32 — WATER FREEZES

Figure 1. Comparison of Fahrenheit and Centigrade Thermometers.

To reverse the procedure and *convert from a centigrade reading to a Fahrenheit reading*, determine 9/5 of the centigrade reading and add 32:

$$100°C. \div 5 = 20$$
$$20 \times 9 = 180$$
$$180 + 32 = 212°F.$$

9. Other Measurements. *Pressure* and *humidity* are measurements of importance to operating room personnel.

a. Both the metric and English barometer scales are used to measure pressure. Thus oxygen, autoclave, and other air pressures are expressed in *pounds per square inch* (psi); blood pressure is measured and expressed in millimeters of mercury.

b. *Humidity* is the *percentage of moisture* in the circulating air and is a big factor in the amount of static eletricity present.

LABOR AND DELIVERY

LABOR is the term given to the entire process of bringing the baby into the world. The course of labor and the expulsion of the fetus is usually considered in three separate stages. For purposes of this article, we will focus on the first stage—from the onset of labor to full dilation of the cervix. Stage II begins when the cervix is completely dilated and ends with the birth of the baby. Stage III is from the completion of delivery of the baby to completion of delivery of the afterbirth, or placenta.

First stage labor is further broken down into three separate categories, and it will help you to know what they are so that you will know approximately how close you are to actual delivery. These three categories are early or inactive labor, active labor, and transition labor.

But before we discuss the progress of labor, it would help to understand what is happening inside of you and the functions of some of the major organs and muscles used during pregnancy and birth.

The **UTERUS** (womb) is a hollow organ which measures about two inches by four inches. By the end of pregnancy, it measures about 10 inches by 14 inches. By volume its capacity increases about 500 times; in weight it grows from about 1½ ounces to almost 30 ounces. The muscle fibers that make up the uterus grow to ten times their original thickness. After pregnancy, the uterus returns to approximately its size before pregnancy.

The uterus is made up of the cervix—the mouth or opening—which is long and thick during pregnancy, and the upper uterine segment. which grows and thins out with pregnancy. The upper segment contracts and retracts. The cervix becomes softer and thinner and dilates as it is pulled upward around the baby's head during delivery.

The uterus is one of the strongest muscles in the body. During the height of a uterine contraction, the pressures created are considerable. Yet this muscle contracts regularly throughout a woman's life. Though most women are not aware of this, the contractions may be noticed as pains associated with the menstrual period.

Throughout pregnancy the uterus contracts at slightly irregular intervals, about every 15 or 20 minutes and lasting for about 25 seconds. They may be felt as tightening of the abdomen, but they are not painful. Many years ago these contractions were described by Braxton Hicks and have since become known as Braxton-Hicks contractions. What they do is exercise the uterus and prepare it for functioning during actual labor. They are also useful in assisting the circulation of maternal blood to the placenta.

Toward the end of pregnancy, these contractions become stronger and more regular. Now it is time to ask the question, "When does labor really begin?" Since each labor is unique, it is almost impossible to give a general answer. But there are three distinctive signs that labor is about to begin, and most women will recognize one or all of them, though not necessarily in this order.

The **first sign** is the onset of regular, strong uterine contractions, occurring every 15 to 20 minutes and lasting from about 45 seconds to a minute. They are uncomfortable, but not necessarily painful. They are accompanied by a definite hardening of the uterus, which can easily be felt by placing your hand on your abdomen.

The **second sign** is rupture of the membranes or the "bag of waters." Also called the forewaters, this is a quantity of liquid which lies in front of the baby's head and is held within the uterus by intact membranes. When these membranes rupture, it is a sign to call your doctor. Rupture may occur slowly by leaking, or in a gush. The fluid is clear and sweet-smelling. But this will not hurt as there are no nerves in the membranes. For many women, rupture does not occur until early or late in labor. In this case, they will be ruptured by the doctor.

A **third sign** is the passage of a small amount of blood-stained mucous or brownish blood, called the "show" or "bloody show." Sometimes you will find this on your underclothes. It is the mucous plug that has been formed during pregnancy to close off the cervix. Its purpose is to keep the uterus free from germs. Many women never experience this "show," while others have an increasing amount all through the first stage of labor, and some have it as early as two weeks before the onset of labor.

Other common signs of approaching labor are diarrhea, backache, decreased movement of the baby, and an increased desire to clean everything in sight! This last so-called "nesting instinct" often occurs on the very day labor begins.

The **INACTIVE** OR **EARLY PART** of **FIRST-STAGE LABOR** is concerned with opening up the mouth of the uterus (the cervix). Before labor begins the wall of the uterus is thin. The cervix is long and thick. The cervical canal is narrow and the membranes are still intact. Now, the bands of longitudinal muscle fiber in the main part of the uterus are contracting and thus gradually drawing up, thinning, and opening the walls of the cervix. The cervical canal thus gets shorter until the cervix is of the same thickness as the uterine wall. This process of shortening the length of the cervical canal and taking it up into the uterus is known as **effacement,** or "taking up of the cervix." (It may help you to visualize a wine bottle with a long, thick neck. Cutting off the neck would be the equivalent of effacement.) Effacement is measured in percentages, from 0-100%, so if you are 80% effaced, that means the opening of your cervix is almost totally thinned out. (See illustrations below.)

Once the cervix is effaced, the force of uterine contractions is devoted to dilating the cervix. **Dilation** (or dilatation) is the term used to refer to the size of the round opening of the cervix. It is measured in centimeters, sometimes in finger widths. Full dilation is 10 centimeters, or five finger widths. Now the cervix is completely open and becomes part of the uterus. Uterus, cervix and vagina then form one canal for the baby to pass through.

Dilation is slow during the early first part of labor. It usually takes much longer to go from one to three fingers dilation than it does to go from three fingers to full dilation.

Some mothers are already one or two fingers dilated when they start labor. The process of dilation has begun without their being aware of it.

Now that you know what labor is and what is happening in your body, the question becomes, "What will it feel like?" No one can answer this question for you because there are so many variables which affect the length of labor and what it feels like. Among them are the pain threshold of the mother, the preparation she has had for labor and delivery, the position and size of the baby, and how quickly the baby moves through the birth canal. However, there are some descriptions of labor which will prove useful.

Once labor is really underway, the

Effacement and dilation of the cervix

(1) The state of the cervix at 36 weeks. The cervical canal is long and the membranes are still intact.

(2) The cervical canal gets shorter as the uterus contracts and gradually draws up, thins, and opens the walls.

(3) The cervix completely effaced, early in labor. The canal has disappeared and some dilation has already taken place.

(4) Partial dilation of the cervix, about three fingers. The intact bag of waters is bulging through the cervix into the vagina.

(5) Full dilation of the cervix. The membranes have now ruptured and the mother is in the second stage.

contractions will become stronger and closer together. Many women describe them as moving like waves, gathering in the distance, rising, breaking and falling on the shore. The pressure in the uterus is rising slowly and increasing in power until it reaches a maximum where there is a crest or plateau, which lasts for about 30-50 seconds, and then disappears rapidly. When it is over, you feel nothing until the next contraction, which may be anywhere from 20 to 5 minutes away. It varies for every woman. What you will feel is a gradual tightening of the uterine muscles and a discomfort or a gripping sensation around the pelvis and a nagging backache.

As the cervix continues to dilate, the strength and frequency of the contractions gradually increase. Now the discomfort is felt over the whole of the uterus. The cervix is now dilated three centimeters, and the longest part of labor is over. This **INACTIVE** first stage is often the most easily handled and the least uncomfortable. But since it may take up to six hours or more, most women stay home until this stage is over. Once you are in the hospital, you are a patient, confined to a room and a bed, and if you arrive there too early, you may be sent home.

Most women are told to go to the hospital when their contractions are five minutes apart and have been that way for a full hour. Or, if the membranes rupture or if there is any bleeding, these are also signs to leave immediately for the hospital.

Once in the hospital, you will have a vaginal examination, and depending on hospital policy, a physical examination and medical history. If you have arrived too early and are discharged, you may have to pay a fee. But if you are in active labor, you will be admitted and asked to pay part or all of the agreed-upon costs.

You will be taken to a labor room and given a partial shave—on either side of the vagina to keep the area clean. (Nowadays in most hospitals, a complete pubic area shave is not done.)

Enemas are given to prevent you from accidentally expelling some feces as you bear down during delivery. But don't give yourself an enema or suppository at home—you don't know how dilated you are. If you arrive at the hospital at 8 centimeters dilated, you will not be given an enema. And once labor has started, don't eat. When labor begins, digestion stops. Drink only black tea or coffee or eat some jello. You don't want to feel nauseous during the later stages of labor. In the hospital, you'll be given only ice chips.

In most hospitals today, you will also be monitored—both for your baby's heart (an electrical impulse) and for your uterine contractions (a mechanical impulse). The monitor gives a continuous picture of the fetal environment. It is attached to you by way of two belts— one is placed just above the pubic hair line to monitor the baby's heart, and another is placed just below your navel to check the uterine contractions. This monitoring will be done from the time you enter the hospital to the time your baby is born. The machine, mounted on a movable table, goes with you from labor room to delivery room. Most hospitals routinely use the fetal heart monitoring, and if you are lucky enough to also have the uterine contraction monitoring, you can see the contraction coming before you actually feel it and can prepare for it. (If the membranes have ruptured, you may have an internal fetal monitor for the baby's heart. A wire, inserted through the vagina, is attached to the baby's head and gives a complete picture.)

Once settled in the labor room, you will be in **ACTIVE** labor, the stage when the cervix dilates from three to seven centimeters. By the time you are six centimeters dilated, the contractions may be very strong and will gradually increase in frequency until they are occurring every 2 to 3 minutes and lasting about 60 seconds. You will probably feel a definitely uncomfortable rise of pressure and tension, and then a gradual lessening of the tension until the contraction is over.

Just as you are reaching eight centimeters and lasting until the full ten, comes the hardest and shortest part of labor. It is called **TRANSITION,** and for most women, this is the part that gives the whole experience a bad name. Contractions are now 2 minutes to 1 minute apart and last for 90 seconds. It is the most discouraging part of labor and often considered the most painful. The closer you get to this stage, the more intense will be your contractions, and the more help you will need to cope with them. But this stage only lasts between 20 and 45 minutes. Some common signs of transition are: irritability, rectal pressure, premature urge to push, bloody show, shaking and chills and/or nausea and vomiting, and leg cramps. (If these signs do not occur during transition, the cold and shaking can occur after delivery of the placenta. It can be quite overwhelming, but it passes quickly.)

Suddenly, just when you feel that you can't go on, you will feel an entirely different sensation. It is hard to describe, but it will be different from any previous feeling of contractions. You will feel a pressure in the pelvis and an almost uncontrollable desire to push or bear down. But unless the doctor says you are a full 10 centimeters dilated you must not push or you might tear your cervix.

With the onset of pushing, second-stage labor has begun, and in 20 to 90 minutes, your baby will be born. The entire first stage may take anywhere from 12-14 hours for a first-time mother. For a second-time mother, the time is between 5 to 7 hours.

THE BABY, before labor begins, has descended slightly into the pelvis and his head is crowding the pelvic organs. As labor begins and progresses, his position gradually changes to accommodate the largest diameters of his body to the largest diameters of the pelvis. As he descends, he rotates and there is increased crowding of the mother's bladder and rectum.

The baby's skull is not hard bone all over, and his skull bones have not yet grown together. There are soft spots, or fontanels, at the front and back of the head, with a narrow gap connecting the two. During the second stage of labor, the skull is molded by overlapping of the bones. By internal examination, the doctor can feel these fontanels through the dilating cervix and can determine which way the baby's head is lying.

The presentation of the baby is usually by the back of the head (vertex), though the face, brow, or breech (buttocks) can present. The most common and most favorable way for the baby to present is with his head down, the nose facing the mother's back, with the back part of his skull (the occiput) toward the mother's front. The baby can be lying on the left side (in medical terms called left occiput anterior or L.O.A.) or on the right side (right occiput anterior R.O.A.). The left position is the more common of these and is an efficient way for the baby to move through the birth canal.

Some babies lie in the posterior position, facing either right or left, and the occiput is toward the mother's back

(called right occiput posterior R.O.P. or left occiput posterior L.O.P.). These positions are less favorable because the baby will try to turn around during labor in order to be born in a more favorable way, facing the mother's back. Labor will be longer and more uncomfortable and will create more severe backache pains. Rarely, the baby begins to rotate but gets stuck in a transverse (across) position, and if it remains in this posterior position, help from the doctor is needed. (See sketches below.)

In a face presentation (very rare), the baby's head is not flexed onto his chest as it usually is, and unless his head is small, labor may be slower and help may be needed with delivery. Brow presentation is also very rare.

The breech (buttocks down or feet first) presentation occurs in about three percent of deliveries. This, too, can cause a longer labor with contractions felt in the back. Back labor involves backaches which increase in intensity during contractions, then lessen, but don't go away totally. The danger in breech births is that the baby will take its first breath as soon as its bottom is born, while the head is still inside. The doctor may use forceps for the head or may insert a finger into the birth canal to clear a passageway for air to reach the baby's face. A Cesarean section is often performed in breech births for fetal safety.

By the combined force of your pushing with the diaphragm and abdominal muscles, and the uterine contractions, the baby's head descends and stretches the pelvic floor so that it comes into contact with the muscular outlet of the pelvis, known as the perineum. There is pressure in the rectum and stretching of the ligaments of the coccyx (tail bone). As the perineum is slowly distended, there may be some discomfort in the back, almost like a

tearing sensation, as if everything were splitting wide open. Actual tearing does not occur because the vaginal opening can stretch to wide proportions. But to enlarge the opening, many doctors perform an episiotomy—an incision of the perineum—between the vagina and the anus. This will not hurt as the doctor will use a local anesthesia.

The baby's head can now be seen at the entrance to the vagina when it begins to distend the perineum. Since it is the crown of the head which will first be visible, this moment is known as "the crowning of the baby's head." At this point—or in some cases, when the doctor can actually see the color of the baby's hair—you will be moved into the delivery room. This is particularly true for first babies; for second, the move takes place earlier—when the cervix has reached full dilation.

In minutes, your baby will be fully delivered.

A discussion of labor would not be complete without an explanation of the various methods of PAIN RELIEF.

There are roughly two sides to the issue of pain: on one is the view that labor pains are the most excruciating that a woman will ever experience, but that it is unfair to tell this to a pregnant woman because it will frighten her and make her experience even more difficult. On the other side is the view that with proper preparation for childbirth, pain and discomfort can be controlled and in some cases, almost eliminated.

We stand somewhere in between. When you consider what the body has to go through to help deliver the child, it would be naive to think that this wouldn't cause discomfort. In fact, it hurts, and depending on the woman and a number of factors, it may hurt a little or a lot. But it is true that with proper preparation in a prenatal class the experience can be less painful.

Positions of the baby as labor begins

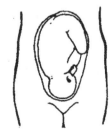

(1) Right occiput anterior. Baby's head down, facing the mother's back; the back part of his skull toward the mother's front. Baby lying on the right side.

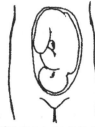

(2) Left occiput anterior. Most common position. Baby facing mother's back, lying on the left side.

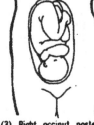

(3) Right occiput posterior. Baby is facing the mother's front; the back part of his skull toward the mother's back, lying on the right side.

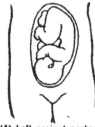

(4) Left occiput posterior. Same as above, but baby lying on the left side. These two positions are less favorable and labor may be longer.

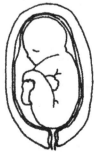

(5) Breech presentation. Buttocks down or feet first. Labor may be longer with contractions felt in the back.

There are essentially four ways to help diminish, control, alleviate, or completely eliminate pain and discomfort during labor. This discussion is not meant to be an exhaustive one, but rather a brief description of the methods and some of the advantages and disadvantages of each.

1) PSYCHOLOGICAL PAIN RELIEF. Psychoprophylaxis (or prepared childbirth) is a method of pain relief by conditioned reflex. As taught by the French obstetrician Fernand Lamaze and his advocates, the approach is twofold: first, the mother learns a variety of breathing exercises to use during labor and delivery which distracts her from conscious awareness of pain and helps her to relax. Secondly, the mother is educated about what to expect during labor and delivery, and this helps reduce the fear and anxiety which can intensify pain. By attending six classes with her husband eight weeks before her due date, she becomes prepared for the experience of labor and delivery.

The advantage to this method is the educational approach. Regardless of which method or combination of pain relief methods you finally use in the labor room, there is no substitute for knowing ahead of time what to expect. Every couple should take these classes, whether they plan to go through with the breathing exercises or not. Sharing the birth experience with your husband is described by many as one of life's most exciting moments. Finally, the Lamaze teaching discourages couples from using drugs and encourages the mother to be fully awake when the baby is delivered. Today in most hospitals, parents are told to go through the Lamaze training, and many of the classes are given in conjunction with the hospital.

Another variation of this method is called "natural childbirth" and was developed by Dr. Grantly Dick-Read before the Lamaze method. The course emphasis is slightly different, but the underlying point is the same—fear and tension lead to pain in labor, and all can be eliminated with proper knowledge and conditioning.

2) DRUGS. There are many drugs and combinations of drugs used today to alleviate labor pains. They may be given by mouth, rectally, or by hypodermic injection directly into a vein or muscle. We can't list all of them here, but a definition of certain terms will help clear up confusion about which drug and which method might be used. An **analgesic** is a drug which relieves or diminishes the sense of pain. Aspirin, for example, is a mild analgesic. An **anesthetic** obliterates all sensation, either through the production of transitory unconsciousness (general anesthetic) or by temporarily interrupting the pathway by which sensory nerves communicate pain to the brain (called conduction anesthesia).

The analgesics used today can be sedatives, which reduce anxiety and induce drowsiness; tranquilizers and narcotics, which reduce anxiety but don't induce drowsiness, and hypnotics, which induce sleep. Demerol and Valium are two of the drugs often used, alone or in combination.

As a group, these drugs are nervous depressants, depressing not only the sensation of pain but other nervous mechanisms, including breathing. The majority of drugs administered during labor will slow the progress of labor and will cross the placenta and therefore enter the baby's circulation, and they will exert an effect similar to that which is exerted on the mother. No matter by what route they have been given, they will gain access to her blood and therefore to her baby's. For this reason, doctors and childbirth educators today caution against the excessive use of drugs. We simply don't know what effects they may have on the fetus. The baby may be drowsy at birth, though he will recover quickly. But the final evidence on drugs is not yet in, and you should be aware of the possible hazards and/or the need for drugs used during labor and discuss this with your doctor.

3) GENERAL ANESTHESIA. This is the method of putting the mother completely to sleep and is done either by inhalation of nitrous oxide, ether, etc., or by intravenous sodium pentothal. The whole body is affected, creating temporary but complete unconsciousness.

This method is not used very often today because of the potential hazards to both mother and baby. The anesthetics will pass across the placenta into the baby's circulation and may make him sleepy, though with careful handling, he will be fine. If this method is used, it is usually not until very late in labor. (Many women argue that this is when pain relief is least needed.) But sometimes the method is needed, as in the case of an emergency Cesarean section.

4) REGIONAL ANESTHETICS (also called local or conduction) are widely used in labor, usually when the cervix is about halfway dilated. Essentially, they work by anesthetizing the nerves in a specific area of the body by interrupting the path from the area of pain stimulus to the brain. Since they act locally, little of the anesthesia is absorbed into the mother's bloodstream, and only small amounts cross the placenta. Still, there are cautions against the use of some of these methods, and in most cases, an anesthesiologist should be present to administer the dose.

The forms of conduction blocks (as they are called) are named for the location where they are given. A **caudal block** is given in the space at the base of the back (sacral canal). It may be given in one shot or continuously—additional amounts are given as soon as the numbness wears off. Or it may be administered through a catheter (tube), which is introduced into the lower back, and the anesthetic is then injected through the catheter.

Epidural anesthesia is injected between two vertebrae in the lower back—into the epidural space outside of the spinal canal and causes numbness from the navel to the mid-thigh area. An anesthesiologist should administer it. It slows the progress of labor and sometimes causes a slight drop in blood pressure. As the effects wear off, additional medication can be given, but you can be up immediately after delivery.

A **paracervical block** is the injection of anesthesia on either side of the cervix and the lower lateral borders of the uterus. A **pudendal block** anesthetizes the nerve fibers in the external organs—the perineum, vagina, and the entrance to the vagina (vulva).

A **spinal** is the injection of the anesthetic into the spinal fluid around the spinal cord, and therefore numbs the birth area from belly to thighs. It is one injection, so when it wears off, there is no more. Following delivery, you must stay flat for 18-24 hours, and spinal headaches are a common side effect.

A **saddle block** is a low spinal—it numbs the area where you would sit if in a saddle. It has the same side effects as the spinal.

There is growing evidence about risks in each of the above methods—the most common being a sudden drop in the mother's blood pressure which can jeopardize her welfare and the baby's. Again, ask your doctor what he might use and when.

The important issue here is not which method or combination of methods you use to deliver your baby, but the baby itself. Nothing should overshadow the experience of having the baby. Your doctor is there to offer you help if you're having trouble, but to keep the right perspective, remember why you're there—to deliver a healthy baby.

This concludes our discussion of first-stage labor. Next month we will discuss delivery and the new baby.

QUICK DICTIONARY OF TERMS

analgesic—a drug which relieves or diminishes sense of pain

anesthetic—a substance that obliterates all sensation, either through transitory unconsciousness, or by temporarily interrupting the path between sensory nerves and brain

bag of waters—(also called forewaters)—liquid which lies in front of baby's head and is held intact by uterine membranes

birth canal—space through which the baby moves in order to be born; formed by uterus, cervix and vagina

Braxton-Hicks contractions—preliminary, painless contractions

cervix—mouth of the uterus

dilation—(or dilatation)—the size of the round opening of the cervix; measured in centimeters or finger widths

effacement—process of thinning or "taking up" the cervix

first-stage labor—from the onset of labor to full dilation of the cervix

occiput—back part of the baby's skull

psychoprophylaxis—method of pain relief by conditioned reflex; the basis for prepared childbirth

second-stage labor—from full dilation of the cervix to birth of the baby .

show—(or bloody show)—blood-stained mucous from the plug that has been at the mouth of the cervix; often a sign of beginning labor

third-stage labor—from completion of baby's delivery to completion of delivery of the afterbirth

transition—labor from eight to ten centimeters dilation; often considered the hardest part of labor

uterus—(or womb) hollow organ which expands to house the baby

---

DELIVERY. The word derives from the Latin *de* (from) and *liber* (free), and at this point in your labor the baby is working his way down the birth canal, so that his "delivery" from the womb is imminent.

During the **transition stage,** you may have experienced an urge to push or bear down. Since your cervix was not fully dilated, the doctor/nurse encouraged you not to push and advised you to pant lightly and "blow out" continuously when the urge to push became overwhelming. (Pushing prematurely will tire you out by expending unnecessary energy and possibly tear your cervix.) Once you reach full dilation, you have completed the first stage of labor.

Many women describe the second stage as the "best" part of labor, as now they can take an active part in their child's birth by bearing down at the appropriate times. For the primapara (woman giving birth for the first time) delivery will begin in the labor room. At full dilation the doctor will tell you that you may now push when you have the urge during a contraction. The onset of pushing marks the beginning of the **second stage of labor.**

The desire to push may be sudden and overwhelming. With each contraction your baby's head is moving lower, aided by your bearing down. You may feel the pressure of the baby's head against the rectum, and the sensation may be an unpleasant one—as if you were splitting open. Actually, the baby is causing the ligaments around the coccyx (base of the spinal column) to

stretch. Some women never feel this pressure and must follow the doctor's direction to bear down.

The primapara must push the baby from full dilation to the opening of the vagina (approximately 4 inches) before she will go to the delivery room. This may take as little as twenty minutes, up to a maximum of an hour and fifteen minutes. Multiparas (women who have previously given birth) will go to the delivery room as soon as they are fully dilated. This is because their pelvic floor muscles have been previously stretched, and the descent of the baby will be more rapid.

With each contraction your baby's head is moving lower, aided by your bearing down with the diaphragm and abdominal muscles. The head will move forward with each contraction and recede slightly at the end of the contraction when downward pressure is no longer being directed.

When a portion of the baby's head about the size of a quarter remains visible at the opening of the vagina, you will be transferred to the delivery room. **The delivery room** is really a fully-equipped operating room with table, anesthesia machine, infant-resuscitation machine, and other items that may be needed. If you have had a hospital tour beforehand (usually included in childbirth preparation classes), the room and equipment will seem not ominous, but reassuring.

The delivery room table is equipped with wrist straps, stirrups, and possibly pistol grips. The wrist straps prevent you from accidentally touching the sterile drapes used during delivery. Often they are not used if the mother is to be awake during the birth and is in control of her contractions. The stirrups can be adjusted to make you comfortable, and they make pushing a bit easier as you are no longer supporting the full weight of your legs.

The most common delivery position is called **lithotomy**: you will be lying on your back with two pillows behind your head and shoulders; your legs will simultaneously be placed in the stirrups. The position is similar to that used during a gynecological exam except that the stirrups support the back of the thighs and legs, instead of just the feet. A very few hospitals are experimenting with a French labor-delivery bed which can be easily adapted to delivery requirements. The laboring woman can thus remain in the same bed (and room) for the entire childbirth process.

After your legs are placed in the stirrups, your hands will be placed on a metal pistol grip on either side of the delivery table to assist you in lifting yourself up during the expulsion of the baby. The doctor will wash you with a disinfectant (prep) and drape you with cloth or paper drapes to cover all areas except for the vagina.

With the next few contractions, the outlines of the baby's head can be seen stretching through the perineum, and it looks like a large grapefruit. This is referred to as the **crowning** of the baby's head and it is a very exciting moment. Usually, your baby's head will be born with just a few more pushes.

If you are going to have a general anesthesia, it will be administered now. During a contraction, the doctor may give the local anesthesia for the **episiotomy**, an incision to enlarge the vaginal opening and to prevent the tearing of the **perineum**, the area between the vagina and rectum. However, if the episiotomy is made during a contraction, it will be painless—the pressure of the baby's head on the paper-thin tissue of the perineum creates a natural anesthesia. Although some people question routine episiotomy, it should be remembered that a straight incision is easier to repair than a jagged tear.

Most babies make their appearance head first, face toward the floor. This **vertex** position means that the baby is leaving the uterus head down. The back of the baby's head (occiput) is toward the mother's abdomen when labor begins; as the baby descends into the pelvis the head turns so the soft cartilage of the nose will be against the mother's tailbone (coccyx). This is the most efficient way for a baby to slip past the pubic bone and into the birth canal. As the doctor gently guides the baby's head out, the head spontaneously turns to the left or right to line up with the baby's as-yet-unborn shoulders. The doctor will next locate the cord. Should it be around the baby's neck, he would try to draw the cord down around the occiput to prevent compression by the shoulder, and when possible, clamp and cut the cord—painless to both mother and baby.

With the next contraction, the upper or anterior shoulder will be delivered and the rest of the baby will slither out, completing the second stage. When the umbilical cord stops pulsating, it is clamped and cut. Your baby is now a separate individual!

Some babies may take their first breath and begin to cry, suddenly turning red even before they are completely born. But often the baby will not begin to cry until the attendant has removed the mucous from his nose and mouth. This is nothing to be alarmed about. In either case, the sound of your baby's first cry is something you will never forget.

Forceps delivery. If for some reason you were unable to expel the baby on your own, your child would be delivered by forceps. The forceps resemble a pair of salad tongs with long, curved blades to fit the shape of the baby's head. Each blade is inserted into the vagina separately and placed carefully on either side of the baby's head. The two handles cross and lock together, and the baby's head is slowly and gently extracted. The delivery of the rest of the baby is the same as in a spontaneous delivery. The primary indication for a forceps delivery is fetal distress, indicated by a slowed heart rate. Other indications are excessive pressure on the baby's head resulting from a short, stormy labor or an extremely long one; incorrect position of the baby's head, and inability of the mother to push the baby out due to use of conduction anesthesia, or exhaustion.

THE BABY'S APPEARANCE AT BIRTH. If your baby has begun to breathe before it is completely born, it may have a normal flush. Otherwise the baby will be a bluish color at first or, in the case of a black baby, gray to black in color. The doctor will suction any blood or mucous from the baby's nose and mouth. (The stereotype of the physician holding the newborn by its heels and giving it a slap on the backside is outdated. Slapping on the back is only done in extreme cases, since it can cause trauma to the baby.) Resuscitation equipment stands by in case it is needed. If the baby has difficulty in breathing, immediate assistance is necessary, as there may otherwise be damage to the brain cells due to lack of oxygen.

The baby will be wet looking and may be covered with a white creamy substance called **vernix,** which has been protecting its skin in utero and has acted as a greasing agent as the baby has moved along the vaginal canal. (Some babies will also be spotted with blood from the birth canal.) Another newborn characteristic observed in some babies is the appearance of a fine downy covering called **lanugo,** which disappears within a few days. You may be surprised by the odd, elongated shape of the baby's head. The molding will help adapt the head to the shape of the birth canal, and it is temporary. Since the skull is not yet completely hard (there are two soft spots called fontanels that overlap as the head comes along the vagina), it will soon take on a normal, rounded appearance, about 12-24 hours after delivery. If the delivery was by forceps, the baby may have red forceps marks, which will also quickly disappear.

At one minute, and again at five minutes after birth, your baby's condition will be evaluated visually by what is known as the **Apgar Score.** This system, developed by Dr. Virginia Apgar, uses the vital signs of heart rate, respiratory rate, muscle tone, cry and color to determine the newborn's status. Two points are given for each of the five categories. The one minute score may indicate that the baby requires assistance. The five minute score is the important one in relation to how a baby will fare later in life. A maximum of ten may be obtained. This procedure simply allows the attendant to quickly assess your newborn's health; it is not a "test."

The nurse will also place a drop of silver-nitrate solution in each of your baby's eyes to eliminate the chance of infection from undetected gonorrhea in the mother, a procedure required by law. The baby is then given a nameband with your name, sex of the baby, date and time of birth, and a duplicate is given to the mother to prevent any mixup. He is then wrapped in a blanket and placed in a warming bed to help maintain his body temperature. If your husband is present, the nurse will usually hand the baby to him for a moment.

A rare exception to this rule is the so-called "modified" Leboyer delivery. This delivery procedure, developed by a French obstetrician, calls for a quiet, dimly-lit delivery room. Immediately after birth, the baby is placed on the mother's stomach and gently massaged. The umbilical cord is not cut until the baby begins to breathe on its own. (The warm water bath advocated by Leboyer is usually omitted in this country.) The aim of all this is to make the birth more pleasant for the baby who, it is claimed, faces the trauma of bright lights and noise after a peaceful existence in the womb. However, at present only a handful of doctors in this country offer this type of delivery.

DELIVERY OF THE PLACENTA. Meanwhile, the delivery of the afterbirth or placenta marks the **third and final stage** of the birth process. During pregnancy, the placenta is attached to the wall of the uterus and connected to the baby via the umbilical cord. It provides the vehicle through which nutrients from the mother pass to the baby, and wastes are removed. After the child's birth, the uterus becomes much smaller and stops contracting to "rest" after the strenuous work of delivery. In a few minutes it begins to contract again. This time the purpose is to free the placenta from the wall of the uterus, then to squeeze the placenta down into the vagina where it is removed by the obstetrician.

As soon as the placenta is delivered, the doctor examines it carefully to be sure it is complete. This organ is composed of twenty or so placentae, sort of like a honeycomb of smooth tile-like pieces. If part of the placenta remains in the uterus, it might cause hemorrhaging. Most doctors perform a manual removal of the placenta if it has not been expelled several minutes after the baby. The placenta is red and "meaty" and its appearance may be a bit shocking to the uninitiated.

Excessive bleeding is usually not a problem after delivery. The blood loss at delivery averages eight ounces. Since the blood plasma volume increases about a quart during pregnancy, the loss of half a pint is easily tolerated. Nature has arranged the muscles of the uterus so that they can "close off" the blood vessels in the lining to prevent excessive bleeding. But it is essential that the uterus remain fairly firm after delivery in order for it to function properly. The doctor may firmly knead the uterus through the abdominal wall, or use hormones such as Oxytocin or Ergonovine to make it contract.

With the birth completed, the doctor repairs the episiotomy using catgut sutures. The stitches will be absorbed in 15-20 days and need not be removed. Some authorities recommend that an ice pack be placed on the episiotomy site immediately after repair to help decrease the tissue swelling and thereby ease the discomfort that is a common postpartum complaint.

The doctor will check your baby carefully, and then the baby will be brought back to you. This is the moment you have been looking forward to for many months, and it will surely be an exciting one. If your husband has participated in the birth, the three of you will have a chance to get acquainted now. Some mothers even nurse their babies for the first time right on the delivery table (ask ahead if this is permitted). Women who are not going to breast-feed will be given medication to prevent engorgement of the breasts. Regardless of whether you are going to breast-feed, you should wear a good bra 24 hours a day for two weeks, starting right away, to also prevent engorgement of the breasts.

Unfortunately, in most hospitals mother and baby are soon separated. Baby will be taken to the nursery to be weighed, bathed and diapered. You will remain in the recovery room for several hours so the staff can monitor your blood pressure and bleeding from the placental site. (A woman who has been heavily sedated may wake up in the recovery room and ask when she is going to have her baby!)

Now that the delivery is over, you may feel euphoric—a bit "high" at the thought of what you've just accomplished. Some women, however, feel a bit "empty" and depressed as they wait for their babies to be brought to them (your baby may remain in the nursery for anywhere from six to twenty-four hours). Many hospitals now offer rooming-in or family-centered maternity plans that allow mother and newborn more time together. Check on the hospital's policy to see if you must keep the baby with you at all times (you may become overtired), or if there is a modified rooming-in plan where you can have your baby taken back to the nursery if you need some rest.

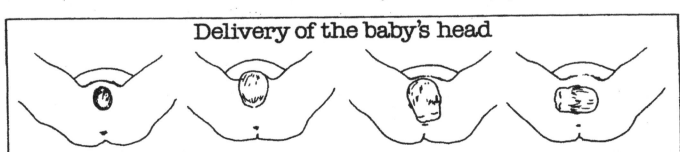

Delivery of the baby's head

The baby's head can be seen at the entrance to the vagina (1) when it begins to distend the perineum. His neck is situated just behind the front bone of the pelvis, and from this time on, the completion of the delivery is by the baby extending his head over the perineum. (2) First the brow and then the nose, face, then mouth and chin are delivered. (3) As soon as the head is delivered, the shoulders rotate (4) so that the baby looks at either the right or left thigh of the mother.

Your hospital stay may be anywhere from two days to a week or more (average is three days), depending on the type of delivery you had and, of course, your rate of recovery. Generally Cesarean patients are hospitalized for a full week, but by the fourth day they may feel as strong as women who have had an uncomplicated birth. If there were no complications, you should be allowed out of bed the day of delivery. (Early ambulation can lead to a quicker recovery and decreased bowel and bladder problems.)

It is, however, a good idea to take it easy even if you think you feel terrific. One way to do this is to pace the number of visitors you have in the hospital (and again when you get home, where you may be expected to play hostess and feed and entertain guests). Your husband can tactfully suggest to friends and relatives that you will be delighted to have them come and see the new baby—just as soon as you feel up to it.

THE IMMEDIATE POSTPARTUM PERIOD. Within a few hours of delivery, you will have already lost about 12 pounds. Your tummy will not flatten out for about a week, although your uterus will have begun to shrink back to its pre-pregnant size. The entire process takes about six weeks, and this period is known as the **puerperium** (from the Latin for "having brought forth a child"). When the puerperium begins, the uterus is a two-pound mass of muscle; by the end of six weeks it has shrunk to three ounces. This is referred to as **involution** of the uterus.

Contractions continue after delivery so that the uterus may involute nor-mally, and they may cause discomfort similar to menstrual cramps (known as "after-pains"). After-pains may last for several days and may be especially noticeable during nursing sessions. This is because involution is stimulated by nursing, thus the uterus of a nursing mother shrinks more rapidly. After-pains can usually be relieved by simple analgesics, such as aspirin.

The lochia is the postpartum uterine discharge. Immediately following delivery, the lochia is bright red and the amount is noted by the nurse. As the uterus shrinks back to its normal size (probably slightly larger than before pregnancy), the lochia will become brown and cease altogether. (It may, however, become red again during the first days at home if you overdo your normal activities. Reduce your activity, and if the bleeding is progressive, call your doctor.) The length of bleeding varies considerably from woman to woman, but the average is about 21 days. There is also no set rule for the reappearance of menstruation after delivery. (Sometimes menstruation is confused with a heavy lochia about one month after delivery.) If you are nursing, you may not resume menstruating until the baby is weaned, although you could begin to ovulate (and accidentally become pregnant) without resuming menstruation.

Increased urination is common between the second and fifth days after delivery. In this way the body rids itself of the extra tissue water (2-3 quarts) that has accumulated during pregnancy. Rarely, a woman may be unable to urinate after a long and difficult labor or a forceps delivery, and may have to be catheterized for a day or two. There is also a tendency to become constipated during the puerperium and hemorrhoids may also occur. As long as you don't strain, you won't tear your stitches. A diet with sufficient fluids will help keep the bowel movements soft. Early ambulation and elimination of bedpan use make constipation far less of a problem than it used to be. Warm baths and soothing ointments can help relieve discomfort from hemorrhoids.

The episiotomy stitches may itch or be painful, and this area may continue to be tender for several weeks. Among the remedies for a painful episiotomy site are: 1) sitz bath—warm, shallow soaking of episiotomy, 2) dry heat from a heat lamp, 3) witch hazel compress, and 4) medicated ointments or sprays.

The breasts will begin to secrete **colostrum** (a sticky, yellow fluid) after delivery. If you are nursing, the colostrum will provide the baby with its major source of nourishment the first few days after delivery. Your baby may not seem interested in nursing at first—he is tired. Don't worry—patience and persistence will pay off. On the third day his interest in eating will increase.

When your milk comes in, on the third day after delivery, your breasts may become suddenly larger, firm, hot, and painful. This is called engorgement, and it rarely lasts more than 24-36 hours. You can avoid it by applying ice packs between feedings. Breast-feeding on demand also helps relieve this situation.

The "baby blues" (or postpartum depression) are a common phenomena among new mothers. Doctors put part of the blame on fatigue and hormone changes, but you may also feel depressed because your tummy hasn't immediately become as flat as you'd hoped it would; because you didn't feel a rush of maternal feelings at the first sight of your baby (this will come in time), or because you feel awkward in caring for your baby.

Usually these blues last only a few days and are accompanied by the **milk letdown reflex.** Some women never feel depressed, while others feel blue for several months after the baby is born. Usually, as you become more confident in your mothering abilities and adjust to your new lifestyle, your emotions will improve. It will also help if you set aside some time for yourself—to read, take a walk or whatever—and for occasional outings with your husband (time to spend as a *couple*, not as parents). If, however, feelings of depression persist, you may need the help of a professional counselor.

Going home with your new baby will be an exciting (and perhaps a bit scary) moment. You may feel overwhelmed by your responsibility for this new life. Try to relax and remember that most new parents have a few doubts. Ideally, you should have someone to help with the housework for the first week or so—a friend, relative or paid help. You'll need plenty of rest. Don't overexert yourself.

If you have any unusual symptoms—particularly increased vaginal bleeding—call your doctor at once. And don't be tempted to skip the six weeks' checkup just because you are feeling fine. It's important that your doctor examine you to be certain that your recovery is going normally.

The first few days and weeks at home with your new baby will be a real time of adjustment. Many parents say they had no idea how much time and trouble it took to care for a baby. They also say they wouldn't have missed having one for anything!

QUICK DICTIONARY OF TERMS

Apgar score—Rates newborn's health on a scale of 1-10 after a visual examination performed at one and again at five minutes after birth

colostrum—thin, yellow fluid secreted by the breasts before the milk comes in. Thought to contain helpful antibodies

crowning—when the top of the baby's head becomes visible at the vaginal opening just before birth

episiotomy—incision in the perineum to prevent it from tearing during delivery

fontanels—soft spots on the baby's head. There are two: anterior (front of the skull) and posterior (back of the skull)

forceps—special surgical applicators sometimes used to deliver a baby

in utero—in the womb

involution—process by which uterus returns (shrinks) to normal size

lanugo—fine downy hair which may appear on the newborn but disappears within a few days

lithotomy position—most common delivery position in this country. Woman is lying on her back with legs up and held apart in stirrups

lochia—postpartum uterine discharge. (Amount and color indicate how involution is progressing)

perineum—muscular area between the vagina and rectum

postpartum depression—(also called "baby blues")—a short period of depression which often follows childbirth. Thought to be related to hormone changes

vernix (also vernix caseosa)—a white creamy substance which covers the newborn skin (provides protection for skin in utero)

BASIC FUNDAMENTALS OF PEDIATRIC NURSING

CONTENTS

Page

———

BASIC FUNDAMENTALS OF

PEDIATRIC NURSING

Section I. INTRODUCTION

1. Definition

a. Pediatrics is that branch of medicine that deals with (1) the diseases of children and their treatment and (2) the child's development and care.

b. Pediatric nursing is considered a specialty area within the field of nursing. The information that is offered will assist the specialist in his care of the pediatric patient; however, he should never proceed in his care of the patient unless directed by the nurse in charge. Irreparable damage can be done by the well-meaning, but poorly informed specialist. Although care of the newborn is usually considered a part of obstetrical nursing, certain aspects of newborn care are presented here in order to maintain continuity.

2. Physical Differences Between Infants, Children, and Adults

The child is *not* a "little adult." As table 1 shows, there are real physiological differences between children and adults.

Table 1. Physical Differences Between Infant, Child, and Adult

	Infant	Child	Adult
Susceptibility to disease	Inherits immunity to some diseases for around 6 months from his mother.	Highly susceptible to respiratory infections. Many minor illnesses of short duration and many contagious diseases. Gradually builds up immunity.	Has developed certain resistance to some infections.
Nutritional needs	Frequent feedings needed	Greater because he is growing and developing.	Less.
Cardiovascular system	Blood loss is more drastic, Differs from adult in blood pressure (higher), blood volume (lower), and cardiac output. Vital signs are unstable.	Heart develops in size less rapidly than body. Its work is increased. Easily damaged by toxins and bacteria and must be protected against strain during convalescence. The blood pressure may fall.	Tolerates a greater blood loss than infant or child.
Central nervous system	Not fully mature. Some reflexes are absent. Temperature fluctuates.	Same as infant. Hand-eye coordination are not complete.	Mature reflexes present in normal person. Stable temperature regulator.
Gastrointestinal system	May swallow air. Thin muscles of abdomen predispose to gastric distention. Vomiting may be dangerous.	Vomiting may be dangerous	Mature system in normal person. Vomiting not usually dangerous if conscious.
Pulmonary system	Often has irregular respiration, chest wall is thin, and pressure or restraint may deter breathing. Artificial respiration is given differently (ch. 8). See statements about child which also apply to infant.	Intercostal muscles that help breathing are not fully developed. Lumen of trachea is smaller and easily occluded by secretions. Large catheters can irritate trachea and cause laryngospasm or cardiac arrest in the young child.	Mature system in normal person.
Urinary system	Not fully developed. Dehydration and overhydration may occur rapidly. Difficult to excrete toxic substances.	Same as in infant	Mature system in normal person.

3. Effect of Illness on Child's Personality and Behavior

a. The developing personality can be affected by illness; for example, "being different" because of illness can definitely change a child's personality. Just being physically separated from his family can cause anxiety. This anxiety can often be helped by letting the child play out his problems. Nursing personnel can also help by understanding the child's feelings. Just when he needs his parents most, he is separated from them and surrounded by strangers in a strange environment where he has to eat different foods.

b. A child patient needs much closer observation than an adult patient. Medical specialists must learn to recognize the types of behavior that indicate specific conditions or problem areas. This recognition includes fear and withdrawal. The specialist must also realize that the quiet good child may be suffering the greatest trauma. Among the causes of behavioral problems are—

(1) The child's response to hospitalization as a threatening situation.

(2) Child's fear that his parents have abandoned him.

(3) The belief that hospitalization is a punishment for previous "bad" behavior. (The child may have been threatened with shots or told that he will become sick if he does so and so.)

(4) Negative attitude of parents, which can affect child. Thus, you can expect tantrums, refusal to eat or cooperate, attempts to "run away," or attacks on other children. You can also expect different reactions on different days. A child may suddenly refuse to eat a favorite food or accept one that he previously rejected. He may also suddenly refuse to accept help from a favorite specialist.

c. The proper psychological approach is necessary to prevent as much trauma to the child as possible and to accomplish nursing objectives. Use as little force as possible and then only that which is absolutely necessary. The following approaches are some that might be helpful in dealing with children:

• Never lie to a child.

• Remember that a child's attention span is short, especially in the very young.

• Keep explanations brief and positive. Don't allow him to be in a position where he can say no.

• Never use treatment, injections, etc., as a threat.

• Do not tell a child of forthcoming treatments or other medical needs until immediately before they are performed, as the child will probably become anxious—but *do* inform him.

• Tell the child that the treatment, medicines, etc., are given to make him well. Offer some explanation even if a child is crying.

• Do not talk down to a child, but be sure he understands you. Use the terms his family uses for going to the toilet, for bottles, etc. Also use his nickname, as he may not recognize his name.

• Reward him for acceptable behavior with your approval.

• Attempt to keep him busy and distracted from unpleasant situations. Try new approaches.

• Make games of procedures if possible (gold stars for drinking a certain amount of fluids, "hero" badges for bravery, saving medicine cups to show his mother).

• Consider each child as an individual with rights of dignity and modesty, and respect these rights.

d. If misbehavior occurs despite everything you can do, his misbehavior must be dealt with, but certain rules can be used for guidance—

Rule 1. Keep discipline firm, just, and consistent.

Rule 2. Deal with misbehavior as it happens. If you ignore the breaking of rules, you weaken discipline and confuse the child. However, do nothing when extremely angry.

Rule 3. Explain the reason for rules. It will help the child (after 2½ years) to understand that he is not just being pushed around—that each rule has a reason behind it

CAUTION
Be sure you do have a good reason.

Rule 4. Keep your voice calm. It does no good to scream at a sick child (his illness is probably affecting his behavior) or to talk in a loud voice to a child who does not understand you.

Rule 5. Avoid bribes; they let a child remain immature and be paid for it.

Rule 6. Whenever possible, give the child a reason for changing undesirable behavior to good behavior.

Rule 7. Make suggestions positive rather than negative. "Put your toys in this box," rather than "Don't throw toys all over the floor."

Rule 8. Do not ridicule a child.

TABLE 2 – NORMAL GROWTH AND DEVELOPMENT

Age	Body development	Mental development and specialist's approach
Infancy (birth to 1 year).	Infant may be long and thin or short and chubby. His head and abdomen are large, his chest is small. Trunk is longer than extremities. Head grows more rapidly than any other time. Soon after bath, usually can arch back and hold head erect for short time in supine position. At 5–6 months, learns to roll over. Learns to stand with support by 12 months.	At first the baby cries the same way, regardless of reason, but by 1 month, parents can tell whether a baby is angry, tired, or hungry. At 3 months, laughs aloud, smiles at mother, babbles. About 6–7 months, tries to talk. Although he cannot be understood, respond. At 9 months, cries when scolded. At 10 months, understands the meaning of "No, No," knows his name and should be called by it. At 12 months, knows about 2 words, plus "ma ma" and "da da." Loves rhythms and rhymes. After 8 months, becomes distrustful of strangers. From then to 18 months, does not like to be looked in the eye by a stranger. Do not smile, frown, or make sudden moves until the child accepts you. If there is a need for immediate treatment, position or hold the baby firmly and gently and speak reassuringly.
Toddler (1 to 3 years).	Body proportions change as child grows. Able to crawl or walk, no longer completely dependent. Develops muscular coordination. Needs to learn to do things for himself but will be very slow. Energetic and restless.	The 2-year-old has a vocabulary from 12 to 300 words. Learns to use words and can use short sentences. Can follow simple directions. Explanations of treatments should be given after 2½ years, but must be simple, direct, and truthful. The 30-month-old has an increased vocabulary and speaks well. He knows something of "yesterday," "tomorrow," and "today" but, if told that something might happen on "Wednesday," he would be confused. Tell him short stories during treament; he will listen and be interested.
Preschool (3 to 5 years).	Gains control of elimination. Achieves physiological stability. Very active, needs exercise for his large muscles. Slower rate of growth. Full set of temporary teeth by 3 years. Large muscles have developed, but development of motor skills is uneven. At 5 years, system is mature enough to have habits of eating, sleeping, and elimination fairly well established. Energetic and restless.	The 3-year-old can carry on a conversation about what he is doing. Also understands more and can be reasoned with. Has some idea of reading and can give his full name and address. Has an understanding of time and can plan where he is going. The 4-year-old is aggressive, boasts; likes to talk about his family and what they do, so get him to talking during treatment. The 5-year-old wants information; he's the one who asks question after question. He likes to talk and is interested in everyone. Do not talk too personally about people; he will parrot everything you say. The 4- and 5-year-old will try to delay anything unpleasant. Don't let this go on too long or you may lose control.
6 to 8 years.	Physically active. Will resent illness because he can't play. Physical growth slows a little, but some changes in height and weight should be expected every 3 months. Has a sense of equilibrium. The large muscles of the arms and legs are more developed than the small muscles of the hands and fingers. Right- or left-handedness has been established and should not be changed. Lungs are very small. Child may indicate fatigue by being cross.	The 6-year-old begins to accept the attitude and beliefs of his friends, not just those of the family. He needs to be best in everything. Encourage a withdrawn child to join action groups, as he needs group play. The attention span is still short. The 7-year-old is quieter than the 6-year-old. He may want to read, think, or play alone. May become absorbed in thought. He is modest, so respect his privacy.
8 to 11 years.	Slow growth in height and weight, (but girls have a spurt in growth at about 10 years). Manipulative skills increase as small muscles develop. Has good muscular coordination. May have poor posture. Watch when playing with more mature individuals as the heart, which develops less rapidly than the body, could be overtaxed. Lungs are still not fully developed. Eyes, however, function as well as an adult's eyes. Has enormous energy.	The attention span is longer. The 8-year-old is more restless than the 7-year-old. Real problems occur when he is on bedrest as he wants to be active and wants company; watch him to be sure he stays in bed. He likes school and friends but is also a good listener. He resents being treated as a child and needs to assume responsibilities within his own capabilities. The 9-year-old is calmer, but will resist adult authority when it interferes with his wishes. Be sure to point out when and where he does well. Encourage him to write letters. Can be trusted to assume responsibility for many of his own affairs and to follow-through on plans. The 10-year-old is even more responsible. He should help plan for his home care. He is courteous but tends to criticize people and ideas. Likes a challenge. Able to think clearly and will challenge your logic, so be sure to explain carefully.
11 to 12 years.	Period of great adjustment. Rapid changes in height, weight, shape. May tire easily. Puberty usually begins for girls at about 12. Secondary sex characteristics appear. Do not push him beyond his physical limits, but he will want real tasks. Body proportions are affected by growth. Awkward. Posture may be slovenly. Heart is not growing as rapidly as the body. More rest is needed. Blood pressure may fall. Muscular growth is very rapid and may be accompanied by restlessness. Children differ widely in physical maturity. Appetite may be ravenous but capricious.	For something one minute and against it the next. May be confused. Little interest in home or his own property. Encourage development of spirit of cooperation. Interest in exploration and adventure.

TABLE 2 *Normal Growth and Development.* (cont'd)

Emotional or personality traits	Toys
Responds toward people's attitudes to him by fear, love, pleasure, or anger. Can even feel insecure. This is the oral period when he gets satisfaction from sucking, needs to belong, and to be loved. Does not like sudden changes, noises, or bright lights. Excitement or bustle may frighten him. Care of child must not be mechanical as he needs mothering, caressing, and fondling.	Rattles, durable, bright colored; large colored beads on heavy cord; toy animals that are easily cleaned; bright hanging objects. At 10 months, likes pat-a-cake, peek-a-boo, and bye-bye.
24-30 months: The 2-year-old cares for those who care for him. Explores his body. Shows definite emotional reactions. May have violent changes in mood and be unable to control himself. May make many unreasonable demands. Requires that every simple routine be repeated in detail and may require that certain persons perform these routines. He is a perfectionist and rigid in his demands. Likes to dawdle. Fusses or fights with other children. Will not share toys. Tries to force others to do what he wants. May be extremely jealous and may attack others. Cannot take turns. Is likely to feel guilty about being ill. Begins to change from dependence to independence. Changes play often.	Push-pull toys; dolls, fabric or rubber doll's eyes tested for safety, whistles removed; kitchen ut sils of wood or smooth-edged pan lids. Small bright bloc! Floating toys for bath, balls, color pegs, bells, simple books.
The 3-year-old is cooperative and anxious to please, so praise when possible. Interested in new and different things. Learns to relate emotionally with others; gets on better with other children. Quarrels may occur but children usually settle them without help. Can take turns. The 4-year-old is social, plays more with others, likes to act out situations. Plays best with only one child and may prefer his own sex. Aggressive but can usually work out differences. Has strong home attachment. Careless and rough with toys. Has a beginning sense of property rights. Tells tall tales, may be defiant or swear—this is the way he learns what others will accept and can establish his own standards. Likes drawing, painting, cutting, pasting, looking at books, story telling, radio, and TV. Often is afraid that parents have deserted him or had a terrible accident. Usually responsible, obedient, and easy to please. Curious and continues to explore own body.	Wagon; wheelbarrow; simple trains; boat and dump trucks; large blocks, sand pile, shovel, pail; rag dolls, doll furniture, carriage; large bright ball; something on which to climb, picture cards (old Christmas cards); bright colored paper and blunt scissors (used under supervision) to make chains, to decorate a space; nests of colored boxes; cuddly animals; large crayons and paper; empty spools, tin dishes.
Sensitive, may become dependent on one specialist, so personnel should be rotated. May be a showoff or defiant. May have tantrums. May alternately play and fight with other children. The 7-year-old is sensitive to the opinion of others. If frustrated, may throw or break objects. May quit playing if he doesn't win. May be a "tattle-tale." More aware of right and wrong.	Needs imaginative play. Likes to imitate adults. Likes fairy tales, rhythm, music, and dancing; scissors, pictures to cut and paste; large beads to be strung; clay; picture books; paper dolls; musical instruments; radio, TV. Also puzzles, riddles, scrapbooks; to make tops, beanbag games, puppets, soap, bubble sets.
The 8-year-old needs others. Interested in adult standards and in game spirit but also has private interests. Has creative imagination. The 9-year-old is competitive, worries when he does not do well, afraid of failure. Has improved social skills and enjoys his own age group. Fair and just with others. Flexible and willing to change ideas if a better thought presentation is made. Has sexual modesty. Needs some freedom in setting up his own rules.	Tops, marbles. Likes hobbies, checkers, crayons and paints, scissors and paper, boxes and boards for building, TV and radio. Membership in a secret club helps fill the need for an assured position in a social group.
Self-conscious and irritable because of physical changes. May have one or two close friends, who are extremely important to his personality development. Disorganized. May be aggressive. May be unable to control himself and may change behavior rapidly. Resents the curb of illness because he likes to be physically and mentally active. Apt to show frustration by withdrawing. Ambivalent feelings about dependence and his struggle for independence. May rebel against routines, washing, dressing, getting to meals. Strives to act like his friends and respects good sports. May be overanxious about his own health. Children differ widely in temperament.	Gangs are still important. Both sexes enjoy earning money. Boy's play is rough. Likes drama, group activities, music, TV, books, hobbies, letter writing, telephone calls. In prolonged cases, provisions should be made for doing school work.

TABLE 2 NORMAL GROWTH AND DEVELOPMENT (cont'd)

Sleep	Food
The newborn sleeps most of the 24 hours. At 4 months, needs 20 to 22 hours; at 6 months, 16 to 18 hours; at 1 year, 15 hours.	Milk, water, juice at first, then supplemental foods. Hold the baby while feeding him, supporting his head, neck, and back. Remove nipple when baby's mouth is open; otherwise, some of the formula might go into his mouth and choke him. Nipple holes should be large enough so he doesn't have to suck too hard but not so large that the fast flow will choke him. Burp baby at frequent intervals, as a minimum at midway point and after feeding. Keep atmosphere restful. Between 6 months and 1 year, the child will try to play, feel, or smell his food. Put only one food at a time in front of him and watch him closely.
Needs 12-13-14 hours, plus a long nap. The 2-year-old will take a nap, but may want his favorite toy. Usually he will be happy and ready to get up when he awakes. Nap lasts about 2 or 3 hours in afternoon. Sometimes he may just play quietly in his bed. The 30-month-old may insist that his bed be loaded with toys and that they be arranged a certain way, or he may follow a particular routine. Daytime naps are variable. If he sleeps too long, he will be irritable when he wakes up. The slightly older child may need more time to wake up; don't rush him. If he has a long nap, he may need to stay up longer that night. He has trouble going to sleep and may begin to develop elaborate rituals to help him go to sleep.	From 2 years to 30 months: Learns to take solid foods. May have strong food likes and dislikes. He may also change these likes without notice. May want to feed himself entirely. Usually wants only one good meal a day. May also require certain dishes or methods of serving. Although he can feed himself, he may call on a special person to feed him.
The 3-year-old is afraid of the dark. His sleep is restless and he may wake up and want water or to go to the bathroom. May also get up and wander around. May whine and want a lot of attention. The 5- or 6-year-old goes to sleep without rituals. May have nightmares. Usually does not need an afternoon nap, but should sleep about 12 hours.	The 3-year-old likes finger foods. Has a better appetite than the 2-year-old. May ask for favorite foods, may or may not be upset if he doesn't get them. May dawdle or want attention at meal time. The 4-year-old may have definite preferences and refuse many foods. Doesn't have a good appetite. May want to plan his own meals. May leave his food and walk around or forget to eat at all. The 5-year-old has a better appetite but the amount he eats may vary widely from meal to meal. Can feed himself. May have definite food preferences but will usually try different foods. Usually is slow but persistent in eating. At 5½ to 6 years of age, give second helping if desired.
He should sleep about 12 hours.	
He should sleep about 10–11 hours. Usually does not get enough rest. A quiet period in the afternoon prevents overfatigue.	
Needs about 9 hours sleep.	

TABLE 2   NORMAL GROWTH AND DEVELOPMENT (cont'd)

Elimination	Bathing and dressing
No control over body function. The first stool, *meconium*, is dark green, thick, and sticky and is passed at any time up to 24 hours after birth. A breast-fed baby has bright yellow and soft stools, with 3 to 6 BM per day. A bottle-fed baby's stools are yellow to brown, firmer, and usually fewer in number—1 to 4 a day. In both cases, the BM's gradually decrease to 1 or 2 a day.	Must be bathed daily (including shampoo) and kept dry and comfortable. In bathing, give special attention to areas of skin that contact each other such as in the neck, behind the ears, in the axillae, and in the groin. Dry well. Powder is not used in hospital. Bathe him lying down. By 6 months, he enjoys splashing in the tub. Use loose-fitting clothes of simple design.
At 30 months, bowel training is usually completed. He can even get to the bathroom fairly well but may have trouble undressing. Usually wants privacy but may ask for help when he is through. May have 2 BMs a day or may skip a day or two and still be normal. Not yet in control completely of his bladder. Wants to be changed if he is barely damp. May wet the bed.	At 30 months, he likes his bath but may have some ritual about the soap, plug, or faucet. May want to wash himself, but he doesn't do a good job. However, he is more interested in playing. Can take off his clothes but has trouble putting them back on. May fight against being dressed or be particular about his clothes.
The 3-year-old has little difficulty with BM's and can usually take care of himself fairly well. Also has fewer accidents and less bed wetting. Usually sleeps through the night. The 4-year-old is able to manage with little or no help from adults. Very much interested in the bathroom proclivities of others. The 5-year-old usually does not need help but may need reminding when he is playing.	The 3-year-old usually does a fair job of washing himself, but he still likes to play in tub and may not want to get out. Does not usually have any ritual. Can put on most clothing and unbutton a garment (unless the buttons are at the back). The 5-year-old usually does a relative good job on bathing. If reminded, he can wash his hands and face before eating. Although he can usually dress himself, he still cannot button back buttons or tie his shoes. Someone must choose and put out his clothes. He may not always *want* to dress himself even when he can.

METHOD OF DEALING WITH MISBEHAVIOR

- Give a child a substitute outlet for anger such as having him pound pegs.
- Isolate the child if possible; it will give him time to calm down and think about his unacceptable behavior and your response to it. Children normally want approval of their actions and will modify them if they feel that these actions are not accomplishing the desired result. This isolation period should be brief and the child should be allowed to resume his normal activities with the other children as soon as he is reasonable.
- Deprive the child of an activity or a toy—but *not* of a highly prized toy such as a stuffed animal that he always sleeps with.

4. Effect of a Child's Illness on Parents

When you treat a child, you must also consider the feelings of the parents. If they are worried and tense, the child will soon sense it.

Parents may be disturbed because of—

- Guilt feelings.
- Fear of
  - _____the unknown.
  - _____improper care for the child.
- Fear that
  - _____the child will suffer.
  - _____others in the family may contract the disease.
  - _____the child may transfer his love to the people who now care for him.

These worries can make parents illogical, unreasoning, and demanding. Although this puts an extra load on the pediatric specialist, he must understand people and their problems and be sympathetic with them.

5. Growth and Development

a. Stages of growth and development are not marked with sharp lines. Mental development, for example, begins long before it is discernible, but the degree of its progress is influenced by the child's environment and his social development. No child will fit within any absolute pattern, but certain norms an be established. The child will change and develop continuously but the growth can be uneven, with wide fluctuations within the normal. *For example,* most children will crawl before they walk, but they will not all crawl at exactly the same age.

b. Pediatric nursing personnel are in contact with a child for only a short time and then only when he is ill. He may not respond as he might if he were well. However, a knowledge of normal behavioral patterns for his age (table 2) will assist in understanding the child. Remember, though, that the child can fluctuate widely from this norm and still be perfectly normal.

6. Heredity Versus Environment

This is the subject of much controversy. The inheritance of an individual can vary widely from that of his parents, since each parent cell supplies one-half of the 46 chromosomes that begin the new cell. Also, some characteristics are dominant and others are recessive. It is possible, therefore, for a family of high intelligence to have a child with low intelligence or vice versa. However, a child is more likely to have traits and intelligence similar to that of his parents. Environment, too, is different and variable. An infant deprived of love and affection from birth will have a slower mental growth than one that is read to, loved, "mothered," and kept comfortable. A child brought up in a family where a foreign language is spoken may seem stupid when he is entered in a school where English is spoken. Even the health of the mother before the child's birth affects his development. There are also physical differences between the sexes and between people of the various nationalities and races. Thus, many factors must be considered by nursing personnel who furnish patient care for children.

7. Admission Area

Within the limits of the hospital environment, the pediatric admission area should be as bright and as cheerful as possible. Toys for various ages, a bulletin board with pictures or posters, well-chosen fresh magazines, small chairs, a small blackboard with chalk and erasers, and animal paintings or murals will all help entertain children during the waiting period. The room should also be well ventilated.

8. Admitting the Child

The medical specialist who assists in admission or admits the child must use every available means to make the child and his parents comfortable and welcome. He must have a friendly, reassuring manner as, in their eyes, he immediately becomes their host and authority figure and thus represents the type of future treatment that they can expect. He must remember, although he may have admitted dozens of children, that this may be the first time for the child and the parents. Superficiality and a real lack of interest will be spotted quickly by the child and his parents. Above all, speed must not subject the child to new experiences to quickly; he must be given time "to get acquainted." A few extra minutes spent in explanation may prevent misunderstanding and unhappiness. If possible, the child should visit the ward before admission. If the parents have not prepared the child, the specialist must take the time to explain what will happen and to reassure him.

a. Obtaining Information. The specialist who admits a child must be a skillful interviewer. The interview is not just a bare recording of facts but a real opportunity for communication with the parents and for quiet observation of them. The parent's address, manner of speaking, and dress can all give clues to their background if the specialist is alert, and he must find out as much as possible in order to give nursing care day and night. If the child speaks a foreign language, it would be wise to write down a few words of that language. If the child has been admitted before, the specialist should look at his old records and try to say something personal like "I see Tom has had a birthday since he was here" or "Betty was allergic to strawberries when she was here. Is she still avoiding them?'

b. Attitude of Parents. In pediatric nursing care, parents and other relatives need much more reassurance and explanation than in adult nursing care. In some instances the parents may be so afraid and worried that they either do not hear or do not remember. This means that explanations must be patiently repeated time and time again. Often a printed list of rules—the visiting hours, special rules for acutely ill children or those with contagious diseases, lists of prohibited food or gifts, etc.—may be given to the parents. Above all, contact between the parent, the hospital, and the child must be maintained. Remember that the parent is worried about the child and about the treatment he will receive.

c. Attitude of Child. You must remember that the child did not come to the hospital of his own free will and that the actual situation can be quite different from what he imagined. He is probably anxious and unhappy. He may feel guilty and think he is being punished by being hospitalized and deserted by his parents. You should place yourself in the child's position; how would you feel if you were sick and didn't understand why, afraid and yet the people you love most seem to desert you, alone in a strange place and surrounded by people in strange clothes? He deserves the utmost understanding because he may not be able to put his fears in words. Watch for signs that he is frightened, lonely, hurting, homesick. Above all, do not ignore a frightened child, scold an overactive one, or talk loudly in English to a child who does not understand it. Watch the faces of the child and his parents to get clues to their feelings. Remember, too, that crying is a way to express fears, so do not discourage it.

9. Consents

Clinical Record—Authorization for Administration of Anesthesia and for Performance of Operations or Other Procedures must be signed by the parent before operations are performed or anesthesia is given.

Section III. SAFETY

10. Accident Prevention and Restraints

Accidents are one of the greatest hazards in the life of children. Negligence on the part of even one person can be disastrous, so all nursing personnel—and particularly those in Pediatrics—must be safety conscious and exercise day-by-day vigilance. Among other things, windows should be barred or well-screened and radiators, heating pipes, and electric wires should be covered or fixed so that children cannot reach them.

a. Bed. Since the child is too young to look out for himself or lacks the judgment and experience to do so, the medical specialist in the pediatric ward must be extraordinarily safety conscious. A child under 9 should be placed in a crib or a junior bed as appropriate for his size. If he must be placed in an adult-sized bed, the bed should have side rails. Children over 6, who normally during the day would not have side rails up on the bed, should have side rails up at bedtime and any time their condition warrants. Side rails should also be used for any patient who has seizures or para-

lyses. A young child can move with a speed that an adult can only estimate, so the crib side should never be left down even for a moment unless the specialist has a hand on the child to restrain him. Even with the sides up, a child can crawl out of bed and fall on his head, often fracturing his skull. If a child even attempts to climb the side, a crib net should be applied immediately. The ties are secured to the frame so that the child cannot reach them and so the sides can be lowered without disturbing the ties (fig. 1).

b. Extraneous Objects. The specialist should constantly watch for any object small enough to put in any body orifice (buttons, parts of toys, money) or for any sharp item and remove it at once. Safety pins should be closed and placed out of the reach of the child during diaper changing, but kept where the specialist can see them. Laboratory technicians must be watched to see that they do not leave such things as capillary tubes or lancets on the bed or bedside table. Bedside tables are kept clear of anything that can be reached by a patient, and special precautions are taken to be

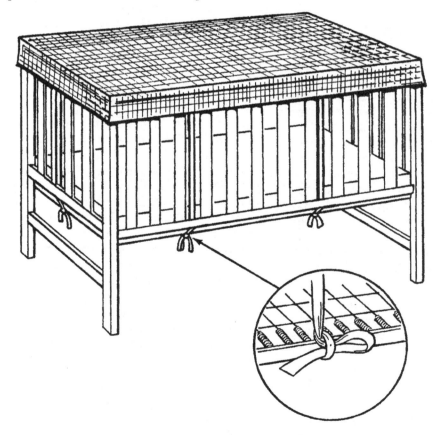

Figure 1. The crib net restraint.

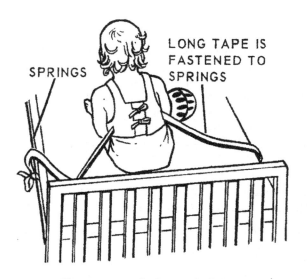

SPRINGS

LONG TAPE IS
FASTENED TO
SPRINGS

Figure   2. Jacket restraint.

sure objects cannot be reached by ambulatory patients. Plastic bags or pieces are not left where children can reach them; they can too easily smother a child. Special precautions are also taken to keep medications out of the reach of children.

c. Restraints.

- *The jacket restraint* (fig.   2). This may be used in place of the crib net restraint. It is put on with the ties in back so that the child cannot untie them.

- *The clove hitch.* This restraint is used when extremities must be restrained. When one arm or leg is restrained, the opposite one should also be restrained so that the child cannot injure himself by twisting or turning. A clove hitch is applied by making two loops and forming a figure eight,   with both ends on top of the figure and pointing in opposite directions. Place soft padding around the part to be restrained, slip the loop on, and adjust to fit. Tie the ends to a part of the bed under mattress (fig.   2) (*never* to the sides of the crib, which might be lowered).

- *The mummy restraint* (fig.   3). Place a sheet or a blanket flat on the bed, then put the child on it with his shoulders at the top of the sheet and the sheet extending about 10 inches beyond his feet. Children who are restrained should be released at frequent intervals to give them respite.

d. Holding Techniques. A child must usually be held to examine his eyes, throat, and nose. The specialist stands at the head of the crib and

brings the child's arms up against each side of the child's head, with the specialist's hands firmly on the elbow joints. Another technique that may be used to examine the ears is to turn the head to one side and flat against the bed. The specialist has one hand on the child's head and then uses the other to hold the child's hands.

e. Miscellaneous Safety Precautions.

- Children should ambulate in approved area of the ward away from places where dangerous supplies and equipment are stored; e.g., treatment or utility rooms.
- Plastic bottles should be used for children who have their own bottles. Glass nursing bottles can be easily shattered against cribsides.
- Strings should not be used to tie bottles or objects to cribs. These are potential strangulation hazards.

11. Identification Bands

As with any other patient, the child must be identified. The clinical specialist must check the child's identification band each time before giving medications or treatment. These bands should list the name, hospital number, unit, and any other required information and be applied so as to avoid restricting circulation. Identification bands must be replaced when broken or lost, or when unable to read.

12. Toys

The toys used in a hospital should be safe—no sharp edges, flaky paint, or removable parts. They should also be clean and, preferably, nonspillable. When used for therapy, they should be durable, be interesting to the child, require a variety of motions to manage them, and provide mental stimulation. Play should be therapeutic. Care must be taken to see that small children do not play with toys intended for older children that are potentially dangerous to toddlers. Marbles, balloons, etc., are all dangerous to have on a ward. A bedridden child could have picture or drawing books, puppets, a ball on a string. Some toys with therapeutic value include toolbox (hand grasp, form perception, hand-eye coordination, supination, and pronation), clarinet (finger flexion and extension for older child), push-pull toys (imaginative play, walking, and crawling), rocking horse (helps maintain sitting balance, reach and grasp, arm movements), tricycle (hand grasp, leg exercise, dorsiflexion of ankle) and wagon (hand grasp, trunk control, dorsiflexion and plantar flex-

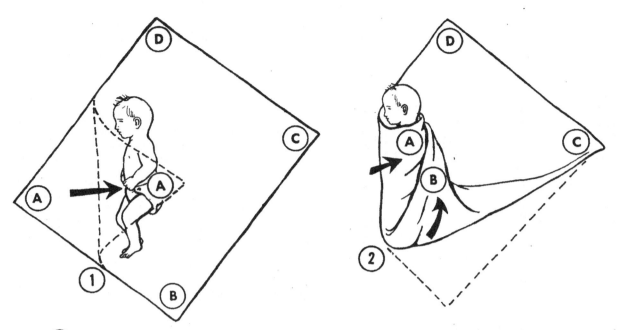

① PLACE CHILD ON SIDE FACING YOU, TUCK "A" CORNER SECURELY UNDER INFANT'S BACK.

② TUCK "B" CORNER BEHIND INFANT'S BACK, MAKING A PLEAT TO BRING BLANKET TO SHOULDER LEVEL.

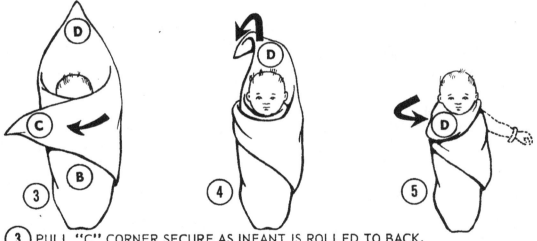

③ PULL "C" CORNER SECURE AS INFANT IS ROLLED TO BACK.

④ HOLDING INFANT UNDER THE ARM AS IN A "FOOTBALL-CARRY," HOLD "C" CORNER WITH HAND SUPPORTING INFANT'S HEAD.

⑤ WITH FREE HAND, PULL "D" CORNER DOWN OVER INFANT'S BACK AND SHOULDERS, SECURING LOOSE END OF "C" CORNER AND FREEING INFANT'S HEAD AND FACE. ARM MAY HAVE IDENTA-BAND OUT OR BOTH ARMS MAY BE SECURED. INFANT CANNOT WRIGGLE FREE, SINCE BLANKET MAY BE LOOSENED ONLY BY FIRST RELEASING "D" CORNER, PULLING IT UP OVER INFANT'S HEAD.

Figure   3.   The mummy restraint.

ion of ankles, and hip and leg extension and flexion). Toys can also be used to teach color, size, and shape discrimination.

3. Shoes

a. Regular Shoes. An infant's foot is flexible, so shoes should not hamper the foot's normal functions. The toddler should wear shoes with firm soles that fit the shape of his foot but are at least ½ inch longer and ¼ inch wider, with securely fitting heels. For the school child, shoes should be sturdy and of the correct size. Particular care should be taken to insure that a diabetic child's shoes are replaced as often as he grows.

b. Shoes for the Pediatric Hospital Patient. Scuffs are not practical for small children. The parents should bring regular bedroom slippers if

at all possible. These should not have smooth soles, or the child may slip and fall. If no bedroom slippers are available, it is best to have the child use his regular shoes while in the hospital.

14. Parents

Parents have been known to bring bags full of candy to the hospital. Check bedside stands frequently to make sure that children are not eating candy to the exclusion of properly nutritious food. Because children will often share these "goodies" with those who are NPO or have diabetes, candy and gum should not be permitted on the ward. Also, parents of older children may bring in potentially dangerous toys for the younger ones. Tactfully explain the danger. Most parents will be cooperative.

Section IV.   BASIC NURSING CARE

15. Temperature of Room

For the newborn, the temperature of the room should not go below 68° F, as he has an unstable heat regulating system. The temperature should be checked each tour of duty and should be fairly constant at 72° F with a relative humidity of about 40 percent.

16. Baths for Newborn Infants

The infant must be protected from sources of infection, so use strict aseptic techniques.

a. Assign a crib exclusively to one infant so that he will not be exposed to cross-contamination.

b. Give routine baths in this crib. Tub baths are given when approved by the doctor but are not given before the cord falls off (usually occurs within 1 week after birth).

EQUIPMENT
Chux, soft cloths, or cotton balls
Thermometer
Diapers
Sterile cotton pledgets
Clean bed linen
Sterile metal prep basins for bathwater
Water at 100° to 105° F
Hexachlorophene solution added to water if ordered

PROCEDURE
1. Wash your hands.

2. Before removing clothes, bathe the infant's head and face. Clean the ears around the fold with sterile cotton pledgets and warm water, but do not enter the ear canal.

3. Cleanse one eye by stroking from the inner canthus outward with a clean damp cotton ball soaked in sterile water. Then use a different one to clean other eye. Do *not* use applicator sticks to cleanse the ears, nose, or other orifices.

4. Expose only part of the infant's body at a time to avoid chilling.

5. Test the bathwater with water thermometer. Temperature should be between 100°–105° F.

6. Wash the skin in the creases of the body daily with tap water, beginning at the neck. Use approved solution to wash any area where dried blood or secretions are present. Soap may be used for older infants.

7. Give special attention to the genitalia.
   a. *Male* (uncircumcised). Gently retract, cleanse, and *replace* the prepuce of the penis. Paraphimosis (impaired circulation to the uncircumcised penis due to the retraction of the foreskin beyond the corona) may result if the prepuce is not replaced.
   b. *Female.* Cleanse labia from front to back to avoid contamination of vagina or urethra with feces.

8. Apply topical application of a prescribed solution to a weeping cord stump. (In this case, be sure the diaper is below the cord so that urine

spreading on the diaper does not reach the cord.) Isolate any child with such an infection.

9. Apply approved baby oil to dry or cracked areas. Do *NOT* use powder, which can be inhaled or which may irritate the skin. Powder is rarely used in hospitals.

10. Use a receptacle for soiled clothing. Do not put on side of crib or on floor.

11. Dress the infant.

    a. *Diapers.* Place one-half of the folded diaper under the infant's buttocks. Draw the rest over his lower abdomen and pin securely at the sides (holding your hand between the diaper and the infant to avoid sticking him). Always point the diaper pins outward (fig. 4); in the event they come unfastened, the chance of injury is lessened. Be sure the diaper is secure around the leg area as feces can contaminate the bed linen and his fingers. In diapers, males need extra thickness in front; females, in the back. Do *not* use plastic or rubber pants as they retain heat and encourage urine stagnation. If a rash is present, leave the buttocks exposed to air.

    b. *Sleeves.* To put an infant's arm through a sleeve, put your fingers through the bottom of the sleeve, grasp the baby's hand through the armhole, and gently pull the *sleeve* up toward the baby's shoulder.

    c. *Socks.* These should be ½ inch longer than the infant's foot and may be advisable not only in winter but all year. Since circulation has not been completely established, the hands and feet may be colder than the rest

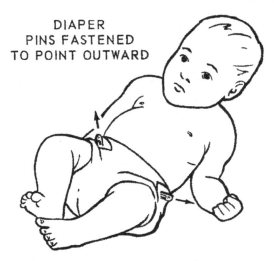

DIAPER PINS FASTENED TO POINT OUTWARD

Figure 4. Diaper pin fastening.

of the body. If not available in hospital, suggest parents bring them in from home.

17. Bathing a Child
OLDER INFANT

1. Use an infant's bathing tub or an oblong enamel tub. A washcloth under his buttocks makes a baby feel more secure if a metal tub must be used.

2. Use tepid (95° F) water, but do not fill too full.

3. Bathe the face, nostrils, neck, ears, and scalp before undressing the child.

4. Remove the diaper and cleanse the buttocks.

5. Remove rest of clothing and cover with a bath blanket. Soap without exposing child.

6. Carefully and gently lift him into tub by grasping both ankles with a finger between the tarsi, supporting head and neck in crook of opposite arm, with hand grasping infant's arm just below the shoulder. His smooth wet skin will be difficult to hold and he will probably be attempting to kick or wiggle. Use extreme care. Do not let him slip or frighten him by plunging him into the tub.

7. Support his head, neck, and body with one hand and forearm.

8. Gently rinse all soap off.

9. Lift the child gently and slowly out of the tub as you held him to put him in.

10. Wrap in a soft bath blanket; gently pat dry. Dress him.

CHILD

1. Up until about 7 years of age, the child requires supervision and assistance in bathing (*for example*, most 6-year-olds can wash their arms, legs, and faces but need help with the rest). He should be helped in and out of the tub and the specialist should remain in the room. Hot water is never turned on after a child is in the tub because of the danger of burning him.

2. By 7 years of age, the child can bathe himself fairly well and does not need much supervision, although boys may dislike baths. A tub bath for the older child is similar to that for an adult.

SPONGE BATH

The sponge bath is generally the same procedure as for an adult but the tender skin is patted rather than rubbed dry. When given to reduce a fever, it does not last over 15 to 20 minutes, and the temperature, pulse, and respiration are checked every 5 minutes. The sponge is terminated when temperature drops to 100°–101° range and is stopped immediately if symptoms of cyanosis, chill, slow shallow respirations, or a weak, irregular pulse appear. The room must be free of drafts, and temperature must be at about 72° F. Tepid (95° F) water should be used unless otherwise ordered by the physician.

1. Uncover only a part of the body at a time; cover the rest with a bath blanket.
2. Put a filled ice cap on his head.
3. Leave enough water in the washcloth to squeeze out a little over the area to be bathed. It is the evaporation of the water that accomplishes the cooling goals.
4. Begin at the hairline, then go down the neck, over the shoulder, and outside of the arm and hand.
5. Turn or rinse the cloth, then bathe the inside of the arm and down the chest.
6. Sponge the axilla and the groin, which have large blood vessels, 4 or 5 times.
7. Pat the skin dry or cover with a bath blanket.
8. Proceed to the other side, then turn the patient prone, if possible, or on his side.
9. Go over the buttocks 4 or 5 times.

NOTE
Procedure 4 through 9 will normally be repeated a couple of times during the 20 minutes.

10. Dry the child, remove bath blanket, and cover.
11. Leave ice cap on for another 20 minutes.
12. Check TPR immediately after the sponge and again 30 minutes after the sponge.
13. Record results.

NOTE
Sponging may have to be reinstituted after a few minutes rest for the child if it is not effective the first time. Once the temperature starts to fall, it will usually continue down a little further after the treatment is stopped.

BATH THERAPY FOR THE BURNED CHILD
The physician may order immersion of the burned child in a bathtub or arm tub (obtainable from the Physical Therapy Section). The tub or tank should be thoroughly cleaned with a detergent-disinfectant cleansing agent such as "A–33, Air-

Kem"* prior to placing child in tub or tank, or burned areas may be washed with soap and water. Perineal care should be given as needed, at least once daily. The procedure for bath therapy is given below.

* Suggested proportions of "A–33, Air-Kem"—dry powder, 1 prepackaged container per gallon of water; liquid, 6 ounces per gallon of water. The tub or tank must be thoroughly rinsed following the cleansing with the detergent-disinfectant solution.

1. Fill tub or tank one-half full with warm tap water or a solution as ordered by the doctor.
2. Place a clean sheet on a litter or wheelchair.
3. Put on a pair of sterile gloves. (It is assumed that the specialist will be wearing scrub-type clothing or a gown.)
4. Lift the child from the bed and place on litter or wheelchair. Be certain that catheter and intravenous tubing, if present, are properly secured.
5. Take child to the tank or tub. If dressings are in place, cut the bandages holding them and remove loose dressings.
6. Change into fresh sterile gloves. Lift child and immerse him in tank or tub. Be certain his head is adequately supported. Reassure the child during the entire procedure.
7. Wearing sterile gloves, remove the dressings gently, after they have been well soaked.
8. Using sterile 4-x 8-inch dressings, gently wash the burned areas and rinse well. Assist the physician as necessary whenever he debrides the burn wound.
9. Complete the bath and shampoo the hair, rinsing well. Lift child from the tank or tub and place on litter or in wheelchair.
10. Return child to bed.
11. If dressings are ordered or an ointment is to be applied, wear a pair of sterile gloves and a surgical mask when doing these treatments.

APPLICATION OF BURN DRESSING
1. Set up a sterile dressing tray with a basin, 4-by 8-inch gauze squares, fine mesh gauze, scissors, and other equipment as ordered by the doctor. Cover tray with sterile towels. Prepare and warm the sterile solution as ordered by the doctor.
2. Place the covered dressing tray, the warm sterile solution, a surgical mask, and a pair of sterile gloves at the patient's bedside.
3. When the patient is ready to have the dressings applied, uncover the tray and place the sterile surface of the towels under the burned area that is to be dressed.

4. Pour the warm sterile solution into the sterile basin.

5. Put on the surgical mask and the sterile gloves.

6. Immerse the roll of fine mesh gauze, if ordered as a part of the dressing, in the solution. Roll the gauze about the extremity and cut it so that single, separate layers of gauze cover the burn wound.

7. Immerse the 4- x 8-inch dressings in the solution, squeeze them fairly dry, and open each 4- x 8-inch dressing lengthwise.

8. Place opened 4- x 8-inch dressings over the burned area.

9. Hold the dressing in place by using 3–4-inch roller bandage (Curlex). Apply without pressure. No elasticized bandages are to be used unless specifically ordered by the doctor.

10. Moisten and change dressings as ordered, using a sterile bulb syringe, a sterile basin, and warm sterile solution. Always be certain dressings are moist before removing them.

18. Care of the Hair

Inspect head thoroughly upon admission and frequently from then on for nits, pressure sores, cuts, bruises, or other abnormalities. Comb the child's hair at least once a day gently. The restless child's hair may mat. If it does, hold a section of the hair near the scalp to prevent pulling and gently untangle the hair below. Give a weekly shampoo to the child and a daily one to the infant, if the child's condition permits. Be careful not to get soapy water in any child's eyes or ears, or over his face as it may frighten him. Quickly dry the hair with warm towels or a hair dryer.

19. Mouth Care

Insure that the older child brushes his teeth daily, using the same technique as for an adult
        unless contraindicated. Offer the infant sterile water between feedings.

20. Feeding a Child

a. Bottle Feeding.

(1) Feeding the newborn depends upon the physician's preference. Feeding usually begins from 12 hours to 3 days after birth. The infant should always be clean, warm, and dry when fed. He is held in the same position, whether breastfed or not; that is, he is picked up and held with his head and back supported. A bottle should never be propped in baby's mouth as this can cause aspiration of the formula.

(2) If he is to be bottlefed, wash your hands. Get the formula from the refrigerator and check the name of the infant with the name on the bottle or insure in some way that the correct formula is given to the infant. The formula should be given at room temperature. Put on a gown before feeding the infant and also put a quilted pad on your lap for protection. Hold the baby, giving sturdy support to the head and back. Infants that are held so that they are partially upright swallow less air. The holes in the nipple should be small enough to prevent choking but large enough to let the milk come through with some sucking. If the infant becomes frustrated and angry when fed, first check the size of the nipple hole. When the bottle is held upright, the milk should fall slowly in drops, not in a steady stream. Also hold the bottle so that the nipple is always filled with milk. The atmosphere must be calm and unhurried during the feeding; you should allow a half hour for each feeding. Watch how the infant takes his formula. If he takes it eagerly and hurriedly, he should be burped for every ounce consumed as a minimum and at the end of the feeding. To burp the infant, sit him up with his head tilted slightly forward and his head and chest supported by putting your fingers over the mandible bone of the face, and gently pat his back. This will permit you to observe him. After feeding, place him on his abdomen or right side to help empty the stomach and prevent regurgitation and aspiration.

(3) Record the type of formula, amount taken, and amount retained.

(4) After use, rinse the nipple and bottle with running water.

(5) Suspect underfeeding if the infant fails to gain weight. In the hospital, babies are usually weighed before their morning baths and a record kept of the daily weights.

b. Transition to Cup Feeding.

(1) Feed the baby from a small cup or training cup for a short interval at the beginning of the feeding period. Never use force to make a child eat; stop the cup feeding when the child gets tired.

(2) Begin any new food gradually. The infant should just be given a taste (1/2 to 1 teaspoon) the first time and then early in the day. A new food is NOT introduced when a child is tired

or fretful nor if the person doing the feeding is a stranger to the infant.

c. Food. Feeding regimen vary greatly according to the doctor's preference and the area of the country, as well as with the current trend. The following general comments can be considered as basic. Vitamins are usually added to the infant's diet the second week. Water and orange juice are soon added and then cereal and baby foods. Solid foods are usually begun with cooked or preprepared cereals (may occur at 3 to 6 weeks after birth). Solid foods are always offered before the formula. Sometimes it may be necessary to mix the cereal with the formula to get a desired consistency. Feed cereal (and other solid foods) with a spoon, not in a bottle. After cereals, yellow fruits are usually added to the diet, followed later by infant pureed vegetables. These foods should be fed individually rather than mixed together, so that the baby will learn the taste of each. When pureed foods can be handled well, junior foods are added to the diet.

CAUTION

Two new foods are not started at the same time; several days should elapse.

Commercially prepared food will be available on the ward, but a specialist may have to mix certain foods. (Before opening a can or jar of baby food, wipe the top clean to avoid contaminating the food when opening the container.) When teeth appear, the infant is usually given crackers, zwieback, or hard toast. By 1 year, he should be getting whole milk, cooked cereal, strained cooked vegetables and fruit, well-ripened banana, egg, meat juice and scraped meat, orange or tomato juice, and additional vitamins. Chopped foods are started about 14 to 18 months when he has enough teeth to chew. He should be encouraged to eat slowly and to chew thoroughly. As soon as he indicates a desire to feed himself, get two spoons. Permit him to lift one spoon to his mouth, but give him help in filling it. He will spill some at first, but he will soon learn how to hold the spoon. Praise his successes. Meanwhile, use the other spoon to feed him while he is experimenting. Serve the food at the moderate temperature he prefers—never hot or cold. Sometime between 2 years and 30 months he should learn to take solid foods. Finger foods such as carrot sticks or bacon are especially good from this age through about 4 or 5 years of age. Older children generally are served adult food in a pleasant, happy environment. Exercise particular care on the ward to see that sweets or large amounts of fluids are not ingested before meal time. However, in certain cases, one of your most important duties may be to see that the child has a high fluid intake. You should offer gelatin, carbonated beverages, Koolaid, popsicles, water, and fruit juices. Vary the container as well as the fluid. Use small different-colored paper cups. Let a girl pour a drink from her doll's teapot. Make use of surprise and novelties. Have a child cut out a glass from colored paper and paste on a large paper for every glass of fluid. For variation, offer fluids in a bottle with a straw, unless contraindicated. Whatever you do, serve fluids and foods attractively and in small servings. Daily personal touches and surprises can also help make a sick child more interested in eating. Ask parents, volunteers, and visitors to encourage the child to drink and to help you devise games to stimulate fluid intake. Even if he needs extra fluids, however, do not give large amounts just before a meal.

21. Observation of Vital Signs

a. Normal signs are as given below:

Age	Pulse	Blood Pressure	Respiration
0–1 year	120–140	80/50	40–60
1–4 years	100–120	94–100/64	24–36
4–10 years	100	100/60	20
10–14 years	80	114/60	15–20

b. Signs and symptoms.

(1) *Pulse.*

- Full and throbbing—fever, patent ductus arteriosus, aortic regurgitation.
- Pulsus alternams (alternately strong and weak) —danger sign of heart failure, tension pneumothorax, cardiac tamponade.
- Rapid, weak, or fluttery—shock, cardiac failure, respiratory trouble, blood loss.
- Weak or absent in lower limbs—coarctation of aorta.
- Irregular, then absent—atrial fibrillation.
- Unusually slow—overdose of digitalis or heart block.
- Less than 40—may have unconscious spells.

(2) *Blood pressure.* (Use a cuff of 1/2 to 2/3 the size of the child's upper arm—the wrong size cuff will give a false reading.) Blood pressure on a child is taken only when specifically ordered by the doctor—generally on children with previous abnormal readings, those with serious heart disease, and those in the postoperative period. Agitation or fright can increase the BP, so the specialist should explain and perhaps demonstrate on another cooperative child how it is done, or dis-

tract the child with a toy. Babies can be given a bottle of milk or a pacifier for calming purposes.

(3) *Respiration.*

- Increase of 10 per minute in a quiet sleeping child—sign of trouble.
- Labored breathing, flared nostrils, restlessness, fear—signs of cardiac failure.
- Tachypnea (excessive rapidity in breathing) in infant—may be only sign of early heart failure.
- Change in rate—important.

22. Fluid Therapy

The normal fluid requirements of a newborn baby are few; he has a higher ratio of water to his body weight than at any other time. However, vomiting or diarrhea will cause dehydration and loss of weight. Symptoms of excessive fluid loss are—

- Sunken eyes and fontanels (unossified spot on the head).
- Poor skin turgor (distention and resiliency).
- Dry mouth.
- Concentrated urine.
- Loss of weight.

a. *Oral Fluids.* The best and the most natural method is to give fluid by mouth. Since infants and small children need help to drink, the specialist must remember to offer drinks often but only in small amounts. Sometimes a bright-colored container will help with a child. The specialist must also keep an accurate record of the child's intake and output. This is extremely important on a pediatric ward.

b. *Intravenous Fluids.* Since infants do not have large veins at the antecubital fossa, two methods are used to give IV fluids to infants up to 6 months of age: scalp-vein infusion (simplest) and surgical cutdown. Both of these procedures are done by the physician. The specialist may assist.

SCALP VEIN INFUSION

Equipment

Syringe, 2 ml., filled with saline
Short bevel needle
Elastic tubing
Antiseptic sponge
Infusion set with 100 ml. bag and microdrip chamber
Fluid (ordered by doctor)
Rubber band tourniquet
Dry 2- x 2-inch sponge

Procedure

1. Attach bevel needle to plastic tubing (fig. 5).
2. Turn infant crosswise and shave head over temporal area.
3. Apply a rubber band about the head just above the ear.
4. Restrain the infant with head held to one side, using the mummy restraint. (The doctor will disinfect the site, insert the needle, and tape it in place.)
5. Cut the rubber band.
6. Express air bubbles from IV tubing and connect to a plastic adapter.
7. Permit a small amount of fluid to run in rapidly to check for swelling at the site.
8. Apply final dressing.
9. Do not permit the infant to lie on the side with the needle. Depending upon the site of the needle insertion, the infant's head may have to be taped in an immobile position or simply positioned with sandbags. This will prevent him from dislodging the needle.

SURGICAL CUTDOWN

NOTE

This procedure requires sterile technique.

Equipment

Commercially prepared cutdown tray or tray prepared by CMS
Splint
Tape
IV stand, tubing with 100 ml. chamber and microdrip, solution as ordered by physician
Sterile gloves

Procedure

1. Open cutdown tray using sterile technique.
2. Be available to help restrain infant and supply material that may be required by physician.

CAUTIONS

1. Start the fluid slowly.
2. Calculate the number of milliliters per hour and the drops per minute. Adjust the flow.
3. Observe the infant for edematous tissues or evidence of infiltration.
4. If the fluid stops running, check the flexion of the limb (straighten it), the tightness of the bandages (loosen them), and the tubing (milk it to try to reopen it).

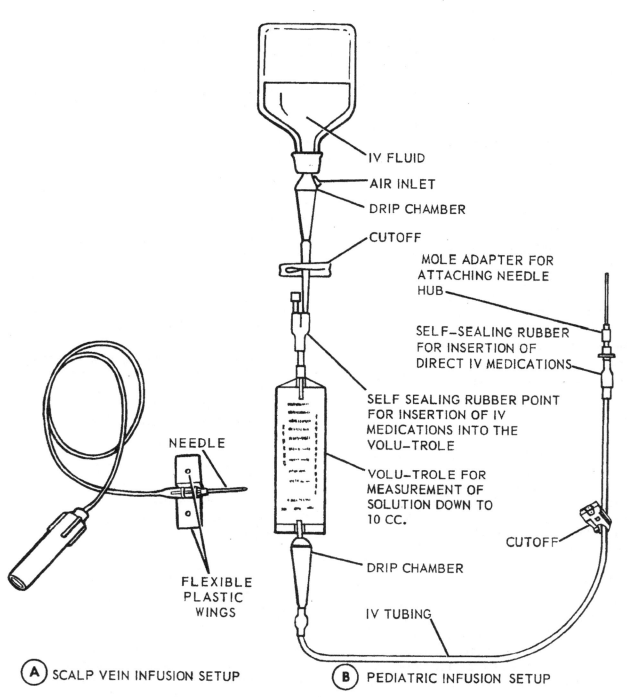

IV FLUID

AIR INLET

DRIP CHAMBER

CUTOFF

MOLE ADAPTER FOR
ATTACHING NEEDLE
HUB

SELF-SEALING RUBBER
FOR INSERTION OF
DIRECT IV MEDICATIONS

SELF SEALING RUBBER POINT
FOR INSERTION OF IV
MEDICATIONS INTO THE
VOLU-TROLE

VOLU-TROLE FOR
MEASUREMENT OF
SOLUTION DOWN TO
10 CC.

CUTOFF

DRIP CHAMBER

IV TUBING

NEEDLE

FLEXIBLE
PLASTIC
WINGS

(A) SCALP VEIN INFUSION SETUP   (B) PEDIATRIC INFUSION SETUP

Figure   5.   Scalp vein infusion setup.

NOTE

The baby does not remain restrained unless the doctors so orders. If he does, put
the baby on his side and change his position frequently.

23. Suctioning and Tracheotomy Care

ESTABLISHING RESPIRATION IN NEWBORN

NOTE

Any step may be omitted as necessity
dictates.

1. Try to remove obvious secretions that might

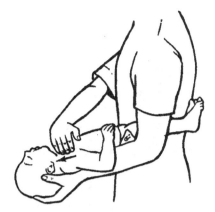

Figure 6. *Trendelenburg position and stroking the trachea.*

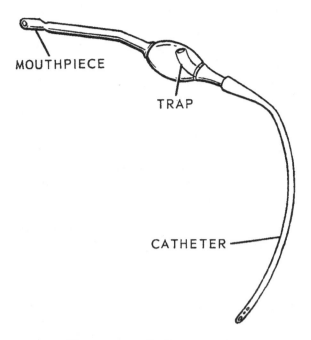

Figure 7. *De Lee mucus trap.*

hinder breathing by wiping the infant's nose and mouth.

2. Place the infant in the Trendelenburg position to promote drainage and gently stroke the neck up toward the mouth (fig. 6).

3. Use a bulb syringe.

4. If the steps above do not work, use a small catheter with a De Lee mucus trap. Hyperflex the infant's neck slightly and place the catheter in his nose or mouth. Insert the mouthpiece (fig. 7), in your mouth and suck. The mild suction will draw mucus into the trap.

5. Use special precautions for oropharyngeal suctioning:

    a. Be sure catheters are sterile. Handle only with gloved hands or sterile forceps. Contamination may cause pneumonia.

    b. Extend the baby's head.

NOTE

Deep aspiration, when required, is done by the nurse.

    c. Insert the catheter into his nostril for 5 to 6 cm., being careful not to apply suction during insertion as it removes much of the oxygen in the airway. Using a different catheter, repeat procedure in the mouth.

    d. Apply suction. Remember suction must be gentle. Excessive pull could damage the infant's mucous membranes.

    e. Withdraw with a twirling motion.

WARNING

Do this all within 10 seconds as this procedure also extracts oxygen from the infant.

f. Rest and repeat as necessary, letting baby breathe oxygen between applications.

6. Use these precautions in a tracheostomy—

    a. If there is time and the child can understand, explain why this tracheostomy must be done; i.e., "To help you breathe better."

    b. In pediatrics the doctor will select the tracheotomy tube. He bases his choice upon the size of the trachea. The specialist may be required to select a suction catheter size that will leave enough space for breathing (table 3).

Table 3. *Size of Catheter.*

If the doctor selects a tracheotomy tube sized—	Then the catheter you use for suctioning would be—
00–1	8 Fr.
1	10 Fr.
2	12 Fr.
3	14 Fr.
4	16–18 Fr.

    c. Since infants and children have short necks, the mital lock on the tracheotomy tube can hurt the skin. Place a small towel roll or padding under his shoulders. You can also pad his chin.

WARNING

Do not use gauze bandages.

    d. Tie the tape on the side to avoid confusion with ties of clothing.

e. Use restraints on the child or get another specialist to help you.

f. Since an infant cannot utter a sound, watch him closely.

g. Report any cough that is followed by swallowing to the doctor or nurse.

h. Be sure not to occlude the tube's lumen with a bib while feeding.

i. Maintain high humidity with atomizer, mask, nebulizer, or steam.

j. When tubes are to be removed, remember that a child may become frightened because he has become dependent on the tube. This will cause respiratory trouble—so give him tender loving care during this period.

24. Retention Catheters

The specialist may assist the nurse in this procedure, but his main responsibility will be in after care. He must watch for kinked tubes and be careful not to pull the catheter when caring for the child. Cleanliness is important, especially after the child has a stool.

25. Intake and Output

The importance of adequate intake and output records has been discussed in this chapter and in chapter 5. It cannot be overemphasized.

a. Urine. Unless the doctor specifies otherwise, "Barely damp diaper—voided small amount" or "saturated diaper—voided large amount" are accurate enough for the record. Sometimes, as in peritoneal dialysis, an hourly accurate intake and output record must be kept and any change in output reported. These records are also extremely important when a patient has been burned, as renal failure can occur. The hourly urine output indicates circulating blood pressure as well as kidney function. Regardless of age, no child's output should be less than 10 ml. per hour. In an infant, the diaper may be weighed before and after urination. The weight in grams is considered equal to mls. for an accurate urine output.

b. Stools. A description of the stool can be important such as "large amount of soft yellow stool" or "small amount of soft formed brown stool." If the stool is green and watery (may have diarrhea) or small and hard (may be consti-

pated), report it to the nurse. The newborn infant will have two to four stools in a day, up to one with each feeding.

26. Enemas

If the hospital does not have a prepared pediatric disposable enema, be sure that enema can or asepto syringe and tubing are sterile.

PROCEDURE FOR SMALL CHILD

1. Position the child. Put a pillow under his head and back to maintain alinement.
2. Use a child-sized bedpan, pad it, and place under his buttocks. (If desired for security, put a diaper under the bedpan and bring over the child's thighs and pin.)
3. Expel air by running solution through tubing.
4. Select a small catheter and lubricate it.
5. Insert 1½ to 3 inches into the rectum (the distance depends on child's size).
6. Elevate the asepto syringe with the measured, ordered solution just far enough to let the solution flow into the rectum. Only a small amount of solution is used.
7. Wait for returns to cease.
8. Cleanse child.
9. Cleanse equipment.

Precautions

- Use a soft rubber catheter.
- Do not inject fluid until catheter is fully inserted.
- Do not use tap water—use normal saline or as prescribed by the doctor.

27. Isolettes

If a baby must be put in an incubator, the concentration of oxygen must be checked with an oxygen analyzer with every change of shift. Oxygen should be maintained at 40 percent because of the harm that can be done to the baby with a higher concentration (blindness or retrolental fibroplasia). *EXCEPTIONS:* When baby has cyanosis or the doctor orders more oxygen for severe respiratory distress. The incubator also has nebulizers (water chambers), which must be removed and cleaned daily. Each week, cultures of the oxygen tubing, nebulizers, and water must be spot checked.

Section V. MEDICATIONS

28. Rules for Medications

Follow the rules for medications given .

29. Administration of Medications

Special knowledge is required to administer drugs to children because they can react quickly and violently to medication. The specialist who is authorized to give medication to children must be aware of toxic side effects that might occur. A specialist never computes nor gives fractional doses of medication.

GIVEN TO A CHILD

1. Be firm, but kind, when you give a child his medication. Never let any doubt creep into your voice. He doesn't have any choice, so say something like, "Timmy, take your pill with this fruit drink." If he is under 5 years, he does not know how to swallow a pill. You can use two approaches to make it palatable:

a. Give it suspended in syrup.

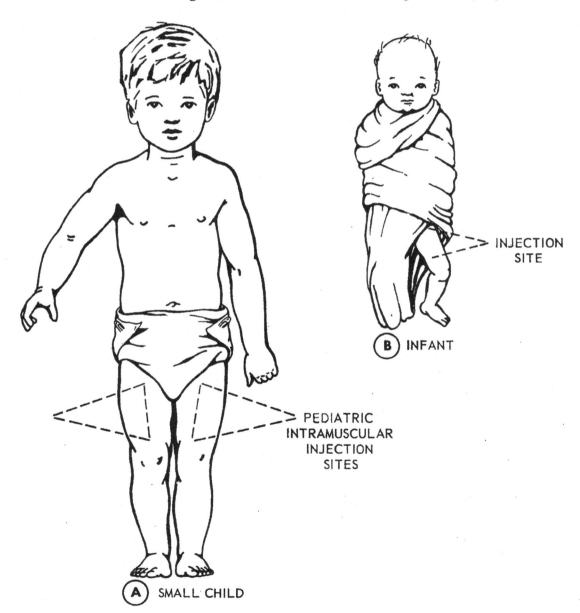

INJECTION SITE

B INFANT

PEDIATRIC INTRAMUSCULAR INJECTION SITES

A SMALL CHILD

Figure   8.   Position for administration of intramuscular injection.

b. Crush the tablet out of the child's sight and disguise it in a large spoon or two of strained fruit.

CAUTION

Do not put medications in a bottle of water or milk. Part of it might be refused and you would not know how much drug was ingested.

2. Identify the patient. If the child can talk, ask him his name (you never say his name yourself because he may say yes to any name). You also check his identification band. If the child is too young to talk, check his identification band and check the location (room number, ward, bed number) and the bassinette or crib tag.

3. Be prepared to answer questions like "Does it taste bad?" Answer honestly.

4. Be prepared to deal with delay. The child will delay you as much as possible. You may have to ask him if he is going to take the medicine or if he prefers that you give it to him.

CAUTION

Do not say this about oral medications which can be aspirated.

NEVER hold a child's nose to give medicine. Do NOT give medication when a child is crying; he might choke.

5. Make sure that oral medications are swallowed.

NOTE

A souffle cup can be used with a toddler. You can compress it slowly and expel the medicine into the child's mouth.

GIVEN TO AN INFANT

Use calibrated eye dropper to give oral medications to infants.

1. Raise the infant's head and depress his chin with your thumb. This will open his mouth.

2. Using eyedropper, drop the liquid slowly on the middle of his tongue. Use a rubber tip on the dropper to avoid contact of the glass with the lip. If this is done, the baby can be permitted to suck and swallow the liquid slowly.

3. Now, raise the infant's chin and let him swallow.

4. Be sure all the medication has been swallowed before putting the baby back in his crib.

RECTAL MEDICATIONS

Children's suppositories are a different shape from the cone-shaped type used for adults; they are long and thin.

1. Put on rubber gloves or a finger cot.

2. Insert the lubricated suppository about one-half as far as the forefinger will reach.

3. Gently hold the buttocks together for a few minutes to keep the child from expelling the suppository.

30. Injections

Important: It is difficult to control the movements of children, especially from 1½ years to 9 years. Even a quiet, cooperative child may jump or move unexpectedly. Safety requires that two people give the injection: one to restrain the child and the other to give the injection.

a. Feed a baby first or he may be too upset to eat.

b. Mix drugs in a syringe when possible in order to cut down on the number of injections. Never draw up an injection where the child can see you. Seeing the needle may increase his anxiety.

c. Inject into the anterolateral (quadriceps muscles of midanterior thigh) aspect of the thigh (fig. 8) for an infant and small child to avoid nerves and to help absorption, which is more effective than by injection into the buttock. However, use the buttocks for older children as the nurse directs.

d. Use same injection technique as for adults but give as quickly as possible.

e. Pick up an infant or small child and cuddle him after the injection.

CAUTION

Never tell a child that an injection will not hurt.

f. Rotate injection sites.

g. Do not exceed the prescribed volume of injection for child's size.

Section VI. CHILDHOOD SURGICAL CONDITIONS AND ILLNESSES

31. Changes in Physical Condition

Changes in a child's physical condition can be rapid and extreme. Nursing care personnel must keep close watch on an ill child for signs and symptoms, especially of the following:

a. Fever. This is probably the most common symptom seen in children. Up to 3 years of age, the greatest danger of prolonged high fever is that it may cause a spasm or convulsion. Even when old enough to talk, children will rarely mention that they feel "hot" or "cold," so the specialist must be ever watchful for signs such as an increase in redness of the cheeks or brightness of the eyes, twitching of muscles, or an increase in radiation of heat from the patient. If these signs occur, the temperature should be taken immediately, as a child's fever can shoot up suddenly and dramatically. Up to 6 years of age, a child's temperature is usually taken rectally, with the child prone and the thermometer inserted 1 to 2 inches (depends on the patient's size) in the rectum and directed toward the umbilicus. Regardless of age, rectal temperatures should be taken on any patient whose condition warrants it, such as patients who are disoriented, have respiratory difficulties, or are mentally incompetent. The specialist holds the thermometer in place for 2 minutes, regardless of how reliable the child appears. Anything above 99.6° F is considered fever. Over 6 years of age, the temperature is taken orally—but even then the specialist must stay with the patient until the thermometer is removed. The normal reading for an oral temperature is 98.6° F. When a doctor orders that measures be instituted to reduce a fever until it reaches a certain figure, the specialist must check with the nurse about the type of cooling measures to institute, as doctors vary in their preference of methods. The specialist must realize that these procedures take precedence over all routines, and he must accomplish them immediately. He must also notify the doctor or nurse if the fever does not go down within 30 minutes to 1 hour. Of special importance here is accurate charting .

b. Chill. The patient has uncontrollable shaking or shivers, and the skin may become blue and mottled. Although goose pimples may occur and the child's teeth may even chatter, this is not always true, especially with infants. Application of heat usually does not help, although it must be tried. The specialist must time the duration of the chill and report its length and severity.

c. Sweating. This is accompanied by a drop in temperature. Excessive sweating all over the body is not generally normal and should be reported. The specialist watches for excessive sweating and, when it occurs, keeps the child protected from drafts and dry, regardless of the work involved.

d. Convulsions. A convulsion occurs much more frequently in a child than in an adult. The tonic type (stiffened position) is most common in an infant. Since a convulsion's onset is quick and violent, a specialist must stay with the patient and call for help, yet be prompt and remain cool in taking the following actions:

(1) If the child is lying down, and if possible, first place a gag between his teeth so that he will not bite or swallow his tongue. If the teeth are clenched tightly shut, do not attempt to insert mouth gag because of danger of breaking teeth or dislodging loose teeth. If the child is not lying down, place him so that he is, but elevate his head a little. If on the floor, support head to prevent trauma.

(2) Note the symptoms and duration. The specialist should know if the convulsion was preceded by an aura (sound, smell, or a sensation of cold air rising to the head—this information can only be obtained from an older child) or an emotional disturbance, the area of the body involved, which muscles were first affected, the type of muscular contractions, color of the patient, relaxation of bladder or anal spincter, degree of consciousness (if any), expression on the face, size of pupils of the eye, frothing from the mouth, and the number of convulsions.

(3) Keep the child warm. If a child is known to be convulsive, his bed should have padded rails and should be placed where he can be observed constantly. A padded gag should be put where it can be easily reached. Oxygen and suction must also be readily available. His toys should be selected carefully to avoid those that might cause him injury during a convulsion.

e. Vomiting. Nausea may precede and follow vomiting, but a small child seldom complains of nausea; however, yawning, sweating, paleness, and restlessness may be signs of its presence. The specialist must observe, record, and report the appearance of the vomitus. Look for the presence of undigested food; presence or absence of bile; odor, especially a fecal odor; and presence of bright red blood or "coffee-ground" vomitus. The type of vomiting should also be reported as projectile (an explosive type where the stream may travel 3 to 5 feet) or nonprojectile (a milder type where the stream does not travel over 12 to 15 inches). Vomiting is always accompanied by forceful contractions which do not occur with regurgitation or "spitting up." The specialist must be aware, too, that some children can vomit at will or when too full, anxious, or angry. Vomiting may also be an attention-getting device.

f. Pain. Children must be observed closely for signs of pain such as frowning, dilated pupils, and drawn lips. If a child insists on a certain position, becomes less active or inactive, presses a particular portion of the body, or shows symptoms of muscle rigidity, pain should be suspected. Pulse and blood pressure can also be indicators, usually rising with pain (exception: *severe* pain). You cannot rely on a child's word description of his pain; ask him to point where it hurts. Even this may not work—often the child cannot identify the area of pain. The specialist must be sure to record the time the pain began and its duration.

g. Respiratory Distress. Another cardinal symptom of trouble is difficulty breathing. It is frightening to be deprived of adequate oxygen and particularly so to a child. This is a common emergency with a child, so suction equipment, laryngoscopes, tracheostomy tubes, etc., should always be readily available on a pediatric ward. Respiratory distress such as dyspnea, cyanosis, sternal retractions (indrawing of the suprasternal notch, epigastrium, and intercostal spaces), grunty respirations, and stridors (harsh, high-pitched whistling sounds) are danger signals, and a nurse or a doctor should be notified at once.

h. Other Signs and Symptoms. These include crying, particularly a weak or inaudible cry; coughing; restlessness, hemoptysis (spitting blood), anorexia (refusal of all or some foods); pulse and respiration; constipation; diarrhea, and melena (dark feces caused by blood pigments); hemorrhage; shock; distention; regurgitation ("spitting up" food) or rumination (intentional regurgitation and reswallowing of regurgitated food); jaundice; and lethargy.

32. Greenstick Fractures

a. These are the most common fractures of children. A greenstick fracture is an incomplete frac-

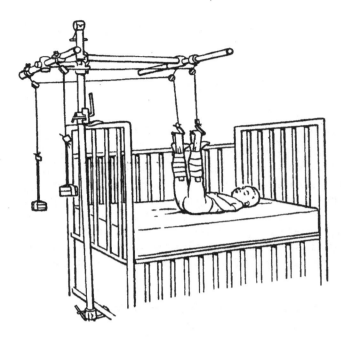

Figure 9. Bryant's traction.

ture with one side of the bone broken and the other side bent. This type of fracture occurs because children's bones are soft and flexible and more prone to splinter. Simple and compound fractures can also occur, however.

b. Breakage of the femur (thigh bone) is one of the most serious breaks. Bryant's traction is used for small children (usually under 2 years of age). It is similar to Buck's extension but the legs are suspended vertically (fig. 9) with the buttocks barely clearing the bed.

CAUTION
Be sure to keep side rails of the crib up. A restraint jacket may be used to keep the child from turning.

The specialist watches the ropes to be sure they are in the pulley grooves. The pull of the weights must not be obstructed, as they must hang free. He checks the child's toes often to be sure that they are pink and warm. He gives the child plenty of fluids and food high in roughage content to insure good elimination. He also entertains with records and stories. Parents are encouraged to visit the child.

33. Eye Conditions

a. Strabismus.

(1) This condition, also known as cross-eye, is a deviation of the eye that the patient cannot

overcome and may be congenital or acquired. One eye or both eyes may deviate. Treatment usually begins before the child is 2 years old; the good eye is covered so the child must use the deviating eye. This eye defect may affect the child's personality, since the other children may make fun of him. If an operation is necessary, the child should be told that his eyes wil be bandaged when he awakes from the anesthetic. Necessary restraints are applied before the child reacts but are removed afterward if he is old enough to understand and follow instructions. The child will usually be released within a day or so after the operation.

(2) With both eyes patched, the child will need much assurance. As you approach the bed, speak to him and explain what you are doing. Do not suddenly walk up to him and lower the bedside rails, as this would startle and frighten him. He will also have to be fed.

b. Cataract. This is an opacity of the lens of the eye or its capsule or it may be of both. It can be congenital or develop as the child grows. The first sign may be strabismus. The only treatment is surgical removal. If a young child has congenital cataracts removed, he will be spread-eagled with clove hitch restraints or will be put in a jacket restraint. Coughing will jar his eyes so, if the doctor wants the head immobilized, sandbags may be used on either side of the head. In such a case, the specialist must never startle, jar, turn, or pick up the child until the doctor's orders add the activity needed. The specialist must also be careful in feeding the child not to choke him and to speak to him before touching him. Petting the child and talking to him in a kind manner may help to soothe him.

c. Infections of the Eye. Among common childhood eye infections are *styes* (an infection of an eyelash follicle or a sebaceous gland of the eyelid), *chalazion* (an obstruction of the meibomian gland in the eyelid), *conjunctivitis* (which is inflammation of the conjunctiva), *keratitis* (inflammation of the cornea), *glaucoma* (an increase in intraocular pressure due to interference in the flow of aqueous humor), and *blepharitis* (an inflammation of the eyelid).

d. Injuries to the Eyes. Among the types of injuries are burns, foreign bodies, lacerations, trauma without entrance of a foreign body (such as a black eye), and sympathetic ophthalmia (where a good eye becomes inflamed after the other eye has been injured).

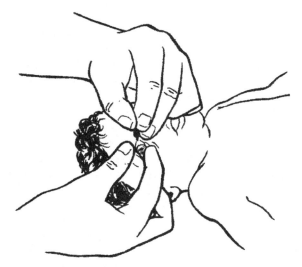

Figure 10. Instillation of eyedrops.

e. Nursing Care for Eyes. The specialist should restrain a young child if necessary to administer eye drops and use the technique shown in figure 10 . If two specialists are present, one should restrain the child's head and arms as necessary. The specialist administering the drops should, with one hand, place one finger upon the child's lids near the upper lashes and another finger near the lower lashes and gently separate the lids (fig. 10). Holding the eye dropper in the other hand, the specialist directs the solution from the inner canthus outward. The specialist holds the eye open for a moment to allow the solution to spread all over the eye's surface. (If only the lower lid is held, the drops may be forced out of the eye by the blinking of the upper lid).

WARNING

Do not force the eyes apart as it can cause trauma.

Remind the child often not to touch or rub his eyes as he will forget.

34. Ear Infections

a. Otitis Media. This infection of bacterial or viral origin is common among infants because their eustachian tubes are almost straight and are wider and shorter than at anytime in their life. Symptoms include elevated temperature, pulling or rubbing the ear, turning the head from side to side, restlessness, vomiting, and crying. If an abcess forms, the eardrum may rupture and pus drain from the ear.

b. Ear Care. In nursing care, the patient is

isolated; antibiotics and pain relievers are given as ordered; and ear drops, nose drops, and ear irrigations are also given as ordered. If ear drops are ordered, they are warmed to body temperature unless the doctor's orders specify differently. When eardrops are applied, the pinna of the ear is pulled down and back, and the warmed drops are allowed to fall on the external canal and run into the ear. Restraints may be necessary. The patient must lie down till the drops are absorbed and is then turned to the affected side to let the ear drain properly. The specialist records the type of drug or oil and the number of drops; the ear in which drops are instilled (right or left); and any reaction, therapeutic or untoward. The skin around the ear is lubricated to keep it from being damaged by the drainage. In older children, ear drops are instilled as for an adult: the pinna of the ear is held back and up.

35. Tonsillectomies

As with an adult operation, the child is admitted the day before the surgery so that he can have a complete physical and the various tests made. He is observed for any signs of an upper respiratory infection or loose teeth. Foods and fluids are withheld (NPO sign may be on bed *and* child). The specialist checks to see that the child's identification band is securely attached. The child should void before leaving the ward. Any strange procedures such as being pushed on a stretcher are explained. After surgery the child is placed in a prone position with a pillow under his abdomen or chest to aid in drainage and to prevent aspiration. He may swallow a great deal of blood if not watched closely. When he regains consciousness, he is turned over and supported in a semisitting position. He is watched for any evidence of bleeding (restlessness, frequent swallowing, etc.) as hemorrhage is the most common complication. Delayed bleeding can occur hours after surgery so his vital signs must be checked frequently. His gown and bed are changed as needed. He is given small amounts of liquids if he is not vomiting and is encouraged to eat cold foods such as gelatin and ice cream after nausea subsides.

WARNING

Do *not* give hot or spiced foods, carbonated beverages, or those with high acidity such as orange juice. They can result in pain or bleeding. Some doctors also discourage sucking from straws.

36. Circumcision

This is the surgical removal of the foreskin of the penis. The care depends upon the doctor's orders. Generally a specialist will look at it every 15 to 20 minutes for the first 2 hours after the operation to check for bleeding. Diapers are kept in place and changed frequently for 48 hours after surgery. Voiding of any type must be reported to the nurse (urination may cause pain at first, and an older child may attempt to avoid it as long as possible). Vaseline gauze is applied and changed p.r.n. to keep dressing moist.

37. Intussusception

This is a condition in which part of the intestine telescopes into another. It is more frequent in males and in children under two years of age. The primary symptoms are drawing up the leg, vomiting, and passing a stool with a mixture of blood and mucus. Postoperative nursing care is the same as for any bowel operation: fluid therapy, frequent determination of pulse and respiration rate, change of patient's position to side, care of nasogastric tube, etc. Suction and oxygen are kept available. The three most common complications are diarrhea, peritonitis, and high fever. The specialist must be particularly careful to prevent exposure to other patients with diarrhea.

38. Cardiac Conditions
(fig. 11)

In postoperative nursing care for heart surgery with general anesthesia, the specialist must be prepared for any emergency. All necessary equipment (oxygen tent, suction machine, tracheotomy tray, 3 large hemostats, emergency drugs, etc.) should be at the bedside when the child returns. The specialist must insure that there are no leaks in the system of chest tubes, see that the tubes are in place, and watch for any obstructions or kinks. He must check to insure that a patent airway exists and then use the oxygen tent in accordance with the doctor's orders. Next, he should check the intravenous and blood transfusion apparatus and see that properly applied restraints prevent thrashing. The level of drainage in the bottles is marked every 8 hours unless drainage is excessive; if it is, then it is marked and labeled every hour. The specialist must also be alert for any signs of bleeding. The pulse, blood pressure, and respiration must be checked as often as the doctor orders. Dressings must also be checked for bleeding or oozing. Most patients are usually turned

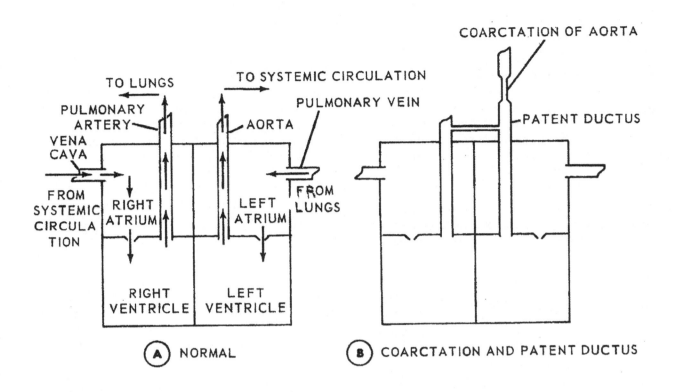

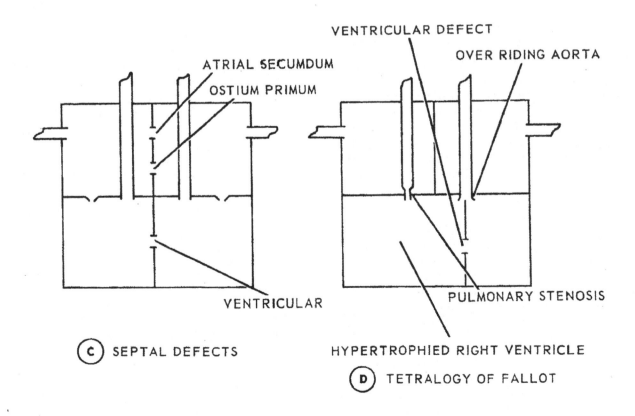

Figure   11.   *Congential anomalies of the heart (schematic diagram).*

every hour as soon as they react, and they are usually made to cough every hour. Some types of congenital heart disorders which may be correctable by surgery are listed below (fig. 11 Ⓐ) shows the normal heart).

a. *Ductus Arteriosus.* This is a normal condition during fetal life. There is a connection between the aorta and pulmonary artery which permits the blood to flow directly to the aorta, thus bypassing the lungs. If the connection fails to close shortly after birth, it may give rise to symptoms of cardiac failure, depending upon its size. It is known as a patent (open) ductus arteriosus.

b. *Coarctation of the Aorta.* The same mechanism that normally affects the ductus areteriosus may extend to the aorta and narrow its lumen (fig. 11 Ⓑ).

c. *Atrial Septal Defect* (fig. 11 Ⓒ).

(1) *Atrial secundum defect.* This is a hole in the atrial septum, permitting communication between the two atria and the shunting of blood from left to right.

(2) *Ostium primum.* This defect is lower in the septum. Involving the areas of the mitral and tricuspid valves, it is more complicated because, in addition to the shunting of the blood, the clefts in the mitral valve permit blood to regurgitate from the left ventricle into both atria. Both types increase the workload of the heart.

d. *Ventricular Septal Defect.* This is a hole in the ventricular septum permitting communication between the two ventricles. In this, the flow of blood is also from the left to the right, because the blood pressure is higher in the left ventricle than the right. Blood sent to the left ventricle from the left atrium and lungs makes a circuit again through the right heart and the lungs.

e. *Pulmonary Stenosis.* Sometimes the pulmonary valves unite together, which narrows the passages from the right ventricle to the pulmonary artery. At other times, the entire ring of tissue around the valve may be narrowed. Muscle bundles within the right ventricle itself may also obstruct the flow of blood to the pulmonary artery.

f. *Tetralogy of Fallot.* This malformation (fig. 11 Ⓓ) includes a defective interventricular septum, a right position of the aortic arch or a biventricular origin of the aorta (overriding aorta), an abnormal increase in the size of right ventricle, and a stenosis of the pulmonary artery. The stenosis will not permit the blood to flow

through the lungs in sufficient amounts, so it goes through the septal opening into the aorta. This condition produces a cyanotic heart disorder, more commonly known as a "blue baby."

39. Diabetes

Diabetes is a condition in which the body cannot oxidize carbohydrates properly because of a lack of insulin. Although the cause and cure of this disease are not known, heredity is a predisposing factor. The disease can be controlled by diet, insulin, and exercise. Common symptoms include polydipsia (extreme thirst), polyphagia (constant hunger), and polyuria (excessive urine, which may cause bed wetting and "accidents" in the day). The overweight that is characteristic in adult patients with diabetes seldom appears in children. Complications include *diabetic acidosis* (also called diabetic coma), where the face flushes, the lips become red, the breath has a characteristic sweet odor, the respirations increase and become labored, and dehydration occurs; *hypoglycemia* (insulin shock) which is caused by too much insulin and is characterized by irritability (temper tantrums in young children), hunger, weakness, double vision, and tremors; and *pyogenic infections*, which are more dangerous to a diabetic child than to the normal child. The specialist will routinely check the urine before each meal and at bedtime for presence of sugar and record the result, and insure that the correct diet is served on time. He then checks the types and amounts of food that the child did not eat, records this, and also informs the nurse in charge (she informs the dietitian who can then determine whether the child will need a snack between meals). Diabetes is much more difficult to control in children than in adults because of the need to compensate for irregular eating habits, expenditure of energy in spurts, and more frequent infections. The doctor prescribes the amount of insulin and the time that it is to be given. It is usually administed *subcutaneously.* The dosage is measured in units and special syringes used only for administration of insulin are used. This medication is usually given by the nurse, but if the clinical specialist does it, he must administer insulin in the exact dosage ordered and at the prescribed time.

40. Epilepsy

Epileptic seizures are usually recurring periods of unconsciousness that are often accompanied by paroxysmal (sudden), tonic (continuous muscular contraction) or clonic (a series of spasms) muscle spasms. The seizures may be mild and brief (petit mal) with little muscular spasm, if any; or they may be generalized, with both tonic and clonic spasms (grand mal). The onset of grand mal is sudden. As it begins, the patient may utter a quick cry and then fall. The face may be pale, the pupils dilated, the extremities stiff or contracted; the jaw muscles may also contract swiftly (this may cause the tongue, lips, or cheeks to be bitten); and incontinence may occur. During a seizure, maintenance of an airway and prevention of injury are the first concerns. (Once a seizure begins, the specialist can do nothing to stop it, but he can prevent injury to the child.) A padded gag or a firm roll of gauze should be inserted well back in the mouth between the teeth. The gag should not be forced between clenched teeth because of the danger of trauma to the gums and teeth. After a seizure has started it may be too late to prevent the child from biting his tongue by inserting a wedge. If on the floor, the head should be protected or cradled. The specialist should record exactly what happens—the time; how it began and in what part of the body; incontinence; position and movement of eyes; duration, severity, and reaction of the child after the attack. Afterward, the child should be made clean, dry, and comfortable and allowed to sleep. When he wakes up, he may be confused and have a severe headache. He should be carefully observed. The specialist must be careful to avoid showing overprotection, pity, or disgust. If anticonvulsant drugs are ordered, the specialist must be sure that they are administered at the correct time and are actually swallowed. Treatment also includes provision of a calm atmosphere and dietary management.

41. Skin

The skin of a child requires special care in diarrhea and in other conditions.

a. *Infantile eczema* is an inflammation of the skin. The lesions form vesicles (small blister-like lesions) and the baby scratches because the itching is unbearable. The infant's arms must be restrained, which causes frustration. He will need cuddling because of this. The doctor will order an ointment and solution to be applied and may order an emollient bath such as oatmeal or a mixture of corn starch and baking soda. The specialist puts the prescribed emollient in the water while it is

filling and stirs it to mix it evenly. Before shutting off the faucets, he runs some cold water through them to cool them so the baby will not get burned if he grasps them. The bath temperature should be 95° F, but hot water is NEVER added after the baby is in the tub. He is usually kept in the tub for about 20 minutes but is NEVER left alone. If wet soaks are ordered, a gauze bandage is dipped in the solution ordered, squeezed gently to remove any excess, and then applied. These soaks must be kept wet. They are *not* covered with towels or rubber sheeting because evaporation cools and helps to relieve the itching. Wet compresses are applied to the face by using a square piece of gauze with places cut out for eyes, nose, and mouth. Four strings are attached to its four corners. The wet mask is then put in place and tied. Ointment, if ordered, is applied evenly and reapplied as needed. This is usually done by using the hand, rather than a tongue depressor.

b. Although *Nephrosis* is a kidney disease and not a skin disease as such, the gross edema which is symptomatological of the disease requires special consideration of the skin. Edema first starts at the eyes or ankles but spreads until it becomes generalized. It shifts as the child changes position while sleeping. The abdomen can become so distended that stretch marks similar to those of a pregnancy may appear. (Vomiting and diarrhea may also occur.) The child is irritable, listless, and pale. Good skin care is especially important during the severe edema. At least one bath daily is required and more may be necessary. Special attention must be given to neck, underarms, groin, and other moist areas. Soothing powder is used on male genitals. The scrotum may need support; if so, a soft pad is held in place by a T binder—adhesive tape is NEVER used. The child is turned frequently, his head may be elevated from time to time to reduce eyelid edema, and a pillow between the knees may help prevent pressure on sore surfaces. Accurate intake and output records must be kept. For a baby in diapers, an accurate record of the urinary output may be kept by accurately weighing the diapers before and after the child urinates. The character, odor, and color of the urine must also be noted.

c. *Pediculosis* is lice infestation. The nits (eggs) of the head louse appear as small, white or grayish flecks which are attached firmly to the hair shafts. Each nit will hatch in a maximum of 4 days. Treatment consists of cutting long hair and administering specially medicated shampoos and baths, as prescribed, to kill the organism. The prescribed medication is also administered. Nits may be removed by combing the hair with a fine-tooth comb dipped in hot diluted acetic acid (vinegar). Bed clothing, hats, caps, and clothing must be cleaned and disinfected.

d. *Ringworm* (*tinea*) occurs on the smooth skin, hands and feet, or scalp. The *tinea circinata* (smooth-skin ringworm) initially appears on the face, neck, or forearms. Usually only one appears at first—it is small, pinkish, round, and covered with small scales. Other lesions spread from this. There is very little itching. Another smooth-skin type, *tinea cruris*, first appears on the buttocks, thighs, or anal fold. It is accompanied by a greater degree of itching. Both respond to half-strength Whitfield's ointment applied daily. *Tinea capitis*, or *tinea tonsurans* is ringworm of the scalp. One type, *Microsporum lanosum*, comes from an animal source and cannot be transmitted to another child. *Microsporum audouini* is the other type, which is readily transmitted to other children. The lesions are round red patches with scales on the scalp of the head. Usually, no hair is present in the area. Topical treatment may be used for both, but X-ray therapy may be necessary with the latter. *Tinea of the feet* (or athlete's foot) is helped by fungicides of the doctor's choice, frequent sock changes, and airing of shoes.

e. *Intertrigo* (diaper rash) is caused by prolonged contact with wet diapers. The treatment usually consists of exposure of the buttocks and perineum area to air and to light from a 25-watt light bulb at least 3 times. This bulb should be high enough to prevent the child from reaching it. Application of ointment may be ordered. If so, a diaper is applied and the heat lamp not used. Intertrigo can be prevented by frequent changes of diapers, washing of skin at the time of diaper change, and correctly washed diapers. Plastic diaper panties retain heat from urine decomposition and can cause or aggravate diaper rash. They should not be used in a hospital unless a physician or a nurse orders them in a special case.

f. *Dermatitis venenata* is a contact dermatitis caused by direct contact with a vegetable irritant, usually poison oak or poison ivy. It is accompanied by a skin eruption, swelling, burning, and intense itching. If the attack is severe with considerable swelling, the doctor may order continuous hot compresses of liquid aluminum acetate.

g. *Scabies* (*itch*) causes severe itching, particularly at night. Secondary infection from scratch-ing is a danger. Treatment consists of destroying the parasite, the itch mite. In treatment with sulfur ointment, the child must be thoroughly scrubbed and soaped in a hot bath before the ointment is applied. The ointment is applied all over the body except for the head, to include neck and soles of feet. Then no baths are given for 3 days, although the ointment is still applied for 3 nights. On the fifth day, the patient is again given a thorough hot bath and all contaminated clothing and bed linen are boiled or dry cleaned.

h. *Furunculosis* is a condition that goes with boils. A furuncle is usually a staphylococcic infection of a sebaceous gland or hair follicle. It is a red, elevated, sore area, that eventually comes to a head. If it does not rupture, it must be incised, but it should *never* be squeezed with the fingers. Hot compresses will hasten the rupture. These patients must be kept away from other patients to prevent the spread of staphylococcal infection.

i. *Herpes simplex* (fever blisters, cold sores) and *herpes zoster* are virus diseases. The latter's symptoms begins with an area of skin that is tender or sore. This area will later erupt into papular lesions which soon become vesicules. The disease is extremely painful. The most common site is along a rib, starting at the spine, although it can occur at the eye.

j. *Burns* consist of tissue destroyed due to exposure to heat, chemicals, or electricity; ultraviolet and roentgen rays; or contact with radioactive surfaces. Over 55 percent of burns occur in children. Burns are classified according to the depth of tissue destroyed. The doctor will decide the degree and the treatment, but the specialist must watch a burned hospitalized child for shock and toxicity (high fever, rapid pulse, prostration, cyanosis, decreased urine volume, and vomiting). The child must be protected from infection. An accurate intake and output record must be maintained, a footboard used to prevent contractures, proper alinement maintained, the bed kept dry, and the child turned every 2 to 3 hours. Care must be taken to prevent contaminating the burned area with feces. Frequent checking of the child is necessary. Burns usually result in prolonged hospitalization, and recreation must be planned for the child. It is as much a part of the treatment as many nursing procedures.

42. Cerebral Palsy

This is a group of disorders that affect the motor centers of the brain. Although not progressive, there is no present cure. Cerebral palsy is caused by birth injuries, anoxia, subdural hemorrhage, or infections such as meningitis. Symptoms range from mild to severe but usually include feeding problems, convulsions but no high fever, and physical retardation (child is not able to sit, crawl, or walk at the normal range for his age level). Mental retardation may also, but not always, be present. Types of cerebral palsy include spasticity (tension in certain muscle groups, particularly those of lower extremities) and athetosis (involuntary, purposeless movements which interfere with normal motion). Speech, sight, hearing, and emotions may be affected. The disability should be explained to the parents, who must learn to accept the child as he is. Good skin care is essential and exercise is necessary to prevent contractures (a shortening of muscles due to lack of use). The specialist must insist that the patient do as much as he can for himself. The specialist must also carry out the physical therapist's assignments and instructions for the child. If braces are used, he checks them from time to time for such things as alinement and wear. A long hospitalization will probably be required. The specialist must avoid focusing his attention on the child's abnormalities and remember that he is an individual— and *accept him as he is.* He should be *empathetic,* not sympathetic. Above all, he must encourage the child during this stage of psychological as well as physical growth to be self-reliant and independent. The specialist may also encounter feeding problems. Often the child must be fed slowly to prevent aspiration. It is hard for such infants to adjust to solid foods, so the specialist must have extreme patience. Since the child tires easily, he should have frequent naps in a quiet room. The child may appear to be emotionally unstable, but this may be caused by frustration because even simple tasks can be overwhelming to him—his continuous failures cause him to despair of ever succeeding. Guidance and patience are absolute necessities to keep the child happy within his capabilities.

43. Pyloric Stenosis

A condition in which the muscular tissue of the pylorus thickens and hardens, constricting the size of the opening from the stomach to the duodenum. As it progresses, partial or complete obstruction may occur. The primary symptom is projectile vomiting with no sign of nausea. Treatment may be medical or surgical but, regardless of the type of treatment, the specialist must keep an intake and output record. The appearance and color of vomitus should be noted. The amount vomited should be measured accurately, especially if a baby is to be re-fed. If atropine or methscopolamine nitrate is used, the specialist must watch for flushing and record it. The techniques for properly feeding a baby (always hold a baby to feed him; never prop a bottle) should be followed, with particular attention to calm, unhurried feeding. These babies tend to eat too fast, so their rate of eating must be slowed. In postoperative care, the child's color, respiration, and pulse are watched.

44. Erythroblastosis Fetalis (Rh Incompatibility)

This is excessive destruction of the red blood cells of the baby because of an incompatibility with the red blood cells of the mother. Symptoms include anemia and jaundice. An exchange transfusion, followed by small transfusions later, may be ordered. The specialist keeps an accurate record of the amounts of blood withdrawn or injected and watches the baby afterward for jaundice, cyanosis, edema, convulsions, lethargy, vital signs, and changes in urine.

45. Leukemia (Cancer of the Blood)

The cause of leukemia is not known, but the disease is characterized by an uncontrollable increase in production of a specific kind of white blood corpuscles and the decrease of other types of white blood corpuscles, red blood corpuscles, and platelets. It terminates in death. The abnormal blood picture is usually the first symptom. At the present time, treatment gives only a temporary benefit; the primary treatment is to keep the patient comfortable and relatively happy. If Aminopterin or A-methopterin is given, the specialist must watch for symptoms of nausea, vomiting, diarrhea, ulceration of the mucous membranes of the oral cavity, alopecia (loss of hair), and high fever. These are signs that the toxic level of these drugs has been reached. If a child is on cortisone therapy, the specialist should see that the child is put to bed 1 hour before each meal; otherwise, he will be too tired to eat (cortisone makes the child feel better, so his activity increases, but it does not dissipate his tendency toward fatigue). When the platelet count goes under 100,000, the specialist must be alert for bleeding. Cotton swabs must now be used instead of toothbrushes. Bleeding can occur at the gums, nose, or rectum and can be so severe that transfusions will be needed. Petroleum jelly must be applied to the lips, which become dry and cracked. Since the child has so little resistance to infection, he must be protected from infection or chilling. Skin care and care of the mucous membrane surfaces of the mouth must be gentle. The doctor will order comfort measures, but he will need the specialist's observations. Because of the pain, some children will prefer to be in bed or in a wheelchair rather than to be held. The child will also resist being bathed because of the pain. The specialist must encourage the child to eat something, so the diet is never forced on the child. He is usually allowed to eat anything he wants. Since death is inevitable, the specialist must show kindness and consideration to the child and his parents.

46. Contagious Diseases of Childhood

Among the contagious diseases of childhood are the common cold; chicken pox; measles (Rubeola); meningococcal meningitis; mumps; pertussis (whooping cough); poliomyelitis; German measles (Rubella); scarlet fever; and pneumonia.

47. Croup

Croup (sometimes called spasmodic laryngitis) is a common childhood respiratory infection. It is characterized by hoarse cough, noisy inspiration, and struggle for breath which may be accompanied by moderate to severe retractions. Attacks occur mostly at night. The doctor may prescribe an emetic to cause the child to vomit, which helps to reduce the larynx's muscle spasms. Electric steam inhalators may be used, but croupettes are preferable from the standpoint of comfort and safety.

STEAM INHALATOR

Equipment

Steam inhalator
Medication, if ordered
Warm water

Procedure

1. Fill the inhalator with the warm distilled water and put medication, if ordered, in the machine's cup.
2. Plug inhalator in; turn switch to high.
3. Close the door and any windows.

4. Position child comfortably. He may be in a semisitting position unless contraindicated.
5. Put the inhalator's nozzle about 18 to 24 inches from the child; if it is too close, you will burn him.

WARNING

Place out of the child's reach. Children have been known to grab the inhalator and pull it over on themselves, with death resulting from the ensuing burns.

Steam should come out of the inhalator's spout until the steam surrounds the child's head.

6. Adjust switch to medium or low, depending on amount of moisture needed.
7. Time the treatment when the steam begins to flow and continue for prescribed time.
8. Refill with water as necessary.
9. Record relief obtained; how patient tolerated the treatment; time and length of treatment; and medication, if ordered.

Care of Equipment

1. Empty the water jug, wash, and dry.
2. Wash medicine cup.
3. Return machine to proper area unless treatment is to be given several times a day.

IMPROVISED CROUP TENT

Equipment

Cotton blanket
Sheet
Piece of screen
Safety pins
Steam inhalator

Procedure

1. First put a cotton blanket, then a sheet over it, until half of the crib's top and sides are covered. (The blanket absorbs the steam and keeps it from falling on the patient.) The other half of the crib is not covered.
2. Pin blanket and sheet in place, with pins on the outside and out of the child's reach.
3. Put the inhalator next to the crib with the spout forward inside the head of the tent.
4. Put a piece of screen or some other protection between the spout and the child.
5. Refill inhalator as necessary.
6. Observe the child frequently.
7. Record the color of child, degree of restlessness, reactions, and time of treatment.

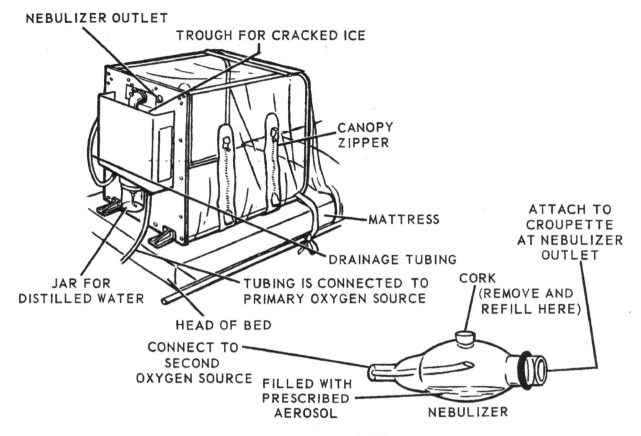

Figure . 12. Croupette humidity tent.

CROUPETTE

(fig. 2)

A croupette may be used for respiratory infections. It uses cool, moist air which liquefies the secretions of the bronchioles and reduces the childs' temperature. Oxygen or air under pressure may be used to provide pressure.

Equipment (With Oxygen)

Croupette
Tap water
Ice
Bucket
Oxygen
Rubber sheet
Cotton blanket
Distilled water

Procedure (With Oxygen)

1. Put a rubber sheet on the crib and then cover with a blanket. (The blanket absorbs moisture and the rubber sheet prevents oxygen from escaping.)

CAUTION

Do not block the lower opening of the recirculation pipe with anything, as this will make the tent warm.

2. Fill trough at back of croupette with ice and tap water to indicated level.

3. Secure the canopy under the frame on both sides.

4. Seal canopy at the front with a folded blanket or sheet tucked loosely under the mattress sides so that carbon dioxide can escape.

5. Fill the jar into which the oxygen flows three-fourths full with distilled water.

6. Refill with ice as necessary. The ice prevents the tent from becoming too warm.

7. Change the child's clothes if they become damp but do not open zippered portholes more than necessary.

8. Use usual precautions with oxygen.

Care of Equipment

1. Empty the distilled water jar, wash, and dry.

2. Drain ice and water from the trough and wash trough with warm water and soap. Do *not* use alcohol.

3. Clean the canopy with mild soap and warm water. Fold neatly.

4. Return to the designated area.

48. Diarrhea

This is characterized by a sudden onset with nausea, vomiting, chills, loose stools, abdominal pain, fever, and prostration. Diarrhea is a severe disease in any child and extremely severe, often fatal, for an infant. The stools usually have mucus and may have blood as the disease progresses. The greatest danger is dehydration and acidosis. A close intake and output record must be maintained. The electrolyte balance must also be maintained, as severe loss of potassium may accompany the disease. The doctor will usually order antibiotics and may order gastric lavage, paregoric, or parenteral fluid therapy. Nothing by mouth except water is also a common order for the first 24 hours. As symptoms disappear, liquids and soft diets are usually ordered. Disinfection procedures must be followed throughout the course of this disease.

49. Rheumatic Fever

Rheumatic fever occurs primarily between 5 and 15 years of age. It frequently follows infections caused by group A beta-hemolytic streptococci. Recurrences are frequent and many deaths because of cardiac involvement are directly traceable to it. Its symptoms are general—malaise, loss of weight and appetite, paleness, low-grade fever (especially in the afternoon), and spontaneous nosebleed. A single attack will last from 1 to 3 months or longer. Successful nursing care depends upon absolute bedrest and lack of excitement. Sometimes a child may not feel ill; then the specialist will have difficulty keeping him in bed. Some children will have emotional difficulty—withdrawal, refusal to admit that they are ill, or a complete rebellion. Mood changes can be extreme, so the specialist must be prepared to be accepting and cheerful no matter what reception he meets. The specialist will probably be required to take the child's TPR every 4 hours and to observe him for lesions, dyspnea, swollen joints, and complaint of pain. Sometimes the child will have diaphoresis (severe sweating); then his skin will have to be bathed and gowns and bed linen changed frequently. An emollient or oil may be prescribed for dry skin surfaces.

50. The Battered Child Syndrome

a. General. The abused child has always been a problem. Although statistics show that this syndrome is increasing in recent years, it may well be that it is only recognized and publicized more. Infants and small children are the usual victims. Suspicion of child abuse is aroused when any one or more of these factors are present—

- There are multiple bruises and lacerations.
- The injuries seem out of proportion to the story told about the accident.
- The parents attempt to conceal information.
- There are obvious signs of neglect and malnutrition.
- The child fails to cry. (The unknowledgeable may think that they are merely being exceptionally good children.)

These battered children arouse strong feelings of indignation, even hostility, but nursing personnel must be careful to remain objective. It is often difficult to prove that the injury was intentionally afflicted; in some cases, it may indeed have been accidental. Even if it seems apparent that the child has been injured by one of his parents, the specialist should report his observations to the nurse or physician, and avoid expressing his indignation to patients or parents.

b. Parents of Battered Children. Such a parent may be like a hurt child, too, and may be incapable of seeing that the infant or child is an immature person. He often looks to a mere infant to satisfy his emotional needs and becomes infuriated when the baby cannot help him. It is a blunder to antagonize the parent because it makes future communication difficult. The majority of parents who injure their children want help. In most cases, they have voluntarily brought the child to the hospital. If help is offered without accusations or threats, the parents may cooperate. The goal is to help the parent and to do what is best for the child. Nursing personnel must remember that some of these parents are mentally ill or mentally retarded; others are emotionally immature persons who were neglected or abused as children; others may be overwhelmed with problems; all have strong guilt feelings.

c. The Specialist. The specialist can best help by observing the parents. What is their reaction to the child? You can suspect abuse and alert the nurse or doctor when parents are critical of the child, angry because he is hurt, seldom touch or look at him, show no remorse nor concern about his treatment, leave the hospital soon after he is admitted, and seldom visit him. These parents usually will not volunteer information and are irritable or evasive when describing the circumstance attending the injury. They will usually maintain that the child injured himself. On the other hand, they may offer much information about the injury; however, much may be false and misleading. Any information obtained from the parents or observation of their reaction to the child should be immediately reported to the nurse or doctor. This information must be considered confidential and not gossiped about with other ward personnel.

d. *The Child.* The child will not cling to his parents for reassurance or comfort. Such children seem afraid of physical contact initiated by the parents or by anyone. They may whimper or try to withdraw from any contact. They seldom cry, seemingly realizing that crying has only brought them more pain. If they cry during treatment, their crying is hopeless, without any expectation of being comforted. Small infants may lie motionless with no expression on their faces. Children who can talk may or may not tell you that their injury was inflicted by the parent.

e. *Nursing Care.* As the child begins to show some awareness of the change in his situation, you should offer some bodily contact. When he responds, you must respond, also. The child will become more active as he improves and may test his relationship with you by such actions as tentative biting or poking with his fingers. He may be extremely anxious and cling to anyone, or he may withdraw completely. Tender, loving care is the key in the approach to the battered child, more so to this child than to any other pediatric patient.

f. *The Health Nurse.* The Health Nurse is usually brought into the case as soon as there is suspicion of child abuse. He needs to establish a relationship with the child and his parents that he can sustain in the home environment. The child may, however, not be returned to his home. He may be removed temporarily or permanently. His safety is the paramount governing factor. Even then the Health Nurse can be of service in his new environment.

Section VII. CONGENITAL ANOMALIES

51. General

Some congenital anomalies cause death or permanent handicaps; others can be corrected surgically. Any part of the body may be affected. There can be a complete absence of a part or a malformation.

52. Malformation of Mouth and Palate

The most frequent of these malformations are cleft palate and harelip, the result of failure of the maxillary, premaxillary, and palatal processes to fuse. One may occur without the other, but they frequently occur together. Although these babies have excellent appetites, they have trouble in sucking and swallowing. They swallow large amounts of air, and need to be burped often. Surgery is the only treatment. A cleft lip can be operated on around the age of 3 months, but a cleft palate is not usually repaired until after the child reaches 2 years of age. Meanwhile the baby must be fed, and the parents must be taught how to feed him. No one method will work for all—some infants can use a special nipple (fig. 13), others must be fed by cup, or by medicine dropper with a rubber tip to prevent injury to his gums, and some require gavage.

NOTE

For infants with cleft lip repairs, medicine droppers with rubber tips or asepto syringes with rubber tips are used. For infants with cleft palate repairs, a cup or asepto syringe with rubber tip is used.

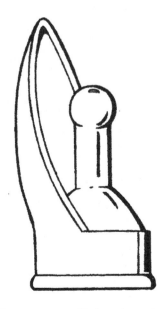

Figure 13. Cleft palate nipple.

CLEFT PALATE NIPPLE

Until a cleft palate is repaired, the cleft palate nippled may be used. The specialist inserts the nipple in the infant's mouth with rubber flange (cut to the size of the cleft in the palate) over the fissure area. This makes it possible to create a vacuum in the mouth and prevent aspiration.

MEDICINE DROPPER

NOTE

The specialist will have to allow more time than the 20 or 30 minutes required to feed a normal baby by bottle.

Equipment

Sterile medicine dropper with rubber tip

or

Asepto syringe with rubber tip
Warmed formula
Bib
Protective covering for specialist

Procedure

1. Wash hands and insure that the infant is dry and comfortable. Mummy-wrap infant.
2. Add the formula to the medicine dropper or syringe.
3. Hold infant in sitting position.
4. Place the rubber tip on top and to the side of the tongue. Fluid should flow from the dropper slowly and in small amounts.
5. Allow the infant to swallow before giving more formula. If possible, do not permit sucking motions.
6. Burp frequently. If the infant can hold his head up strongly, sit him up, support his chest with one hand, and gently pat his back with the other. Otherwise, burp as described in paragraph 20a(2).
7. After feeding, put the infant in his crib on his right side with his back supported by a rolled infant blanket or small pillow.
8. Record results of feeding.

GAVAGE

Equipment

Small catheter or polyethylene gavage tube or No. 8 infant feeding tube
Syringe, 30 ml. or 50 ml.
Cup of water, 1
Small towel
Adhesive tape
Warmed formula

Procedure

CAUTION

This can be a dangerous procedure for the inexperienced specialist and should be performed only under the supervision of the nurse or physician.

1. Using the catheter to be used for the gavage, measure the distance from the bridge of his nose to a point halfway between the xiphoid process (base of breastbone) and the umbilicus. Mark the tube.
2. Put the infant in a mummy restraint and put a small towel roll under his shoulders to hyperflex his neck.
3. Hold the infant's head with one hand to keep him still, and genly pass the catheter through his nose or mouth, depending on the physician's orders, until the preselected mark has been reached.
4. Stop and remove catheter at once if the infant chokes, coughs, or becomes cyanotic. Reinsert the tube only on the direction of the nurse or physician.
5. Secure the inserted tube to the infant's face with nonallergic type tape.
6. Depending upon local policy, the tube may be permitted to remain in place between feedings. If so, before each feeding, test the position of the gavage tube (to assure that it is not in the respiratory tract) by one of these methods—
   a. Attach a syringe to the gavage tube and withdraw a small amount of stomach contents. This insures that the tube is in the stomach.
   b. Place a stethoscope over the epigastric region, insert 0.5 ml. of air through the tube with a syringe, and listen to see if the air enters the stomach.
   c. Invert the gavage tube in a glass of water. If bubbles appear, withdraw the tube, as it is *not* in the stomach.
7. Attach a syringe barrel to the tubing.
8. Pour a small amount of warmed formula into the barrel.
9. Raise the syringe barrel about 8 inches above the *mattress* and let it flow by gravity slowly.
10. Just before the syringe empties, pinch the tube to prevent air from entering the stomach and add more formula to the syringe barrel. Do *not* overfeed, or the infant will vomit.
11. Follow feeding with a small amount of sterile water.

12. Remove gavage tube by clamping it, removing adhesive tape, and withdrawing quickly and smoothly.

PATIENT CARE TREATMENT AFTER SURGERY TO CORRECT MALFORMATION OF MOUTH AND PALATE

1. Aspirate nasopharynx to keep it clear.
2. Give adequate nutrition. Keep the suture line clean after feeding by using water from a cup or medicine glass.
3. Put the infant on his *back* and apply restraints to prevent him from rubbing the sutures.

CAUTION

Close observation is necessary due to danger of aspiration. Head and shoulders should be elevated slightly.

4. Keep the suture line clean at all times, using sterile applicators for cleansing and drying and applying hydrogen peroxide. Clean *toward* the suture line to avoid putting tension on it.

53. Malformation of Trachea and Esophagus

The most common malformation is *atresia* (absence or closure of a normal body orifice) of the esophagus with tracheo-esophageal fistula. In the most common type of this particular malformation, the upper portion of the esophagus terminates in a blind pouch in the upper chest, the lower portion is a closed tube extending above the diaphragm, and the tracheo-esophageal fistula is connected with the lower section of the esophagus. An infant with this malformation wil have saliva flowing from his mouth because he can swallow only a small amount before the pouch fills. If the upper portion of the esophagus fills and there is overflow in the trachea, the infant may get pneumonia. Early surgical correction is necessary since the infant cannot take his formula because of instant regurgitation, choking, coughing, and cyanosis. This operation requires entry into the chest wall, so the infant will require water seal drainage (para 5–113), with the number of bottles determined by the physician. The specialist must change the child's position frequently, and coughing and crying are desirable. (The baby can be made to cry if the sole of his foot is tapped gently.)

54. Malformation of the Epiglottis

Among these malformations are those of the epiglottis and structures around it, collapsing larynx and trachea, and deformities of laryngeal cartilages or vocal cords. These are characterized by laryngeal stridor. Such infants need slow and careful feeding by small nipple or medicine glass and sometimes by gavage. There is contant danger of aspiration and of respiratory infections. Cysts and tumors of the throat are also common. Generally, such surgical patients need about the same nursing care as adults with laryngeal difficulties.

55. Hydrocephalus

This is a congenital anomaly where there is an increase of cerebrospinal fluid in the ventricles of brain which results in an increase in head size and pressure changes in the brain. The main symptom is the enlarging head size, but the scalp may also be shiny, the veins dilated, and the eyes crossed. The infant is irritable, vomits, has anorexia, and may have convulsions. The position of the patient without surgery must be changed frequently to prevent pressure sores and hypostatic pneumonia as the infant or child cannot turn himself because of the increasing size of the head. When the infant is turned, the specialist must support the head in the palm of one hand while rotating the head and neck together to prevent a strain on the neck. The specialist must also support the baby's head when lifting or feeding the baby. A calm quiet atmosphere is necessary when feeding the baby. Afterward he is put on his side and left undisturbed for a time after feeding. This child needs tender loving care like all other children. Do not neglect him.

56. Malformation of the Pylorus

The symptoms of pyloric spasm and pyloric stenosis (para 43) include projectile vomiting without any sign of nausea and with visible peristaltic waves traveling from left to right, and loss of weight, obvious abdominal bulges, and few stools. A child with this malformation is usually tense and needs a quiet, relaxed environment. Attempt to meet his needs for adequate warmth and for cuddling, particularly before and after meals. Do not excite him or handle him vigorously.

57. Intestinal Obstructions and Imperforate Anus

a. The most common anomalies of the bowels are intestinal obstructions—atresia (a complete block), stenosis (a partial block), volvulus (incomplete anchoring), and meconium ileus (meconium is so thick that it cannot pass through the intestinal tract). Most of these require surgical treatment. Even then, there is always danger of chronic nutritional disturbances and pulmonary disease.

b. An imperforate (no normal opening) anus is normally discovered when the baby is examined at birth, and surgery is done immediately. It is often accompanied by fistulas of the perineum, urethra, bladder, or vagina.

c. Infants with intestinal obstruction are in poor condition and suffer from dehydration before surgery. High fever must be reduced to at least 102° F (R). After surgery, the specialist takes and records the respiration and pulse rates every 15 minutes until reaction. If the child becomes cyanotic, the doctor is called, and these procedures are performed every 5 minutes. Afterward, rectal temperatures (except for operations on rectum or anus*) are taken every 2 hours if fever is over 102° F; otherwise, it is taken every 4 hours. If a vein on an arm or leg has been cutdown for continuous intravenous therapy, the arm or leg is put on a well-padded splint and wrapped securely. The child may need to be restrained by clove hitches and is usually turned every 2 hours. Intake and output are totaled every 8 hours and every 24 hours and recorded.

* Axillary temperatures are taken on patients having rectal or anus abnormalities.

58. Spina Bifida

This is a congenital malformation that results in imperfect closure of the spinal canal, usually in the lumbosacral region. Because portions of the bony spine are missing, the membranes may protrude through the opening (called a *meningocele*). If the membranes *and* cord protrude, it is called a *meningomyelocele*, which is often accompanied by leg paralysis and some loss of control of the functions of the bowels and bladder. Surgery may be used for either but in a meningomyelocele, rehabilitation is needed to teach the child to use a wheelchair and to walk on crutches, when possible. This rehabilitation period also requires extensive nursing care to prevent infections and provide for correct positioning, careful skin care, and accurate observations and charting.

59. Congenital Cardiac Disease

This paragraph will list a few of the numerous congenital cardiac conditions, most of which were discussed in paragraph 38. If further information is needed, an up-tp-date pediatric text should be consulted. In general, children adapt themselves readily to the limitations of their disease, and sudden death rarely occurs in these types of cardiac conditions. The main thing that must be guarded against is infection. The heart defects that are congenital are generally divided into cyanotic and noncyanotic.

a. Cyanotic. The children with cyanosis generally have a shunt that lets the venous blood travel by abnormal channels from right to left. Circulation through the lungs, which oxygenates the blood and gives it its red color, is bypassed. The types include—

(1) Tetralogy of Fallot (para 38f) whose symptoms are deep cyanosis, polycythemia (too many red corpuscles in the blood), and circulatory failure. A child with this defect is often below normal physically and is overdependent, insecure, and immature. The specialist must accept the child as he is.

(2) Transposition and displacement of the great vessels. There can be many faulty arrangements of the great vessels. This may be accompanied by pulmonic stenosis. In the Taussig-Bing syndrome, the aorta leads from the right ventricle and overrides the pulmonary artery. In Ebstein's malformation of the tricuspid valve, the abnormal valve is displaced into the right ventricle.

b. Noncyanotic. Among this group are the following: interventricular septal defect (one of the most common), atrial septal defect, patent ductus arteriosus, pulmonary stenosis, and coarction of the aoerta (a constriction of the lumen of the aorta at any point).

c. Postoperative Nursing Care. All nursing care for cardiac patients is under the supervision of a nurse. Immediately after surgery (during the first few minutes), the child is checked for vital signs, skin color, respiration, level of consciousness, and movement of extremities. The team will then carry out the surgeon's orders, which may include the following:

(1) Start oxygen therapy.

(2) Connect water seal bottle drainage.

(3) Connect the urinary catheter to a sterile closed drainage system.

(4) Prepare medications and intravenous fluids.

(5) Check vital signs every 15 minutes until

bleeding from chest tube stops and child has fully reacted.

Once these emergency care procedures have been accomplished, the team will review special problems with the surgeon. If a child has a tracheostomy, the team will verbally assure him that its members will be with him constantly.

d. Postoperative Nursing Care in Heart Survery With Hypothermic Anesthesia. In this type of surgery, the child is immersed in crushed ice or ice water until the body temperature is reduced to 86° F. After the incision is closed and the chest tubes secured, he is gradually warmed, usually by being wrapped in an electric blanket heated to 90° F. He should warm up 1° every 10–15 minutes. At this time, bleeding risk increases, so blood pressure and pulse are taken every 15 minutes after his temperature reaches 95° F. When the temperature reaches 97° F, the electric blanket is removed, and he is covered with a sheet and cotton blanket. He is placed in an oxygen tent with the usual rate of flow for the oxygen, but no icing unit, until his temperature reaches 98° F. Then the ice unit is inserted in the oxygen tent. After this, his temperature is taken every 30 minutes. In 2 hours, he will begin a fever which must be controlled. At 102°, cool sponges for 15 minutes at a time are used until the temperature is taken again. If it is still rising, aspirin is given. The specialist must watch for cyanosis, paleness, very dry mouth, bleeding in the chest, and shock. It usually takes about 14 days for the temperature to return to normal.

e. The Cardiac Patient. The cardiac patient is more apt to have pressure sores, so his skin must be kept clean and dry, and frequent changes of

position must be made. Since there may be a reduction in urinary output, accurate intake and output records must be kept. Any change in pulse, temperature, respiration, color, or blood pressure must be reported at once. The specialist must also help the child accept his condition. This will be difficult as the child will be mentally upset and hate bedrest. The specialist must plan quiet activities.

60. Undescended Testes (Cryptorchidism)

Before birth, the testes of the male descend into the scrotum. If this does not happen and the testes remain in the abdomen, inguinal canal, or other structures, they are called undescended testes. Treatment is important to preserve fertility. When there is no hernia, endocrine therapy is usually tried. If unsuccessful, surgery is used. The specialist will notice that upon the child's return from surgery a rubber band is attached to the suture and anchored to the midthigh with adhesive tape. This is necessary to apply tension to the testicle to hold it in place, and it must be protected from any disturbance until its removal. The child will attempt to walk in a stopped position in order to relieve the discomfort. Encourage him to walk upright and remind him when he forgets. An indwelling catheter may or may not be used to prevent contamination of the suture line.

61. Other Malformations

a. Genitourinary Tract. There can be defective or displaced kidneys or exstrophy of the bladder.

b. Genital Organs. In females, the most common are imperforated hymen, incomplete epispadias, or adhesions of the clitoris or labia. In males,

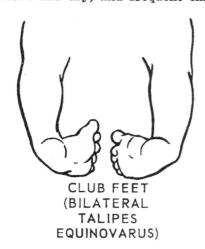

CLUB FEET
(BILATERAL
TALIPES
EQUINOVARUS)

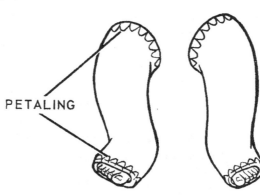

PETALING

CHECK TOES FOR WARMTH AND PINKNESS
AFTER CAST IS APPLIED

Figure   14. Clubfoot (inward) and one type of casting.

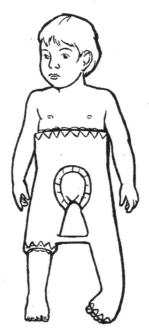

Figure 15. One type of unilateral clubfoot cast.

there can be malformation or abnormal location of urethral openings, phimosis, and hydrocele. An individual may also be afflicted with hermaphrodism—in which both ovaries and testicles are present—but this is rare. It is more common to see an individual possess the signs of one sex and have the gonads of the other.

c. Liver, Gallbladder, and Bile Ducts. There can be tumors of the liver, two gallbladders or none at all, and atresia of the bile ducts.

d. Skeletal System.

(1) Clubfoot is common. The foot may be twisted inward (fig. 14 Ⓐ) or outward (fig. 15). Two types of casts used are shown in figures 14 Ⓑ and 15.

(2) Polydactylism is an excess of fingers or toes.

(3) Syndactylism is a fusion of two or more fingers or toes.

(4) Congenital amputations are those where all or a part of an extremity is missing.

(5) Congenital dislocation of the hip is due to a malformation of the acetabulum which allows the femur's head to be displaced. If treatment begins before the child is a year old, a Putti splint (fig. 16) is usually used.

PUTTI SPLINT

Two boards are hinged together at one end with a wheel-like pulley at the opposite end. The hinged

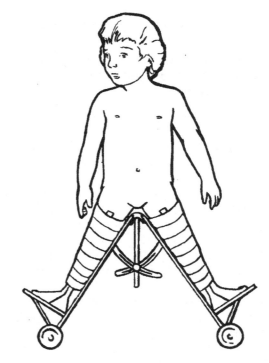

Figure 16. The Putti splint.

point is padded, and then waterproof material is placed over that. This waterproofing material must be washed and dried a MINIMUM of once a day.

Procedure

1. Place the child's perineum on the hinged point with a diaper over the perineum in loin-cloth fashion. The interior of the legs lie along the board.

2. Apply traction as ordered, starting above each knee. This traction extends to the pulley on each side.

3. Attach four straps to each leg: one above the ankle, one below and one above the knee, and one near the groin. Thread each strap through felt or sponge rubber to reduce pressure on the skin.

• Frequently inspect the outside wrapping to be sure it is not telescoping (the bandage bunching over knee, ankles, or foot) and is dry; look at the feet for color and edema and touch for temperature; and test the traction ropes to see if they are taut.

• When the child is supine, be sure there is a board under the mattress and a firm pillow under the buttocks to maintain alinement. To keep the child from falling out of the crib (since both crib sides must be down), tie the *splint* on both sides to the lowered crib sides. Do not permit the patient's heels to touch the bed—use sandbags or rolled towels to elevate them.

4. Turn the child three times a day. Turning requires two people, one on each side of the crib.

   a. The child is pulled to the edge of the bed *away* from No. 1 specialist, who is to receive the child.

   b. No. 1 specialist slips one hand and arm under the patient just below the shoulders and uses the other hand to grasp the splinted leg that is the farthest away.

   c. No. 2 specialist, who is nearest to the child, places one hand under the buttocks and the other hand on top of his chest.

   d. The specialists lift together and turn the child in midair, being sure the splint does not touch the bed.

   e. The toes are checked to be sure they are not pinched or bent under.

   f. If the child is placed on his abdomen, a pillow is put under his chest and a thinner pillow under his abdomen near the hips to maintain alinement.

5. To place the child upon a bedpan, use extreme caution as the skin in this area is easily damaged.

   a. Release the top straps near the groin.

   b. If the patient is female, place one hand on the mons veneris and labia, and then push them back and up toward the abdomen. With the opposite hand on the Putti, push down and pull the point of the Putti up.

   c. If the patient is male, the top of the Putti rests behind the scrotum, so lift up the scrotum and penis toward the abdomen and push down and pull the point of the Putti up to place the child on the bedpan.

   d. Inspect the perineum when the Putti is released. Wash the perineum and genitalia with clear water each time the bedpan is used. (The skin is also inspected after a bath and the perineum and genitalia are thoroughly washed.)

Section VIII. OBTAINING SPECIMENS

62. Urinary Specimens—Clean

These are collected in the morning and are among the most important specimens obtained. They are examined for sugar, specific gravity, and blood cells. Because of their importance, it is necessary to obtain a clean specimen, a requirement that necessitates use of special equipment for a chiild in diapers or any young child. After an operation, output must be observed carefully because it is an index of kidney function and fluid balance. Former methods involved using test tubes for boys (fig. 17 Ⓐ) and a spicer urinal or birdseed cup for girls (fig. 17 Ⓑ). Now, commercially available, sterile, plastic bags that are disposable are generally used (fig. 18).

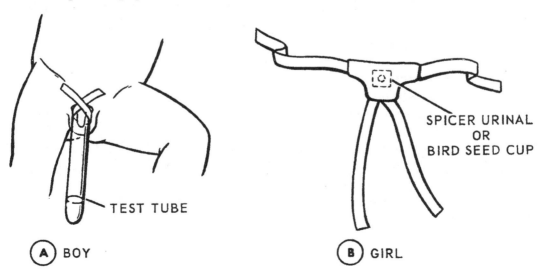

Ⓐ BOY TEST TUBE

Ⓑ GIRL SPICER URINAL OR BIRD SEED CUP

Figure 17. Methods of collecting urine specimens.

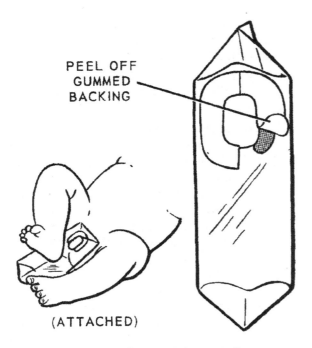

PEEL OFF
GUMMED
BACKING

(ATTACHED)

Figure · 18. Commercial urine collector.

PROCEDURE FOR COMMERCIAL URINE COLLECTORS

1. Cleanse with soap and water or hexachlorophene, using normal precaution of washing away from the urethral meatus.
2. Dry. If collection is to be prolonged, paint with tincture of benzoin.
3. If the child is active, get someone to hold the child's legs in abduction.
4. Peel off the gummed backing from the disposable collector and press the adhesive portion firmly against the perineum of the infant around the urethra (fig. 18). For girls, be sure to make the adhesive adheres to the strip of skin between the anus and vagina.

63. Urinary Specimens—Sterile

If the child is old enough to understand and under close supervision, a clean voided specimen can be obtained by "midstream catch."

CAUTION

Be sure to cleanse the urethral orifice first. Clean catch urines can be used for female infants if good technique is used. Catheterization should be avoided, if at all possible.

64. Stool Specimens

Specimens should be collected in the morning. The infant's perianal area should be cleansed before collection of a stool specimen. The procedure for an adult would be used for an older child who can cooperate. The infant's stool may be scraped from the diaper with tongue blades and placed in a covered specimen cup. It must not be contaminated by urine, so special precautions may need to be taken. Place the soiled tongue blade in trash receptacle. Do not attempt to flush down hopper. Freshly passed specimens should be taken to the laboratory as soon as possible.

65. Blood Specimens

Blood specimens are obtained from children by the same method used for adults however, the site of the puncture and the veins used are different. The veins used for infants and young children are normally the external jugular or the femoral. In the jugular venipuncture, the child is usually put in a mummy restraint and his head lowered over the side of the bed. The specialist holds the infant's head steady with his hands (fig. 19). When the procedure is finished, pressure is maintained on site and the child is elevated to a sitting position until the bleeding stops. In the femoral venipuncture, the infant is put on his back with his legs spread out as shown in figure 20 and his legs restrained by the specialist. After the procedure, pressure is maintained on the site until the bleeding stops. The specialist only assists with this procedure.

66. Lumbar Puncture

When an infant must be positioned for a lumbar puncture, the child's lower limbs must be put in a sheet restraint. He is held as shown in figure 21, with his neck and knees flexed.

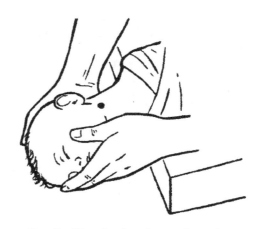

Figure 19. Position for jugular venipuncture.

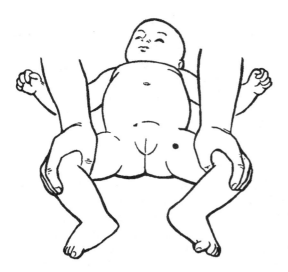

Figure 20. Position for femoral puncture.

67. Subdural Tap

Before the anterior fontanelle has closed, a needle may be inserted directly into the subdural space on the brain's surface for diagnostic or for therapeutic purposes (when abnormal fluid is removed).

EQUIPMENT

Tray with—
Local anesthesia
Sterile 25-gage hypodermic needles
No. 22 needle with stylets
Sheet
Antiseptic

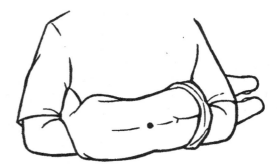

Figure 21. Position for lumbar puncture.

PROCEDURE

1. Put the infant in a mummy restraint.
2. Shave and wash the infant's head as directed by the doctor or nurse.
3. Hold the infant across the treatment table facing the doctor. Support his head firmly.
   (The doctor will apply the antiseptic, infiltrate the skin, and insert the needle to remove fluid, if any, from the subdural space.)
4. Measure and record the volume removed.
5. Obtain specimens for culture and chemical analysis.

NOTE

Pressure on the scalp is usually enough to seal the puncture, so dressings are not normally required. Collodion may be used to insure the closure of the wound.

6. Observe for any leakage.
7. Watch vital signs.

Section IX. PREOPERATIVE AND POSTOPERATIVE CARE

68. Surgery

a. General. If surgery must be performed, the danger of psychological trauma to the child is even greater than that for hospitalization for illness. He requires special care and attention. In an emergency, there is no time to prepare the child or his parents, but a calm, reassuring attitude on the part of hospital personnel will help both parent and child. However, if the operation is elective, he must have intelligent preparation and explanation. A friendly relationship should have already been established with the doctors, nurses, and specialists, and perhaps a tour of the hospital has been made. But no matter what preparations have been made, he will sense tensions and respond to them, particularly those of his parents,

whose fears are easily communicated to their child. The length of time the parents are permitted to remain with him may have to depend on their own emotional states. Attention to the child's needs come first and are always a matter of judgment, as well as a sympathetic attitude.

b. Preparation. The child should be told if he is not allowed to eat or drink for a period before and after the operation and that his temperature may be taken rectally. He should also be told about blood pressure readings, enemas, anesthesia, the operating room, and people in masks. Try to make a game of wearing a mask, the child listening to the stethoscope, etc. *For example,* have a child try on a mask and perhaps tell him he looks like a jet pilot. The anesthesiologist or nurse anesthetist will probably visit him and explain what will happen in the operating room. Minimize pain as far as possible and do not initiate use of the word. Words such as "pain," "shot," "hurt," etc., are anxiety producing; substitute "smart," "sting," "uncomfortable," etc. If he mentions pain or suffering, assure him that he will not be allowed to suffer and that he will be returned to the same room and bed after the operation, even if he spends some time in intensive care. Unless reassurance is given skillfully, your relationship with the child and even the relationship between the child and his parents may be damaged beyond repair. What you should tell the child and when will depend upon the child—his age, condition and intelligence—but he should be told that he will be given all the help he will need. Above all, nursing personnel must respond truthfully (but not bluntly—choose your words with care) to any question and make simple explanations such as, "We are going to fix that place so it will quit hurting in a few days." Older children should have more detailed explanations. These children may be undergoing something similar to a combat neurosis, and every effort should be expended to explain what they will see, what will happen, and where they will be when they wake up. Make every attempt to assuage their anxiety. If the admitting specialist finds out the child's favorite food, perhaps he can surprise the child with it in his last meal before the operation. A young child might be permitted to carry a favorite toy or other "security" object to the operating room.

69. NPO

An NPO order requires special effort where a child is involved. Because the child lacks judgment, the specialist must be ever watchful to be sure the child eats or drinks nothing. The child should be kept in bed and accompanied to the bathroom by a specialist for supervision. Because a child will be fretful without water or food, his parents' pity may be aroused to the point where they will slip him water—or other children may share their breakfast trays. If you find out that food or water has been given to him, notify the nurse in charge, who will notify the operating room so the operation can be postponed. The order is so important because fluid can regurgitate silently and be aspirated during anesthesia, which would result in postoperative pneumonia. The child might vomit, too, and aspirate it. Age is also important in this order. The stomach of an infant under 1 year normally empties in 4 hours,

but even an infant should be limited to clear liquids with sugar added for several hours longer than this. The stomach of a child above that age, as well as an adult, requires a minimum of 8 hours to empty. This time can be extended by fear, trauma, or gastrointestinal disease, which may require use of a Levin tube to empty the stomach.

70. Special Care

a. *Day of Operation.* The usual hospital procedures are followed. Any signs of a cold must be reported to the nurse immediately. The child should be inspected for skin rash or a nasal discharge. If an older child is thirsty, he might be permitted to rinse his mouth, but be sure he swallows no water. The specialist might wipe the lips of a small child. He should be made comfortable and be supervised by someone he knows and trusts.

b. *Postoperative Day.* A child chills easier than an adult and is more susceptible to exposure and to trauma, so he will need expert nursing care. When he awakes, he should see someone he knows and trusts, preferably the same person who accompanied him to the operating room. When he wakes up, he may be frightened and try to tear off dressings or climb out of bed, so he must be watched constantly. After surgery or during a period of illness, he must also be watched for changes in his physical condition.

71. Postoperative Positioning

After an operation, the child is placed on his side or abdomen to allow secretions to drain and to keep the tongue from going back and obstructing the pharynx ——— except that his arm will be *under* his head.

72. Dressings

Dressings are generally used only on open wounds, infected incisions, or incisions that might be contaminated by excrement. A clean surgical wound usually has hidden stitches and is sprayed with plastic or covered with a lightweight bandage that does not adhere. If a dressing is used, select only individually packaged sterile gauze squares or pads. Do not change dressings on an open ward—do this only in a treatment room or private room. The patient must be protected from infection; however, if infection is already present, nursing personnel must insure that it is not spread. Two specialists are needed in addition to the doctor or nurse. One specialist gently holds the child while he tells stories or offers toys. The other specialist scrubs his hands and dries them with a sterile towel. The older child is asked to remove his own adhesive tape, but if he will not, the specialist picks up one edge and pushes the skin down and away (it is never torn off rapidly). Any gauze that is stuck is soaked in saline. The contaminated dressings are put in a plastic bag within a foot-operated wastebasket with *gloved* hands or with an *instrument*. The skin around the wound is washed with warm water and soap; the wound is irrigated, if ordered; and re-covered. If the dressing must be changed often, Montgomery strips are used or nonallergenic tape.

CAUTION

This entire procedure must be done with kindness and care.

73. Bleeding

Bleeding may occur after an operation, so the child must be watched carefully for 24 hours. Just 20 percent loss of blood—a very small amount—in a child can result in shock. Watch for changes in vital signs, for shock, for cyanosis, and for evidence of bleeding.

74. Traction

a. Bryant's Traction. In this type of traction, skin traction is applied to both legs (fig. 9). Just enough weight is used to barely lift the buttocks off the mattress; the child should not be unduly elevated. A diaper can be placed underneath (but NEVER between) the legs. The front

of the spreaders can be taped together to keep the toes pointing straight ahead.

b. Dunlop's Lateral Traction. This type of traction is used for supracondylar (above the elbow) fractures of the humerus. The elbow is either bent at a right angle or slightly extended, and the lines of pull are along the elbow at a right angle to the body's trunk. The forearm is held up by a second weight; another weight hangs from a padded cuff on the arm (fig. 22). The bed is tilted away from the injured arm or the child's body rests against heavy side rails—this overcomes the sideway pull.

75. Special Care for Patients in Casts

a. Circulation. Since swelling is always associated with injury or surgery to a bone, the doctor will pad the cast inside and order elevation of an extremity. He may also order that a bedboard be placed under the mattress to prevent sagging. But nursing personnel bear a special responsibility to see that circulation is not impaired. As soon as the cast is applied, the specialist should observe the color of the fingers or toes and if any pulse is exposed, palpate it. Another good test is to press on the nail beds and watch for blanching and prompt return of color. Swelling, pallor, or numbness of the digits are also signs of trouble. The

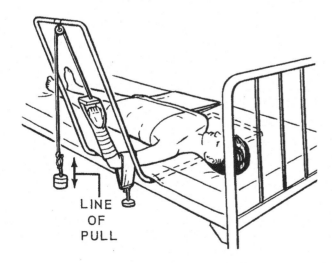

Figure 22. Dunlop's lateral traction.

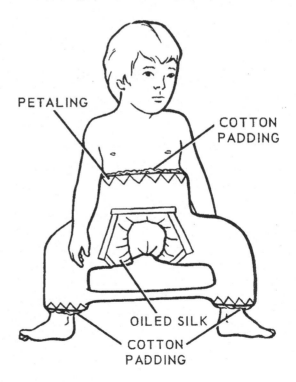

Figure 23. Cotton padding, spica cast.

ability to detect sensation can be checked by lightly drawing a small piece of gauze against the exposed skin. Pain is a symptom of a tight cast, particularly a general or burning pain. Pain severe enough to wake up the child or that is increased by attempts to move the digits should be checked immediately. But pain in children is not easy to evaluate—the cutaneous nerves can be destroyed and pain will lessen, or the child may be complaining just to get attention. That is why extra vigilance is necessary. Two other clues to possible trouble are local soreness or tightness of the cast and failure to find a previously palpable distal pulse.

b. Care of the Cast. In addition to the information on cast care previously discussed, special precautions must be taken with children. The rough edges of a plaster cast may injure the child's skin, so petalling is used to prevent irritation. Waterproofing of the cast and of the petalling are required for infants and for young children who cannot control elimination, and the head of the bed is also elevated a little to prevent seepage. Foreign particles can be put into a cast by the child, so toys small enough to be pushed under it are not used. Fluffy cotton padding tucked at the edges of the cast (fig. 23) will help prevent the child from putting objects under the cast. The exposed skin should be checked every day for irritations, as the child may devise ingenious ways of scratching the itching skin under the cast. Areas at the edges of spica and body casts at the top and back (and at the groin with long leg casts) must be washed with soap and water as far inside the cast as can be reached and then massaged with alcohol, followed by a rub with an emollient cream. A small hand vacuum cleaner can be used to remove some crumbs. Turning the child will give him exercise and prevent pressure sores. Pillows or sandbags must be rearranged with each position shift. Help may be needed. Feeding may present problems where casts extend from the abdomen to the neck, because the child is unable to swallow while supine. If he is placed in a prone position and his chest propped up with pillows, the older child may even be able to feed himself. As for toilet care, casts on infants should have the additional protection of plastic tucked under the cast's edges in the perineal area and then covered with a diaper. Disposable paper, plastic-backed diapers will help, or the infant can be put in the prone position on a small frame over a diaper or bedpan, with some elevation of the infant's head. Older children may have trouble with elimination when in a supine position. One way of helping is to elevate the head of the bed and to lift him on a bedpan while he holds himself up with an overhead bar. Considerable tact may be required because of an older child's shyness and aversion to exposure.

Section X. EMERGENCY CARE

76. Mouth-to-Mouth Resuscitation

The correct technique for infants and small children is covered.

77. Closed-Chest Heart Massage

This may be done in combination with mouth-to-mouth resuscitation, preferably with an assistant. This procedure is modified for an infant or small child. Another method is to use a firm support which is slid under the child and to compress the sternum with both hands, with the arms held straight. Minor force is used with an infant, but an older child's sternum is depressed $1\frac{1}{2}$ inch. As soon as possible, a doctor should be sent for, and emergency drugs and a cardiac defibrillator should be at hand ready for his use.

78. Using the Isolette Infant Incubator

Refer to figure 24.

1. *Lights.* The orange light is on until the desired temperature is reached. The clear light indicates the incubator is working. The red lights comes on if the incubator overheats.

2. *Temperature control.* This is calibrated in numbers, *not* degrees. Higher numbers on the dial are for higher temperatures. Read the thermometer *inside* the incubator and take the infant's body temperature before changing the setting.

3. *Thermometer.* This accurately registers the temperature in the mattress area in degrees F.

4. *Oxygen inlet.* Connect the tube from the oxygen source here.

5. *Ice chamber.* Use ice in this chamber only when the incubator temperature should be lowered to *below* the room's temperature. Use cracked ice (15–20 pounds) and 1 quart of cold water.

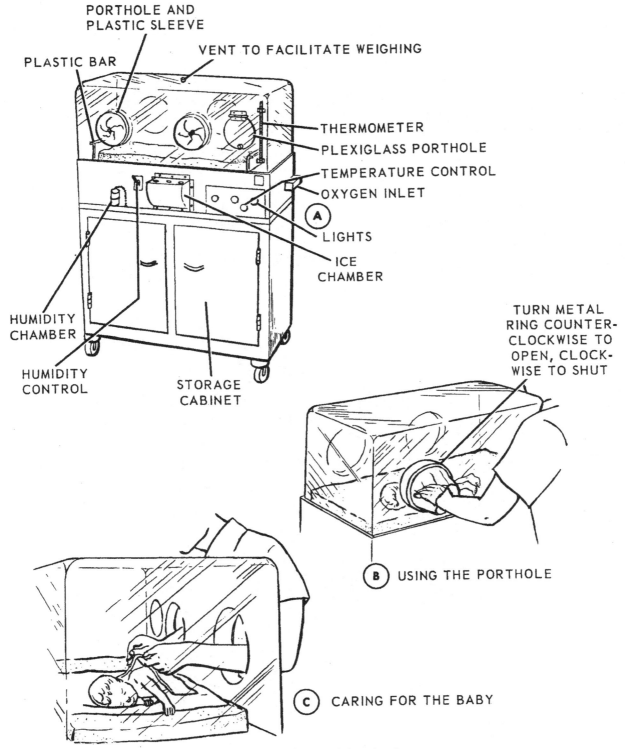

PORTHOLE AND
PLASTIC SLEEVE

PLASTIC BAR

VENT TO FACILITATE WEIGHING

THERMOMETER
PLEXIGLASS PORTHOLE
TEMPERATURE CONTROL
OXYGEN INLET

(A)

LIGHTS

ICE
CHAMBER

HUMIDITY
CHAMBER

HUMIDITY
CONTROL

STORAGE
CABINET

TURN METAL
RING COUNTER-
CLOCKWISE TO
OPEN, CLOCK-
WISE TO SHUT

(B) USING THE PORTHOLE

(C) CARING FOR THE BABY

Figure 24. Isolette infant incubator.

a. Turn the humidity control to open.

b. Check the incubator's temperature frequently.

6. *Humidity control.* Turn to off, midway, or full humidity in accordance with the doctor's orders.

7. *Humidity chamber.* Keep filled with distilled water up to the black line. Invert to dispose of water.

8. *Portholes and plastic sleeves.* These are used to care for the infant (fig. 24 (B) and (C)).

9. *Weighing vent.* This is used when weighing the infant. A special scale is used inside the incubator so the infant does not have to be removed.

10. *Plexiglass porthole.* Remove contaminated linens or other articles through here.

11. *Plastic bar.* Hook the raised end of the mattress board over the plastic bar to get a Fowler or Trendelenburg position.

WARNING

Mattress *must* be flat when the plexiglass hood is lifted to open the incubator.

12. *Storage cabinet.* This can be used to store the weight scale, linens, or other supplies.

Points To Remember

- Place the Isolette with an end to the wall, making it possible for two persons to have simultaneous access to the baby.

- Avoid placing the Isolette near a radiator or in direct sunlight. They will cause the unit to overheat and start the safety alarm buzzer.

- Allow 1 hour, if possible, to preheat the Isolette to approximately 90° F.

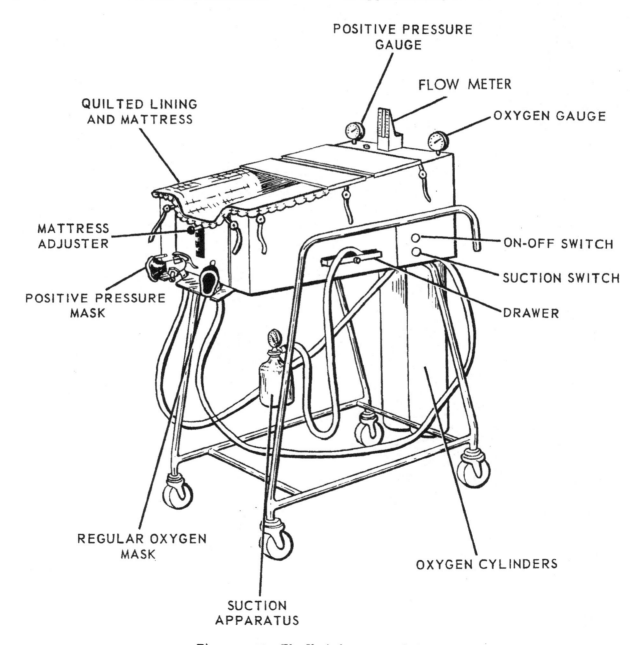

Figure   25.   The Kreiselman resuscitator.

- In addition to these precautions, **see** that the—
    - —Hood is properly seated on the gasket.
    - —Portholes are closed.
    - —Six safety vent holes are open.
    - —Access door is fastened securely, with the door gasket in place.
    - —Filter screen in air intake valve is thoroughly clean at all times.
    - —Drafts directly on the Isolette from fans or open windows are avoided.
- If the Vapojette is attached to the Isolette to saturate the atmosphere higher, fill the jar with distilled water only. After every use, empty the water jar, wipe dry, remove the water filter, and clean.

Cleaning the Isolette

Wash the hood with soap and water only; polish with soft flannel cloth. NEVER use alcohol or tinctures. Isolettes must be thoroughly dismantled and cleaned between patients or as necessary for long-term patients. Isolettes should be cultured periodically since they provide an ideal environment for the growth of organisms.

79. The Oxygen Analyzer

To use, place a paper barrier on the incubator hood. Put oxygen analyzer on top of the paper barrier. Put the long tubing through one of the open vents into the incubator. Pump the bulb about 15 times. Press the button and read the meter, which should not exceed 40 percent unless the doctor orders otherwise.

80. Resuscitation Equipment

a. *The Kreiselman Resuscitator.*
   (fig. 25)

(1) *On–off switch.* This switch is turned on to give warmth for the body.

(2) *Suction switch.* This controls the electric suction apparatus.

(3) *Oxygen cylinders.* These fit into a groove at the foot of the unit. The supply of oxygen must be checked at the beginning of each shift.

(4) *Oxygen gauge.* This indicates the pressure in the cylinder that is connected to the regular *oxygen mask.* Turn the handle clockwise and oxygen will flow from the tank.

(5) *Positive pressure gauge.* The oxygen pressure in the cylinder attached to the positive pressure mask is shown by this gauge. The handle of the mask *must be depressed* before the oxygen will flow.

WARNING

A specialist should never administer this positive pressure to a child unless under the supervision of a physician or nurse.

(6) *Mattress adjuster.* The handle can be moved to other grooves to change the mattress to the Trendelenburg position.

(7) *Flow meter.* This controls the rate of oxygen flow to the oxygen mask.

(8) *Suction apparatus.* The meter on top of the jar, which can be unscrewed for cleaning, shows the amount of pressure used during suction.

(9) *Drawer.* This stores suction catheters and intubation tubes.

b. *Other Resuscitators.* Other resuscitators are shown in figures 26 and 27. The portable resuscitator has an automatic valve that prevents rebreathing expired air. The mask may be used with oxygen or air. To use the Emerson bellows

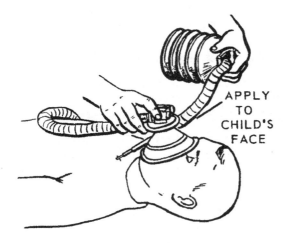

Figure 26. The Emerson bellows resuscitator.

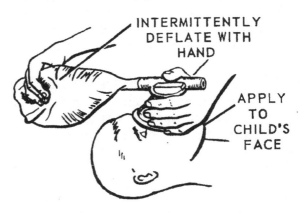

Figure 27. The portable resuscitator.

resuscitator, open the valve, blow into the tube, and close the valve to inflate the rubber face cushion. Put the narrow end over the child's nose and press firmly. Hold securely with one hand and compress the bellows rhythmically and gently (less than full capacity); rate will vary with the child's age. Bellows can be held against the body or put on a flat surface.

Section XI. DEATH OR DISCHARGE OF CHILD

81. Death of a Child

Death is always sad wherever it occurs, but the death of a child in the hospital will have a traumatic effect on the parents, on other children, and on nursing personnel.

a. Parents. Nursing personnel must give emotional support and comfort to the parents of a dying child. They will have many fears and may particularly feel that they need to confide in you. It is absolutely necessary that nursing personnel know what the doctor has told the parents. You may well become the person who translates the care and procedures to the parents.

CAUTION
Under no circumstances should a specialist be the first to inform a parent that a child will not recover or that he is dying. Go no further in your translation than the instructions given to you.

Explanations may need to be repeated again and again, and even then misunderstandings may occur. The parents must be reminded of the need to give other children, if any, as normal a home as possible under the circumstances. Above all, any possible feelings of guilt by the parents must be assuaged. Parents should be encouraged to enliven the child's days with small gifts and surprises. If at all possible, both from the doctor's and the parents' point of view, permit the parents to participate in the care of their child. When death comes, they should be reassured that everything possible was done for their child. Many parents will appreciate a chaplain of their faith being summoned when the childs' death seems imminent.

b. The Dying Child. The child himself must neither be overprotected nor ignored, but during night hours, you can comfort a frightened child with your presence and perhaps close physical contact. He may want to know if he is going to die —and probably already knows, whether you tell him or not. Although the truth is generally best, the decision is made by the doctor and parents. The specialist must follow the direction of the nurse in caring for the dying child. Each situation will probably be handled in a different manner, depending upon the age of the child, the reaction of the parents, or the child's previous experience with death. The specialist can anticipate questions, and he should seek guidance from the nurse. It should be remembered that death is a natural thing—that everyone dies, but no one knows when he will die. Surely, all children will appreciate a reaffirmation of the values of life and living. Many of them can meet death calmly and courageously. If the child is a Roman Catholic, a priest must be notified when death seems near in order to have the Last Rites performed. Death of an older person is more easily accepted, yet the dying child needs the support and mature understanding of the specialist. A calm acceptance will enable both the child and his parents to face the inevitable.

c. Other Children. A child's death, if known, usually results in considerable concern among other children on the ward. Days after his death, they may ask about him and may want to know if they are going to die too. Usually, after the death of a child, the ward atmosphere is strangely quiet; the other children tend to be very helpful and unusually good. Questions about the dead child should be answered truthfully; *for example,* "Yes, Johnnie died. He doesn't hurt any more. He's with God."

d. Procedures After Death. These nursing duties are covered in other manuals.

82. Discharge of a Child

a. The doctor writes the order for discharge and the nurse or specialist, if so directed, notifies the admitting office of the discharge.

b. The nurse obtains the information on followup care from the doctor, writes out instructions for the parents, and also explains them orally. The specialist assists as directed.

c. The child must be returned to his own family. If custody is controversial, court orders may be involved. Check the identification of the parents and the identification band of the child before discharge.

83. Referral to a Health Nurse

a. A child may need the care of a   Health Nurse after discharge. The child's Case Referral Record   should be completed and forwarded to the   Health Nurse prior to the actual discharge of the child, if at all possible. Where feasible, the   Health Nurse may wish to discuss the referral in greater detail with members of the pediatric ward team. The specialists who have cared for the child should be included in this conference.

b. Indications of need for referral are—
  (1) Newborns with—
    • Congenital anomaly
    • Birth weight under 5½ pounds
    • Birth injury
    • Health problem
    • Parents who need guidance.
  (2) Infants and children—
    (a) Who require—
      • A special diet (Diabetic, P.K.U., etc.)
      • Dressings
      • Medication by injection
      • Rehabilitation exercise
      • Colostomy care
      • Urine testing
    (b) Who have—
      • Cerebral palsy
      • Paralysis
      • Cleft palate
      • Battered child syndrome